W9-AWE-058

WILLIAM H. PARKER, M.D., is clinical professor of obstetrics and gynecology at UCLA School of Medicine. He is the former chairman of obstetrics and gynecology at Santa Monica–UCLA Medical Center and is in private practice in Santa Monica. He is the author of numerous publications in professional journals on his research findings in the areas of gynecologic surgery and laparoscopic surgery and has authored several chapters for textbooks standard to the field of gynecologic surgery. Dr. Parker is past president of the American Association of Gynecologic Laparoscopists and an editor of the *Journal of the American Association of Gynecologic Laparoscopists*. He is a board-certified fellow of the American College of Obstetricians and Gynecologists. Dr. Parker has been selected for both *Best Doctors in America* and *America's Top Doctors*.

RACHEL L. PARKER is a middle school English teacher with a love for both teaching and writing. She has also been a community health educator and outpatient mental health program coordinator in New York.

AMY E. ROSENMAN, M.D., is a board-certified Fellow of the American College of Obstetricians and Gynecologists. She is codirector of the UCLA Urogynecology Fellowship Program and is in private practice in Santa Monica. Dr. Rosenman has been selected for both *Best Doctors in America* and *America's Top Doctors*.

INGRID A. RODI, M.D., is a board-certified specialist in reproductive endocrinology and infertility and an assistant clinical professor at UCLA School of Medicine. She is in private practice in Santa Monica. Dr. Rodi has been selected for both *Best Doctors in America* and *America's Top Doctors*.

A
GYNECOLOGIST'S
SECOND OPINION

The Questions and Answers You Need to Take Charge of Your Health

Revised Edition

William H. Parker, M.D.
with Rachel L. Parker

Contributions by Ingrid A. Rodi, M.D.
and Amy E. Rosenman, M.D.

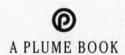

A PLUME BOOK

Every effort has been made to ensure that the information contained in this book is complete and accurate. However, neither the publisher nor the author is engaged in rendering professional advice or services to the individual reader. The ideas, procedures, and suggestions contained in this book are not intended as a substitute for consulting with your physician. All matters regarding your health require medical supervision. Neither the author nor the publisher shall be liable or responsible for any loss, injury, or damage allegedly arising from any information or suggestion in this book.

PLUME
Published by the Penguin Group
Penguin Putnam Inc., 375 Hudson Street, New York, New York 10014, U.S.A.
Penguin Books Ltd, 80 Strand, London WC2R 0RL, England
Penguin Books Australia Ltd, 250 Camberwell Road, Camberwell, Victoria 3124, Australia
Penguin Books Canada Ltd, 10 Alcorn Avenue, Toronto, Ontario, Canada M4V 3B2
Penguin Books (N.Z.) Ltd, 182–190 Wairau Road, Auckland 10, New Zealand

Penguin Books Ltd, Registered Offices: Harmondsworth, Middlesex, England

First published by Plume, a member of Penguin Putnam Inc.

First Plume Printing, July 1996
First Plume Printing (revised edition), January 2003
10 9 8 7 6

Copyright © William H. Parker and Rachel L. Parker, 1996, 2003
All rights reserved
Line illustrations by Peggy Firth, medical illustrator

Ⓟ REGISTERED TRADEMARK—MARCA REGISTRADA

LIBRARY OF CONGRESS CATALOGING-IN-PUBLICATION DATA
Parker, William H., M.D.
A gynecologist's second opinion : the questions and answers you need to take charge of your health / William H. Parker with Rachel L. Parker ; contributions by Ingrid A. Rodi and Amy E. Rosenman.—2nd ed.
p.   cm.
Includes bibliographical references and index.
ISBN 0-452-28362-0
1. Gynecology—Miscellanea. 2. Gynecology—Popular works. I. Parker, Rachel L. II. Title.
RG121 .P286 2002
618.1—dc21   2002031264

Printed in the United States of America
Set in Cheltenham Light
Designed by Jesse Cohen

Without limiting the rights under copyright reserved above, no part of this publication may be reproduced, stored in or introduced into a retrieval system, or transmitted, in any form, or by any means (electronic, mechanical, photocopying, recording, or otherwise), without the prior written permission of both the copyright owner and the above publisher of this book.

BOOKS ARE AVAILABLE AT QUANTITY DISCOUNTS WHEN USED TO PROMOTE PRODUCTS OR SERVICES. FOR INFORMATION PLEASE WRITE TO PREMIUM MARKETING DIVISION, PENGUIN PUTNAM INC., 375 HUDSON STREET, NEW YORK, NEW YORK 10014.

This book is dedicated to our children,
Aaron, Evan, and Brian,
who bring joy and love to each day.

ACKNOWLEDGMENTS

Many people helped during the writing of this book, and I am enormously grateful to them. First, I would like to thank my partners, Dr. Ingrid Rodi and Dr. Amy Rosenman, for their support to me and their valuable contributions to the book. A number of my teachers, colleagues, and friends took the time to review the manuscript and offer their special expertise, which proved to be invaluable: Dr. Beth Meyerowitz, Department of Psychology, University of Southern California; Dr. Howard Judd, Department of Obstetrics and Gynecology, Olive View Medical Center; Dr. Jonathan Berek, Department of Obstetrics and Gynecology, UCLA School of Medicine; Dr. John Bornstein, Department of Anesthesiology, Santa Monica–UCLA Medical Center; Dr. Andrea Rapkin, Department of Obstetrics and Gynecology, UCLA School of Medicine; Barbara Kass-Anesse, NP, Regional Family Planning Center; Carla Dionne, National Uterine Fibroid Foundation; and Joyce Selden, Department of Genetics, UCLA School of Medicine. I would like to express gratitude to our agent, Arielle Eckstut, of James Levine Communications, for her advice, enthusiasm, and friendship.

I would also like to thank all of my teachers over the years, who have given freely of their time and knowledge, and all of my patients who have allowed me to provide their care and who have taught me so much.

CONTENTS

INTRODUCTION

Knowledge about the female body grows by leaps and bounds every year. In the last few years, these gains in science allowed for the development of exciting new medical and surgical treatments for gynecologic problems and made this second edition of *A Gynecologist's Second Opinion* necessary. Ironically, while our gains through research are blossoming at a rapid pace, our nation's doctors face a health-care environment that leaves them little time or incentive to learn about the new medical developments. They have even less time to explain medical problems and treatment alternatives to their patients. That terrible situation has led me to believe it is now more important than ever for women to educate themselves about available treatment options, about what questions to ask their doctors, and about when to seek a second opinion.

I am a practicing gynecologist and clinical professor of the Department of Obstetrics and Gynecology at the UCLA School of Medicine. The surgical techniques covered in this book are part of what I have been teaching for the last fifteen years as past president and continuing faculty member for the American Association of Gynecologic Laparoscopists. I am also an editor for the *Journal of the American Association of Gynecologic Laparoscopists* and a reviewer for the journal *Obstetrics and Gynecology*. My research has been published in those journals and others. Teaching, research, and private practice all enable me to stay in the forefront of the rapidly changing field of gynecology. I have tried to bring you the best state-of-the-art medical information available in a readable form in *A Gynecologist's Second Opinion*.

In my practice, I often have the opportunity to see women for a second opinion regarding gynecologic problems and view my role as both a doctor and an educator. I offer each woman a clear explanation of all the medical information regarding her problem; I make myself available for all questions and concerns. The goal is for each woman to make her own informed, educated decision about the best course to follow for her problem and her body. This book follows that model.

The first edition of *A Gynecologist's Second Opinion* was born out of frustration. There were simply no good books for women to read that provided compassionate, in-depth yet understandable information about the gynecologic problems I often treat in my practice. When my patients asked where they could read about the issues they faced, I had little to recommend. The books were either so broad that they only provided brief descriptions of a large range of women's health issues or they were focused on only one subject, usually hysterectomy, and failed to cover the range of difficult gynecologic issues women sometimes face. Many books contained incorrect medical information or lacked the careful analysis of the risks and benefits of treatment that each woman needs to know to make the right medical decision.

We have written *A Gynecologist's Second Opinion* to help you understand both how your body normally works and what has gone wrong when a problem arises. Arranged in a Q&A format, this book provides clear descriptions of common gynecologic problems, up-to-date thinking regarding causes of medical problems, and state-of-the-art information about treatment. Multiple options for treating each problem with medication or surgery or both are covered. The option of no treatment is discussed when appropriate, and current research that may lead to new alternatives in the foreseeable future is discussed. *A Gynecologist's Second Opinion* is also filled with the personal stories of women who have had these problems. The stories make the medical facts come alive and allow the reader to experience examples of an individual's search for treatment.

A Gynecologist's Second Opinion is not meant to be a substitute for an appointment with a doctor. It is intended to help you comfortably gain information and understanding without time constraints or outside pressures. Reading the book may help you to plan your questions before you go for a scheduled doctor's appointment. It may convince you to make an appointment you've been avoiding, or it may be an educational resource to consult after you've seen your doctor.

Your intelligence, curiosity, and skepticism are needed in any search for good health care. A person facing a serious medical problem should be urged to get a second opinion. This book is a companion in that quest for answers and good health care. We hope it becomes a trusted reference for you, and we wish you good health.

A
GYNECOLOGIST'S
SECOND OPINION

1

NORMAL BODY, NORMAL EXAM

The human body is a fascinating and complicated creation. There appears to be such intentional and intricate design in a woman's body. Just look at the changes that accompany monthly hormonal events, pregnancy, and childbirth. A dazzlingly effective system operates: Hormonal changes heighten a woman's sexual desire around the time of ovulation, the most optimal time for fertilization. This intensified desire for sex by the female occurs at the perfect time to increase the chances of conception. In addition to increased desire, the thick mucus produced by the cervix normally hinders the passage of sperm up into the uterus. However, at the time of ovulation the mucus becomes thin and watery to easily allow the sperm entry.

It is only over the last hundred years that the functions of a woman's body have begun to be studied and understood. Medical drawings from the 1700s show the anatomy of a woman's pelvic organs resembling the pelvic organs of farm animals. The ignorance behind this assumption is understandable, since church law prohibited human dissection. The anatomists did the best they could based on the animals that were on hand at the time. The medical world spent many years working from these incorrect assumptions.

Before the 1900s, the hormonal processes of a woman's body were not recognized at all. Menstruation was believed to result from irritation to the "fallopian tube nerve," a structure that we now know does not even exist. Women were thought to bleed because they had too much blood, more than men had, and more than they needed. When an adolescent girl began to menstruate, people considered her susceptible to weakness, lethargy, and disease. The two female hormones, estrogen and progesterone, and the hormonal events that trigger menstruation were not discovered until the 1920s.

In the 1870s, the uterus was believed to be the physical control center of a woman's body, acting through nerve connections to every other part of her body. Symptoms related to the heart, lungs, liver, and the intestines were considered the consequence of uterine disease. And one strong belief about the source of uterine disease held that reading romantic novels led to the "evil of masturbation," which then resulted in problems with the uterus and abnormal periods.

The ovaries were thought to be the main influence on a woman's emotions, and disease of the ovaries was felt to cause insanity. "Ovariotomy," or removal of the ovaries, was commonly performed for a variety of emotional problems, including overeating and erotic tendencies. The removal of supposedly diseased ovaries seemed to produce a "better" woman—more orderly, industrious, and clean.

It is no wonder that doctors were rarely able to diagnose true gynecologic diseases. Pelvic examinations were almost never performed, lest the woman and the doctor suffer from embarrassment. Often, the doctor made a diagnosis entirely based on reported symptoms sent by the patient via messenger. If an examination was felt to be absolutely necessary, it was performed with the woman covered entirely by drapes, so that the doctor was unable to see anything. Needless to say, a woman's sense of her own ailment or physical condition was rarely respected, and women were not considered stable enough to be physicians themselves.

While medical research sometimes seems annoyingly slow and plodding, there has been a steady march toward understanding of a woman's reproductive system. With each step, we solve more problems and treat more illnesses.

In 1597, Francis Bacon said, "Knowledge is power." That statement is particularly true today with regard to your own health. If you understand your own body, you will be in a better position to take care of it in times of sickness as well as health. Staying healthy is always the best medicine. But if you have a medical problem, getting to the right doctor and getting the appropriate treatment all involve choices. Put some power into your decisions by being well informed. This will help you feel stronger and more capable if you need to make decisions about your health care.

This chapter will describe what the normal female reproductive system looks like and how it works. We will also describe what a doctor looks for during an exam. Getting a brief education about the normal working of the body seems to be a good base from which you can become an informed user of health services. You'll also learn some proven strategies to keep you in good health.

What Does the Uterus Look Like?

The uterus is the largest of a woman's reproductive organs but is still normally no larger than a small pear. The uterus is even shaped like a pear, with the smaller portion pointing down. It extends downward from below the pubic bone to the top of the vagina, where the cervix (the opening of the uterus) attaches (see fig. 1.1). The uterus is a reddish pink color, much like the color of the inside of your lips. Most women, when viewing videotapes or photographs of their uterus, fallopian tubes, and ovaries, are surprised to see the beautiful colors within their bodies.

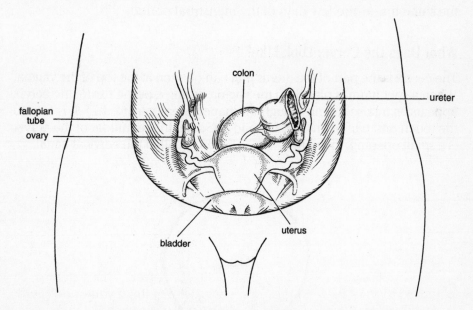

Fig. 1.1.   Position of the uterus, fallopian tubes, and ovaries

How Does the Uterus Work?

The main function of the uterus is to provide a place for a pregnancy to develop. As such, the uterus is capable of a remarkable achievement—the ability to grow from its normal size to a size large enough to accommodate a full-term infant. The uterus is composed mostly of muscle, and this muscle has the ability to stretch. In fact, during pregnancy, no new muscle cells are added to the uterus. The growth is accomplished entirely by the expansion and stretching of the cells that are already there. Since the uterus is a muscle, it also has the ability to contract and, therefore, is able to push a baby out during labor and delivery.

Unlike many creatures that are fertile and menstruate only during mating season, women are fertile for a few days every month. The inside lining of the uterus provides the place where the fertilized egg attaches and develops. The lining (endometrium) is composed of tall cells that are arranged next to each other in rows. These cells appear slightly darker and redder than the muscle wall, mostly because the cells are richly supplied with the blood vessels that are designed to provide for the placenta and pregnancy. Under the influence of the hormones produced by the ovaries, the cells all grow together at the same rate. And if a woman does not become pregnant, all the cells die and are shed at the same time—the few days of the menstrual period.

What Does the Cervix Look Like?

The cervix is the part of the uterus that can be seen at the top of the vagina. When a speculum is placed in the vagina during a pelvic exam, the cervix appears as a raised, pink, doughnut-shaped area (see fig. 1.2). It is firm to the touch and can be moved by mild pressure. In the middle of the cervix is a small opening, the entrance to the uterus, called the cervical canal.

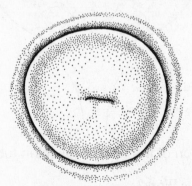

Fig. 1.2.   Cervix

Despite being part of the uterus, the cervix has entirely separate functions from the uterus and may be susceptible to entirely different diseases. For example, the virus HPV (see chapter 9) can cause cervical cancer, but does not affect other parts of the uterus. And while the Pap smear is an excellent way to detect cervical cancer, it is almost never able to detect uterine cancer. Therefore, while the cervix and uterus are connected, they should be thought of as two separate parts of your body.

How Does the Cervix Work?

The cervix is the entrance into the uterus and contains cells that regularly make mucus. The mucus is normally thick and helps to keep bacteria and even sperm out of the uterus for most of the month. As the time nears for an egg to leave the ovary (ovulation), hormonal changes cause the mucus to become thin and watery for just a few days. While still forming a relatively good barrier against infection, the thinner mucus now allows sperm to enter the uterus. Within a day or two after ovulation, the mucus is once again thick and resists the passage of the sperm. Thus, this precise timing permits the sperm access to the egg only at the time the egg is most receptive to being fertilized.

What Do the Fallopian Tubes Look Like?

The fallopian tubes are flexible, soft wands of pink tissue that extend from the top of the uterus outward and toward the ovaries on either side (see fig. 1.3). The tube is open at the end near the ovary, where feathery, short tentacles are present, which are responsible for picking up the egg at the time of ovulation. The tubes are loosely attached to the uterus all along their course by thin, soft tissue that allows them to move back and forth.

How Do the Fallopian Tubes Work?

The freedom of the fallopian tubes to move is a necessary design. Just at the time of ovulation, when the egg is released from the ovary, muscles between the tube and ovary pull the tube closer to the ovary. The fallopian tube then drapes its feathery tentacles over the ovary so that the egg is captured. This movement of the tube toward the ovary has actually been caught on film and is an incredible sight.

Once captured, the egg can begin the journey through this passageway to the uterus. The cells that line the inside of the tube have tiny hairlike extensions that actively push the egg down the tube. Fertilization

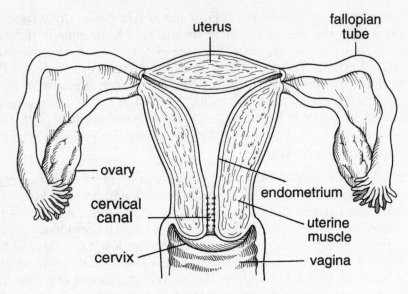

Fig. 1.3.   Reproductive system

by sperm takes place in the middle of the tube, and the tubal cells continue to push the fertilized egg into the uterus. The egg's journey down to the uterus takes about six days.

What Do the Ovaries Look Like?

The ovaries are small, walnut-sized lumps of tissue that are about one inch away from the top of the uterus on either side. They are off-white and, in young girls and adolescents, smooth. After the onset of menstruation, however, the ovaries begin to go through a series of events that leads to a change in their appearance.

Just prior to ovulation, a small (half inch) clear collection of fluid forms around the developing egg and becomes visible below the surface of the ovary. This combination of the fluid, hormone-producing cells, and the egg is called a follicle. During ovulation, the surface of the ovary bursts open, and the egg is carried away in a surge of fluid. The surface cells of the ovary heal quickly, leaving behind a yellow-appearing pocket of cells called the corpus luteum. The corpus luteum produces the hormone progesterone until the developing placenta takes over. If no pregnancy occurs, it will disappear shortly after the menstrual period. As time goes on, the surface of the ovary becomes pitted and irregular, evidence of many ovulations and subsequent healings. After menopause, the monthly formation of follicles and ovulation cease. The ovaries decrease in size to that of an almond and become a pale white.

How Do the Ovaries Work?

At the start of a normal menstrual cycle, the pituitary gland, situated at the base of the brain, releases a hormone called follicle stimulating hormone (FSH) into the bloodstream. When the FSH reaches the ovary, it stimulates an egg and the cells around the egg (the follicle) to develop. The follicular cells surrounding the egg then begin to produce estrogen, the main female hormone.

Around the middle of the cycle, the pituitary gland produces another hormone, called luteinizing hormone (LH). LH causes the cells on the surface of the ovary to break open and release the egg. After the egg is released, the ovary begins to produce progesterone, the other main female hormone, in addition to estrogen. If you become pregnant, the ovary continues to make these hormones for about three months, until the placenta is able to take over hormone production for both itself and the developing fetus.

If you don't become pregnant, the ovary stops making both estrogen and progesterone about two weeks after ovulation. Without these hormones, the uterine lining cells can't survive; they die and are shed as the menstrual flow. Then the cycle starts all over again. These finely balanced hormonal events are crucial to controlling the changes in your menstrual cycle and the normal pattern of bleeding that you expect.

Although the ovary produces eggs and estrogen to enable a pregnancy to take place, the ovary also produces estrogen as a necessary supporting hormone for many other parts of your body. Estrogen has effects on a vast array of tissues. Your bones, heart, bladder, vagina, breasts, and skin all need estrogen to stay strong and healthy.

What Does the Doctor Feel When Your Pelvic Examination Is Performed?

The manual part of the pelvic examination allows the doctor to feel the size and shape of the uterus, fallopian tubes, and ovaries. During this part of the examination, the doctor pushes the cervix upward from the inside of the vagina. This moves the top of the uterus closer to your abdominal wall, where the size and shape of the uterus can be felt between the doctor's two hands (see fig. 1.4). Thus, the doctor should be

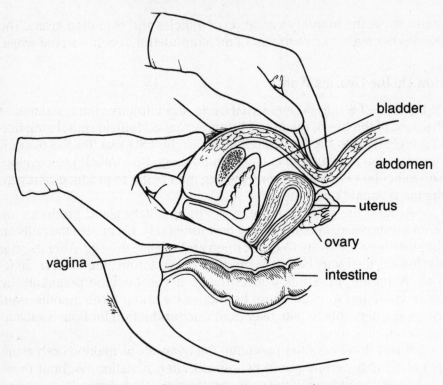

Fig. 1.4.   Performing the manual exam

able to detect conditions that increase the size of the uterus, such as fibroids.

Prior to menopause, the ovaries are normally about the size of a small walnut and, during the examination, can be felt on either side of the uterus. Abnormally large ovaries usually indicate the presence of cysts, benign tumors, or, very rarely, cancer. The fallopian tubes are so soft and mobile that they are normally not detected during the examination. Tenderness in the area of the fallopian tubes sometimes indicates infection. If endometriosis or scar tissue exists from previous infection or surgery near the tubes, tenderness may also be present during the examination.

How Often Should You Have a Pelvic Examination?

The pelvic examination should be performed yearly, starting at the time a woman becomes sexually active or by the age of eighteen. This will allow for the early detection of uterine abnormalities such as fibroids and ovarian abnormalities such as cysts or tumors. The Pap smear is performed at the same time. Pelvic pain, abnormal bleeding, or abnormal vaginal discharges are all reasons to see the doctor for an immediate pelvic examination.

How Is the Pap Smear Performed?

The cervix is the opening of the uterus, and it can be seen at the upper end of the vagina. Your doctor uses a speculum, a duck-bill–shaped instrument, for this part of the examination. When opened, the speculum spreads apart the walls of the vagina, and the cervix is visible at the top of the vagina. This examination should be performed gently and should not hurt.

Using a small plastic or wood spatula shaped somewhat like a Popsicle stick, your doctor carefully scrapes the surface of the cervix to remove some skin cells (see fig. 1.5). A small, soft brush is then inserted just inside the cervix to sample cells from that area. All the cells are spread on a glass slide and sprayed with a solution to keep them preserved. A newer method uses a liquid-filled container into which the cells are placed. This liquid-based method is more accurate because the cervical cells can be separated from mucus, blood cells, and bacteria that sometimes cloud the slide. In either case, the cells are sent to a lab where a pathologist or specially trained technician examines them under the microscope for any abnormalities.

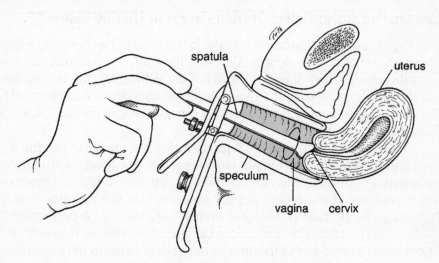

Fig. 1.5.   Performing the Pap smear

How Often Should You Have a Pap Smear?

The Pap smear is used to find cervical abnormalities long before they are actually a threat to your well-being. The major cause of cervical cancer appears to be a virus, human papillomavirus (HPV), that is transmitted sexually. Therefore, once you become sexually active you should start having Pap smears performed. Whether you are sexually active or not, a Pap smear should be performed annually along with a pelvic examination beginning at the age of eighteen.

Cervical cancer starts as dysplasia, a precancerous phase, that is detectable on the Pap smear (see chapter 9). The progression of dysplasia into cancer usually takes many years. Therefore, *yearly* Pap smears should detect changes in the cells long before they become cancerous, while the abnormal cells are easily treatable.

After three normal annual Pap smears, you and your doctor may discuss the possibility of having the test every two or three years. Since dysplasia is usually a slowly progressive disease, it is unlikely that cancer would develop within a three-year period of time. While that is the official policy of the American College of Obstetricians and Gynecologists, I still recommend annual Pap smears to my patients. Cervical dysplasia and even cancer can, on occasion, develop rapidly. Since these changes are easy to detect, an annual Pap smear will usually allow early detection and treatment.

Can the Pap Smear Detect Ovarian Cancer or Uterine Cancer?

The Pap smear is performed by scraping the cells of the cervix to examine them under a microscope. Although there is a continuous channel from the ovary, down through the fallopian tubes, into the uterus, and out the cervix, cells from the ovary never make it down that channel to the cervix. Therefore, the diagnosis of ovarian cancer cannot be made from the Pap smear.

The uterine lining cells are high up inside the uterus; consequently, they are not removed during the Pap smear. On occasion, uterine lining cells may fall through the cervix, and the pathologist will see them on the Pap smear. If these cells appear abnormal on the Pap smear, a dilatation and curettage (D&C) (see chapter 11) should be performed to evaluate whether uterine precancer or cancer is present. However, it is uncommon to find any cells other than cervical cells on the Pap smear, and the test is basically designed for the detection of cervical dysplasia and cervical cancer.

How Is the Breast Examination Performed?

Your physician should perform a breast exam at the time of your annual checkup. There are a number of ways to do this, designed to ensure that all areas of the breast are examined. The breast exam should be performed in the sitting or lying position with your arms over your head to make your breast tissue easier to feel. I start the examination by feeling, with the flat part of my fingers, the area of the breast closest to the armpit. Breast cancers most commonly occur in the upper, outer part of the breast. I then move across the breast in a straight line until I feel the breastbone. I then move my fingers down an inch or so and go back in the opposite direction. I follow this back-and-forth pattern until all of the breast tissue has been examined.

What Does Breast Cancer Feel Like?

Many women get nervous when they feel a slight lump or irregularity in their breast and assume it is cancer. However, most lumps are not cancer. Breast cancer is usually not a subtle finding. It usually feels obviously different from your normal breast tissue. Prior to menopause, normal breast tissue is soft but often has irregular, firm, lumpy areas. In addition, since your breasts are influenced by hormonal changes, they may feel more irregular, firmer, and more tender just before and during your menstrual periods. After menopause, breast glands are somewhat replaced by fat, and the breasts feel less firm and less irregular. This accounts for the change in the appearance of the breasts that women notice after menopause.

Breast cancer usually feels like a distinct and hard lump. More often than not, breast cancer is not tender to the touch and often, if pushed, will not move within the breast. However, new lumps that persist for more than a cycle should be reported to your doctor, even if they are not tender and move when pushed. Since cyclic changes in the breast don't occur after menopause, postmenopausal women should report *any* new lump. Many women will detect a breast lump at some time in their lives, and nearly all of these lumps will be benign. But, if a new lump is causing you anxiety, see your physician. That will help end the worry, and you will know for sure that you are all right. Further evaluation by mammogram and biopsy will be recommended for any suspicious lump that may be cancer (see page 14).

Should You Perform a Monthly Breast Self-Examination?

It is a good idea for you to perform a breast self-examination every month. Although the idea of self-examination makes some women uncomfortable, doing it will allow you to get familiar with the normal appearance and feel of your breasts. Then if any changes occur in your breast, you will be aware of them. Your breasts change as you age and will feel different as the years go by. Self-examination will keep you aware of these subtle changes.

Your doctor will only examine your breasts once or twice a year and may examine a few hundred women between your visits. For even the most attentive doctor, remembering exactly what *your* breasts felt like a year ago is difficult, if not impossible. However, you are examining one person, and you're doing the examination twelve times a year. You are much more likely to know if a lump has always been present and is, therefore, not worrisome. Or, if a significant change occurs, you will be aware of it and can discuss it with your doctor.

When and How Should You Do a Breast Self-Examination?

It is probably best to do a breast self-examination after your period is over, when your breasts are less likely to be tender or lumpy. If you are postmenopausal and are taking hormones, it may be best to do the exam right after the hormonally induced monthly bleeding stops. If you are taking hormones in a continuous fashion, where no bleeding occurs, or if you do not take hormones, then plan to do the self-examination around the same time every month.

There is no magic way to examine your breasts. The important thing is to get a solid sense of how your breasts usually look and feel. If you are familiar with your own body, you'll know if it has changed. It is a good idea to start by looking at your breasts in a mirror, first with your hands at your sides, then with your hands behind your head. Look for any lumps or dimples in the skin and gently squeeze the nipples to look for any discharge. The second part of the examination involves feeling your breasts for any lumps or irregularities. Some women prefer to check their breasts in the shower, some in a chair, some lying down. Some women examine their breasts in a circular motion, others use an up-and-down technique (see fig. 1.6). In general, breast cancer feels like an obvious lump and is often firm, irregular, and nontender. However, if you are premenopausal, any lump that *persists* for a cycle or two should be reported to your doctor. If you are postmenopausal, *any* lump should be reported right away.

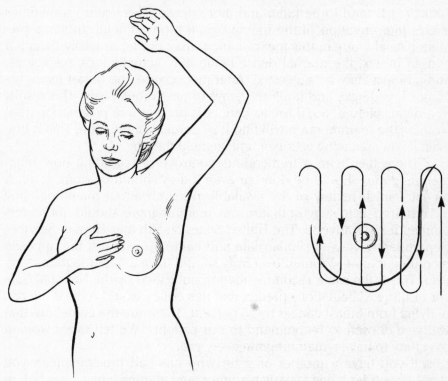

Fig 1.6.   Breast self-examination

How Often Should You Have a Mammogram?

The mammogram is an X-ray of the breast designed to detect breast cancer at an early stage, often before the woman or her doctor can feel it. Early detection of breast cancer with screening mammography appears to improve chances for a cure. The recommendations regarding the frequency of mammogram screening seem to change every year or two. Some physicians have called into question whether they have any value at all.

Without question, the techniques and X-ray machines used for mammograms are more accurate and much safer than they were years ago. Now the X-ray dose you get from one mammogram is less than the radiation you would get flying in an airplane from coast to coast. The risk to your health from the radiation exposure during one mammogram is equivalent to the risk of smoking *one cigarette* in your lifetime.

The accuracy of the mammogram differs in pre- and postmenopausal women. The mammogram is less accurate before menopause because your breasts tend to be fuller and more dense. This texture sometimes makes interpretation of the mammogram more difficult. In some premenopausal women, this means cancer may not be as easily detected and, in others, the normal dense tissue may actually look suspicious, and a biopsy may be suggested. After menopause, the breast tissue becomes less dense, and it allows X-rays to pass more easily. This results in a better picture. So, if breast cancer is present in a postmenopausal woman, the mammogram will find it 90 percent of the time. This is true even if you are taking estrogen replacement therapy.

There has been a tremendous controversy regarding how often mammograms should be done or even if they should be done at all. A recent Danish review of the available research about mammography led researchers to suggest that *routine* mammograms should not be recommended for anyone. The United States Health and Human Services Department reviewed similar data and came up with just the opposite recommendation: Women over forty should have a mammogram every year. This is the same recommendation published by the National Cancer Institute. Calculations predict that this policy would reduce the risk of dying from breast cancer by 23 percent. These are the guidelines that we have chosen to recommend to our patients. We tell every woman over forty to have a mammogram every year.

If you have a mother or sister who has had breast cancer, you should consider having yearly mammograms starting a few years before the age at which your relative was diagnosed with the disease.

Some women avoid mammograms because of the discomfort involved. Most women report that they don't feel any pain, but they do find the procedure to be awkward and briefly uncomfortable because of the pressure that is applied to the breast by the plates of the mammography apparatus. In addition, the plates are frequently cold, and the pose you are expected to hold is undeniably awkward. Some radiologists now use thin pads on the mammogram plates to make them warmer and a little more comfortable. Most women find that the good feeling of relief resulting from being told "all is well, see you next year" is worth the cold squeeze for a few unpleasant moments. Think of the long-term gain, not the short-term unpleasantness. That makes the mammogram well worthwhile.

What Happens If a Suspicious Breast Lump Is Detected?

If a suspicious area is detected in the breast on either examination or mammogram, further evaluation will be recommended. Gynecologists and family doctors are not usually trained to manage these problems beyond the initial examination, and you should be referred to a general surgeon for the detailed evaluation.

Based on the surgeon's examination and evaluation of your mammogram, cells from the suspicious area may need to be removed (biopsied) and examined under the microscope in order to determine if cancer is present. There are a number of different ways to get these cells, and the type of technique used will depend on the size of the abnormal area and the degree of suspicion of cancer.

One biopsy technique uses a fine needle attached to a syringe to draw out cells from the area. This fine-needle aspiration is performed with local anesthesia by either the radiologist or a surgeon. The aspirated cells, however, are sometimes difficult for the pathologist to interpret. If the cells look like cancer, then the test is usually correct. But, if the test is negative, a larger biopsy may need to be done to make certain that cancer is not present.

Another technique, called a stereotactic core biopsy, uses a larger needle placed with the guidance of a special mammography machine. This biopsy is performed in the radiologist's office with local anesthesia. The machine uses a computer to guide the needle directly into the area that looks suspicious. The larger needle is able to remove more tissue, making it easier for the pathologist to interpret. If the suspicious area is easily seen on the mammogram, radiologists frequently use stereotactic core biopsy.

If a lump can be felt, but not easily seen on the mammogram, then another technique, the excisional biopsy, is the choice of many surgeons. This procedure may be performed in the doctor's office or outpatient area of the hospital. Using a scalpel, the suspicious area of the breast is completely removed. If the area to be removed is small, local anesthesia can be used. Removal of larger areas may require general anesthesia in the hospital. The incisions are small, and the stitches dissolve by themselves. If cancer is diagnosed by any of these techniques, other tests will be performed to determine appropriate treatment. The complex issues that involve the treatment of breast cancer are described in a number of books listed at the end of this chapter.

Do You Really Need a Rectal Examination?

Most women find the rectal examination to be their least favorite part of a visit to the gynecologist. But the rectal examination is important because it enables the physician to detect signs of precancerous and cancerous polyps of the rectum and colon. In the intestines, unlike the uterus, polyps can lead to cancer. If polyps are found and removed in the precancerous stage, colon cancer can be prevented.

After the age of fifty, the rectal examination should be performed *yearly* at the time of your annual examination. The doctor performs the test by placing a gloved finger inside the rectum to feel for any hard areas that might represent a tumor. The stool that remains on the examining glove is then spread on a chemically treated piece of paper and tested for the presence of blood. Colon cancer, like some cancers in other areas of the body, causes tissue to become fragile and bleed. The blood can become mixed with stool and may not be visible to you. This chemical test on specially treated paper can detect even small amounts of blood. Sometimes the test may detect blood from food you have eaten or blood from common hemorrhoids. Therefore, a positive test should not be alarming but should be further evaluated by your doctor.

How Often Should You Be Tested for Colon Cancer?

The guidelines for routine colon cancer testing depend on whether you are at high or low risk for developing this disease. The greatest risk factor is the history of colon cancer in a close family member. For women who do not have a close relative who has had colon cancer, testing for blood in the stool should start at age fifty. If these tests are negative, then the stool should be retested every five years. Alternatively, some doctors recommend colonoscopy starting at age fifty and then every ten years thereafter for low-risk women.

For women who have one close relative who developed colon cancer after the age of sixty, testing the stool for blood should begin at age forty and be repeated every year. Sigmoidoscopy should also be performed at age forty and every ten years thereafter. Alternatively, colonoscopy can be performed at age forty and every ten years thereafter.

For women who are at high risk because they have more than one close relative who developed colon cancer before the age of sixty, colonoscopy is recommended starting at age forty or ten years before the age of your affected relative's age at diagnosis, whichever is earliest. Thereafter, colonoscopy should be repeated every three to five years based on the recommendation of your doctor.

A sigmoidoscopy is a test that allows your doctor to see inside your lower intestine, using a long, flexible telescope. Colonoscopy uses a longer telescope to see further up into the entire colon. Truthfully, these are tests most of us would prefer to avoid because the process of preparing for them is so unappealing. However, cancer of the colon is a *pre-*

ventable disease. The very temporary unpleasantness of a colonoscopy or sigmoidoscopy is minor when you understand that these tests literally can save your life.

Virtually all colon cancers start in polyps present in the colon. These polyps can be visibly detected by your doctor. Sigmoidoscopy is performed in the doctor's office in about thirty minutes, while colonoscopy is usually performed in a surgicenter or hospital because it requires sedating medications administered by an anesthesiologist. For a day prior to the test, you must clean out your intestines by drinking a medication that causes diarrhea. Needless to say, that day of preparation is not anyone's idea of fun. No anesthesia is given prior to sigmoidoscopy, and it is common to feel some cramping in the lower abdominal area during the procedure. Because colonoscopy involves inspecting higher up into the entire colon, sedating medication needs to be given to prevent pain. The medication is very effective, and most people do not feel, or remember, anything.

Following the guidelines for screening with sigmoidoscopy and colonoscopy can drastically reduce the incidence of colon cancer. These diagnostic tests have saved many lives and should not be avoided simply because they are unpleasant. Comfort yourself during that day of preparation by knowing that for most people, the preparation is the worst part. Think of something fun for yourself to do once it is over, and you've gotten a clean bill of health. Celebrate your good judgment and good health.

How Often Should You Have a Pelvic Sonogram?

A sonogram may be a useful test if a doctor thinks he or she feels something abnormal during your pelvic examination. The sonogram can confirm if an abnormality is really present and can determine its size and composition. For example, ovarian cysts and fibroids can be accurately diagnosed this way.

However, as discussed fully in chapter 10, the regular use of pelvic sonograms for *healthy* women is *not indicated.* This test often will suggest that something is wrong, when in fact no cancer is present. Any abnormal finding may then lead to unnecessary surgery, as well as to unnecessary anxiety. Experimentally, the use of yearly sonograms is being tested on women who are at high risk for developing ovarian cancer, women with a mother or sister, or both, who have had ovarian cancer (see chapter 10). Even for these high-risk women, the results have not been very encouraging. Some women at high risk have developed ovarian cancer despite a normal sonogram, and others with abnormal tests have been found, at the time of surgery, to have a benign cyst in the ovary.

It is clear that a test for the early detection of ovarian cancer is imperative to reduce mortality from this frightening disease. Some of the newer, promising research regarding ovarian cancer screening tests is discussed in chapter 10. However, while much time and money are being invested in this research, annual pelvic examinations by your doctor may still be the best way to diagnose early.

How Often Should You Have Your Blood Tested?

Your blood can be tested for an almost infinite number of biochemicals and hormones. Obviously, if you have any medical conditions, your doctor will check your blood periodically, depending on the particular condition and its severity. However, even if you are well, you should probably check your cholesterol and the HDL and LDL lipid levels every five years. These tests check for the biochemical that carries fat in your blood. The blood should be taken in the morning after you've fasted for about twelve hours. A high cholesterol and LDL level increases your risk of heart disease, the leading killer of women today, and stroke. Low cholesterol and high HDL levels are linked to a low risk of heart disease and stroke. If the test is elevated, exercise and dietary changes may be prescribed in order to lower the level. Medications may also be used in some women who have a very high level of cholesterol, which is resistant to diet and exercise regimens.

Women have an increased risk of developing an underactive thyroid gland, so after age fifty it is also a good idea to check your thyroid gland function with a blood test. The thyroid gland affects almost all of the functions of your body, so awareness of an underactive thyroid and treatment with thyroid hormone medication is important for your health.

What Else Can You Do for Your Health?

We all want to lead long, healthy lives and then peacefully die in our sleep when old, but not yet declining. You and I both know that, at present, there are no ways to guarantee that for ourselves. But keeping our bodies strong and healthy is something that we do have some control over. People feel better, both mentally and physically, when their bodies are fit. But getting there is sometimes a struggle. We are blessed with a wealth of food in this country, but much of it is too high in fat, sugar, salt, and calories. We are also blessed with the finest health-care services in the world, but some of us are unable or unwilling to use them.

I can only urge you to do the very best you possibly can for yourself. If you hate exercising, just make sure you walk around a bit. Walking for thirty minutes a few times a week can be beneficial to your health. Pick up the pace if you're strolling through the mall or in your neighborhood. Take the stairs occasionally instead of the elevator. Lift one- or three-pound weights while watching your favorite television program. Every little bit helps, and once you get started you may find you actually enjoy the exercise.

If you smoke, try hard to stop. This is the most significant thing you can do for your health! In addition to the well-known effects of smoking—lung cancer, respiratory disease, and heart attacks—smoking also increases your risk of cervical cancer (see page 255).

If you have trouble keeping the fats and calories to a minimum in your diet, begin with small steps toward healthier eating. Have fruits and vegetables with your meals each day. Switch to low-fat milk and cheeses. Give whole grains a try. Hold the mayo. There are many great foods out there that are healthy and truly delicious. We all can't look, eat, or work out like the latest celebrity with an exercise video. But we can do a little better for ourselves than we do now, and it won't take that much effort. When the small changes in exercise and diet start to make a difference in the way you feel or look, you may do more. Don't strive for perfection; just strive for improvement.

While we know that there are limits to our control over our health, we can do our best to stay healthy. For a woman, a Pap smear, a mammogram, and an annual pelvic and breast examination can go a long way toward gynecologic health. If you have questions or problems, be sure to get them answered. Do the very best you can for yourself. Be informed. We hope this book will provide you with the foundation to help you make decisions about your health that you may need to make. Use preventive health strategies and seek the best care possible when you need it. We wish you good health!

REFERENCES

Bettman, O. 1956. *A Pictoral History of Medicine.* Springfield, Ill.: Charles C. Thomas.

Byers, T., B. Levin, D. Rothenberger, G. Dodd, and R. Smith. 1997. American Cancer Society guidelines for screening and surveillance for early detection of colorectal polyps and cancer: Update 1997. *CA—A Cancer Journal for Clinicians* 47:154–60.

Love, S. 1990. *Dr. Susan Love's Breast Book.* Reading, Mass.: Addison-Wesley.

Morra, M., and E. Potts. 1994. *Choices—Realistic Alternatives in Cancer Treatment.* New York: Avon.

National Institutes of Health. *What You Need to Know About Breast Cancer.* Call 1-800-4-CANCER (422-6237) for a free copy.

Singer, C. 1962. *A Short History of Medicine.* Oxford: Oxford University Press.

2

CONTRACEPTION

Most women of childbearing age face the contraception issue at one point or another. What should I use? How effective is this method? Will it have any effect on my health or future fertility? Could I deal with being pregnant if the method doesn't work? While most people regard their children as the light of their lives and their greatest accomplishment, a poorly timed pregnancy can strain a marriage, a family's finances, the care of other children or relatives, or the plans for an education or career. There are also the larger issues we encounter when we stop considering pregnancy on a solely personal level and look at it as a global concern, one with enormous consequences. In most countries of the world, contraception is either unavailable or unaffordable. Both accurate information about contraception and access to qualified medical personnel are often limited. Some women choose, or are subjected to, cultural or religious constraints against preventing pregnancy.

Even in developed countries, contraception may not be easily available to women. The ramifications of the birth control issue are especially compelling in the United States, the richest country in the world, where about 50 percent of all pregnancies are unintended, and 50 percent of those pregnancies end with abortion. Among adolescents, nearly 80 percent of pregnancies are unintended. More than one-half of abortions are obtained by women under age twenty-five, and 80 percent of these women are not married. In many developed countries other than the Untied States, contraception is more easily available to women and less expensive. Other countries allow contraceptives to be advertised on TV and provide better sex education for their children in school. In Sweden, 95 percent of women at risk for an unintended pregnancy use some form of contraception.

In the United States, unintended pregnancy creates economic problems as well as moral ones. For each dollar spent on public funding for contraception and family planning, calculations show that $4.50 is saved on prenatal care, welfare and nutritional services, maternal child health services, and education. This, of course, does not even touch the emotional issues of unwanted pregnancies to mother, child, and family. On all levels, it makes good sense to avoid unintended pregnancy.

If you need contraception, this chapter provides you with a review of the birth control options currently available and the associated risks and advantages for each method. We hope you will get enough information to help you make an educated decision to meet your needs. As always, discuss your questions and your particular situation with your health-care provider.

How Does Pregnancy Occur?

For a woman to become pregnant a number of things must occur. First, there must be an egg available from a woman's ovary to be fertilized; sperm must be available to fertilize the egg; and the fallopian tube must be open so that the egg and sperm can meet. The egg is fertilized in the middle of the fallopian tube and then travels through the tube to the uterus. The uterine lining must be healthy so that the egg can attach (implantation) and develop properly (see fig. 2.1). All contraceptive methods work by interfering with one or more of these processes.

How Likely Are You to Get Pregnant?

If 1,000 healthy women under the age of thirty had intercourse during the mid-portion of their monthly cycle without contraception, about 850 women would get pregnant during one year. Contraceptive methods can substantially decrease that risk.

As women get older, the chance of getting pregnant decreases. By age thirty-seven, fertility starts to decline, and by age forty, it is even more difficult to get pregnant. However, pregnancy is *possible* until menopause, and contraception should be used until that time.

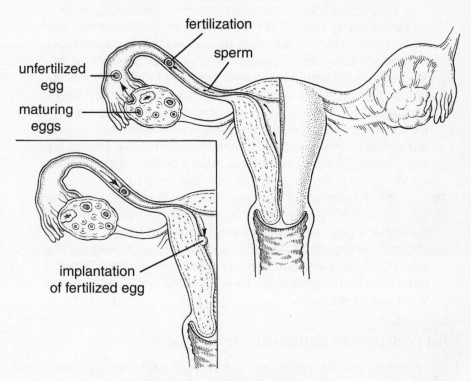

Fig. 2.1. Normal fertilization

Alanna's Story

Alanna is a twenty-year-old sophomore at an Ivy League college where she is studying political science with the intention of going to law school. She came to see us for a routine gynecologic examination. As part of taking her medical history, I asked her if she was sexually active. She said she had been dating another student for a few months and had been sexually active for about one month. When I asked what type of birth control she was using, she casually answered, "We haven't been using anything." I was taken a bit by surprise and asked whether she wanted to get pregnant. She answered with an emphatic "No!" When I asked how she could explain neglecting birth control when she clearly did not want to be pregnant, she had no answer. She said she "kind of thought pregnancy would never happen unless I wanted it to."

It is illogical, but surprisingly common, for intelligent, well-educated young women to either skip over this important issue or be completely misinformed. In our practice, we sometimes experience this "oops" mentality. Alanna and I reviewed her medical history, and I emphasized her need for both contraception and STI (sexually transmitted infection) prevention. After reviewing all of her options, she chose to start birth control pills. I gave her a few months' worth of samples to help her get started immediately. We performed routine testing for STIs during the examination. She also planned to make sure her boyfriend used condoms until they were sure neither had any STIs.

When I saw her for her annual exam one year later, she was still seeing the same boyfriend and had stopped using the condoms since they were both monogamous and free of STIs. But she had continued to take the birth control pills, without any side effects and without any unwanted pregnancies. "When I think back on the chance we took," she told me, "I just shudder. What was I thinking?"

What Contraceptive Methods are Now Available?

No method of contraception is perfect, and each has its own set of advantages and disadvantages. The currently available means of contraception are:

- Birth control pills
- Emergency contraception pills
- Intrauterine devices (IUDs)
- Barrier methods, such as condoms, the diaphragm, sponge, or cervical cap
- Spermicides in the form of foam, film, or cream
- Rhythm (periodic abstinence)
- Abstinence
- Withdrawal
- Hormonal injections (Depo-Provera, Lunelle)
- Hormonal implants (Implanon) beneath the skin
- Hormonal vaginal ring
- Hormonal patch
- Female and male surgical sterilization
- Male hormonal injections

One of these methods may be very reasonable for one woman but unsuitable for others. The goal for you and your doctor is to find out what will work best for you.

Here are the factors to consider when choosing a contraceptive method:

- Effectiveness of the method
- Frequency of intercourse—more often increases your risk of pregnancy
- Relative importance to you of not becoming pregnant
- How careful you are likely to be using the method (Will you remember to take a pill *every day*? Will you insert a diaphragm *every time*?)
- Availability and cost of the method
- Your age and general medical condition (some methods may have increased risk with age or medical diseases)

Sara's Story

In appearance, Sara is the perfect California girl. She's a tall, willowy blonde with deep blue eyes. Our practice attended at her birth twenty-two years ago, and we have been delighted to see her grow into a down-to-earth, kind young woman. During her last visit to the office, Sara excitedly told us about her boyfriend—a young man who is trying to make a living as a tennis instructor. They have been sexually active for the last six months and were using foam and condoms. "I think he might really be *the one*," Sara told us. "Even my dad really likes him. We're probably going to wait to get married, but we are thinking and talking about it!" Since they were having sex regularly, Sara asked about changing to some birth control method that involves a little less hassle than the foam. Her main goal with this office visit was to go over her options. We asked questions about whether she was smoking (no), had any prior STIs (no). We suggested she ask her boyfriend, Eric, to get tested for HIV and STIs before they stopped using a condom. Since Sara knew taking a pill every day was something she would be diligent about, we recommended birth control pills. "I'm hoping Eric will be the father of my kids someday, but we are so far from being ready now. The pill sounds perfect."

What Are Birth Control Pills?

Birth control pills are made of a combination of synthetic hormones—forms of estrogen and progesterone (called progestins) that when taken daily prevent the ovary from releasing an egg, thus preventing pregnancy. Birth control pills come in packages designed to make taking them easy, and they must be taken daily to be effective. When they were first made available in the 1960s, researchers did not know how much hormone would be needed to reliably prevent pregnancy. Those first pills contained very high doses of hormone, as much as eight times the amount found in the low-dose pills of today. However, further research showed that much lower doses of estrogen and progestins were sufficient to prevent pregnancy, and the low doses were fortunately associated with fewer side effects. There are now about thirty types of pills available, differing in the amounts, types, and combinations of hormones.

How Do Birth Control Pills Work?

For an egg to develop in the ovary and then be released, a complicated symphony of hormonal events must take place. An area of the brain, called the hypothalamus, is responsible for regulating the hormonal signals that start this process. The hormones in the pill shut off these signals from the brain that tell the ovary to develop and release an egg. Without these signals, the egg does not develop and is not available to be released (ovulated) and pregnancy cannot occur. In addition, the pill has a few other effects on your body that decrease the likelihood of pregnancy. One of the hormones in the pill, the progestin, makes the mucus thicker in the cervix and tubes so that it is more difficult for sperm to pass into the uterus and more difficult for the egg to move down the tube. Also, the pill causes changes in the uterine lining that hinders implantation of the fertilized egg.

Birth control pills contain synthetic hormones, somewhat different from their natural forms so that they can be taken orally and not be destroyed by the digestive juices in the stomach and intestines. All the pills now contain the same estrogen, ethinyl estradiol, but slightly different types of progesterones called progestins. Different brands of pills contain various doses of both estrogen and progestins to meet the needs of a range of women. While you may find one birth control pill suits you perfectly, another woman may have undesirable side effects from that same pill.

The pills originally made in the 1960s contained about 80–150 micrograms (mcg) of estrogen. Today's pills contain either 50 mcg of estrogen, called high-dose; 35 mcg, called low-dose; or 20 mcg, called very low-dose.

Very low-dose pills are just as effective as high-dose pills for prevention of pregnancy. It is best to take the lowest dose pill, so that side effects are less likely. However, some women notice bothersome breakthrough bleeding on the lowest dose pills. Switching to a slightly higher dose pill often resolves this bleeding. Women's bodies are different, so you may need to try a few types of oral contraceptives to find the one that is right for you.

HOW EFFECTIVE ARE BIRTH CONTROL PILLS?

If taken properly, one pill swallowed every day, the birth control pills are 99.9 percent effective in preventing pregnancy. Some women may occasionally miss pills during a cycle, reducing the general effectiveness to about 97 percent. Using our previous example, if 1,000 women taking birth control pills have intercourse during one year, only 30 would get pregnant. So, when taken properly, the effectiveness of the pill is extremely high.

Pills are packaged with twenty-one pills that contain hormones, called active pills, and these are taken daily for the first twenty-one days of the month. Packages usually also contain seven pills of another color, containing either iron or placebos, to make it easier to remember to take a pill every day of the month. The iron also helps to replenish iron lost in the blood at the time of menstruation. Missing active pills, especially two or more, can make the pills less effective. Missing placebo or iron pills has no impact on the effectiveness of the pill for contraception.

Jennifer's Story

Nadine, a longtime patient of ours, was aware that her daughter Jennifer was sexually active, and she wisely convinced Jennifer to come to the office to discuss contraception. Jennifer, a nineteen-year-old college junior, told us that most of her friends were taking birth control pills, and that's what she wanted to do too. Nadine, however, had serious concerns about the safety of the pill and came to us for "the final word." After examining Jennifer to make sure she was a good candidate for oral contraception, the three of us sat down to talk about the safety issues. "So many women my age talk about strokes and heart attacks being related to the pill," Nadine told us. "And you hear so much about the pill and breast cancer. It scares me. Until my daughter is married, I don't want her pregnant, but her safety and health are my main concerns right now." During our conversation, we realized that Nadine's friends might have been referring to the high-dose birth control pills that were used in the seventies. We discussed the new low-dose pills and the extremely rare risk of serious side effects and also the very rare risk of even minor problems such as nausea or weight gain. Jennifer was happy to hear about the new advances in the pill and decided that this was the best method for her. Learning the facts about the pill reassured Nadine that her beloved daughter was making a sound decision.

What Are Mistaken Beliefs About Birth Control Pills?

There are many mistaken beliefs about the pill. Some of these beliefs stem from the early days when very high-dose pills were used. A recent survey found that 50 percent of women college students mistakenly believed that the pill is associated with a substantial risk to health. Forty-seven percent mistakenly believed that birth control pills cause breast cancer, and 9 percent think that the pill causes heart attacks. Current research shows that *none* of this is true. Birth control pills provide very safe and very effective contraception for millions of women.

There is a common misconception that birth control pills increase the risk of strokes, heart attacks, and blood clots. They *do not*. The risk of a heart attack for a woman on the pill is about 1 out of 10,000. For comparison, the risk of heart attack for a pregnant woman (the placenta makes high levels of estrogen) is 6 out of 10,000, or six times the risk. The only exception to these statistics is for women who smoke, who are older than thirty-five, and who take the pill. If you wish to take the pill after age thirty-five, you must stop smoking for twelve months before you may safely take the pill. Women who use other forms of nicotine, such as the patch or gum, are subject to the same restrictions. Low-dose pills very rarely may cause a slight increase in blood pressure, so your doctor will check your blood pressure every year at the time of your annual visit.

Jody's Story

"That was the worst pain of my life," twenty-five-year-old Jody told us. "I thought I would just die. And going to the hospital in the middle of the night was horrible. I hated the whole thing." Jody has had three ovarian cysts in the last two years. It seems as if every four or five months she feels a dull pain on one side near where her ovaries are. The last cyst resulted in a late-hour visit to the emergency room. An ultrasound done by the emergency room doctor showed a two-inch cyst on her left ovary, and she was sent home with pain medication and told to "wait it out." The pain did get better over the next few days, but she had to miss a few days of work and then pay a whopping emergency room bill. She wondered if there was anything she could do to stop the cysts from forming in the first place to prevent a repeat of that night. The most common type of ovarian cysts usually forms from overproduction of fluid by the cells that surround a developing egg. Because birth control pills work by stopping the development of the eggs in the ovaries, the pill can also be very effective in decreasing the risk of forming this type of cyst.

We discussed the pill with Jody, and she was delighted to know that there was something she could do to prevent another painful cyst. She has taken the pill now for about two years and has not had another cyst or any trips to the emergency room.

What Are the Benefits of Taking the Pill?

In the same study of college women discussed on page 28, less than 20 percent of the women knew about the long-term health benefits of taking the pill. The most obvious benefit of the pill is that it is a very reliable and safe way to prevent pregnancy. In addition, the pill also effectively reduces the risk of tubal, or ectopic, pregnancy. Taking the pill also reduces your risk of developing benign breast cysts and fibroadenomas, both common reasons for breast biopsies. The pill decreases the risk of forming benign ovarian cysts, which sometimes require surgery. Many women on the pill experience lighter and shorter menstrual periods than their prepill periods. With less blood lost through menstruation, a low blood count—called anemia—resulting from previous heavy bleeding, can be improved. Also, many women with irregular periods will find that taking the pill makes their periods very regular and predictable.

The ovary makes testosterone, the predominant male hormone. All contraception pills reduce the level of testosterone present in women. These lower levels of testosterone help prevent acne and oily skin. In addition, the pill makes the cervical mucus thicker, and this acts as a barrier to bacteria. The risk of uterine and pelvic infection is, therefore, lower for women on the pill.

There are also important disease-prevention benefits for women who take the pill for a few years or longer. The risk of getting ovarian cancer decreases by 10 percent for every year of pill use. This means if you use the pill for five years, you have a 50 percent reduced risk; eight years of oral contraceptives reduces the risk of ovarian cancer by 80 percent. And the protection lasts for fifteen years after you stop taking the pill. Likewise, the risk of uterine cancer decreases 50 percent after five years of pill use. The reduction in these cancers is an important, and largely unknown, benefit of taking the pill.

Some women get migraine headaches around the time of their periods. The cause of these menstrual migraines is uncertain, but the fluctuation of your hormones has something to do with it. Many women who take the pill notice an improvement in the frequency and severity of their migraines. Taking the pill continuously, as discussed on page 29, is a good way to prevent menstrual migraines.

Can the Pill Help Relieve Acne?

A few birth control pills advertise that they have been proven to help relieve acne in young women. The ads make it sound like these are the only brands that provide this benefit. However, *all* brands of pills decrease the amount of the hormone testosterone in the bloodstream, and all have a beneficial effect of reducing oily skin and acne. However, under FDA rules, only companies that spent the money to do these specific studies are allowed to advertise this benefit. Other companies that chose not to finance a study about acne are not allowed to advertise complexion enhancement as a benefit of their product. Certain brands of pills may work better for one woman than another, so you may need to try more than one type before finding the one that is best for you.

What Are the Side Effects of Birth Control Pills?

The low doses of the presently available pills are associated with very few side effects. However, some women may experience mild nausea, water retention, or breast tenderness for a short while (a few weeks to a few months) until their body gets accustomed to the pill. Rarely, women may need to switch pills or even change to a different contraceptive method because these side effects are too bothersome or persistent.

Irregular bleeding or spotting is common in the first few months of taking the pills, until your body gets used to the new levels of hormones. This bleeding should also resolve after the first few months. The lower the dose of estrogen in the pills, the more likely this irregular bleeding will occur. Even if you experience irregular bleeding, as long as you are taking the pills properly, one every day, they will work to prevent pregnancy. Also, bleeding or spotting does not mean anything is wrong with you. If the bleeding persists for more than three months, call your doctor to discuss switching to a different pill. If you have heavy or persistent bleeding, an ultrasound of the uterus may be performed to see if there is another cause for the heavy bleeding, such as fibroids, polyps, or overgrowth of the uterine lining.

On very low-dose pills, some women may not have any period at the end of the cycle. This is not a worrisome situation. The low dose of hormones in the pill may not be enough to make the uterine lining cells grow, and, therefore, there may not be enough cells to be shed as the menstrual flow. However, some women worry that lack of bleeding means they are pregnant and end up performing home pregnancy tests every month. If this applies to you, we would recommend changing to a slightly higher dose of pills for peace of mind.

Does the Pill Cause Weight Gain?

Most of the studies that have tried to find a relationship between pill use and weight gain have come up empty-handed. Some women do note a pound or two of water retention the first few months of taking the pill, but this usually goes away by the third month. Despite the lack of evidence from the research, we occasionally see someone in our practice quickly gaining about five pounds on the pill and losing the weight fairly soon after the pill is stopped. Sometimes switching to another pill will avoid the weight gain. One of the newer pills, containing the progesterone drospirenone, has a diuretic effect that prevents this water retention. This pill may be a good choice for women who have had a weight gain problem with the pill. Sometimes switching to another type of contraceptive is the best answer.

What Are the Uncommon Side Effects of the Pill?

One of the infrequent, but unpleasant, side effects of taking the pill is the development of dark spots or discoloration on the face. This increase in facial pigment, called chloasma, occurs in less than 5 percent of women on the pill. There is usually a gradual disappearance of the spots within a few months after the pill is discontinued. Rarely, the pigmentation remains but can be treated with bleaching agents by a dermatologist.

Some women notice a change in mood while on the pill. In the rare individual, depression can occur. So if you notice (or your friends or relatives notice) a change in your mood, discuss changing to a different pill with your doctor. Most women can find a pill that does not alter mood, but some women cannot use any pill for this reason. On the other hand, some women with premenstrual syndrome (PMS) notice that the pill makes the PMS better. In our experience, one-third of women feel there is an improvement in their PMS, one-third notice they feel worse, and one-third will not feel any different. Some women may note a decrease in their sex drive while on the pill. Again, changing to a different pill may make a difference.

What Are the Long-Term Risks of Taking the Pill?

On low-dose pills, the risk of serious problems is extremely small, and studies show us that the pill is much safer than was once thought. In some women the pill may cause the liver to change the way it makes blood-clotting factors, resulting in slightly thicker, more easily clotting blood. This is such a minor change that you will not be aware of anything different. However, a very uncommon consequence is a *very slight* increased risk of blood clots in the lungs. The ordinary risk of developing a blood clot is about 1 in 40,000 women per year. If you are taking the pill, the risk increases to 4 in 40,000, still a very, very small risk. On the other hand, if you get pregnant, the very high amounts of hormones made by the placenta during pregnancy increase your risk of a blood clot in the lung to 24 in 40,000. Therefore, while the pill may increase the risk very slightly, it prevents you from getting pregnant, which would result in a higher risk. Remember, though, that the risk of a blood clot while taking the pill is very small—4 out of 40,000 pill users.

For women who do not smoke cigarettes, the risk of having a stroke or heart attack while using the low-dose pill is no higher than the risk for women not taking the pill. Smoking cigarettes, however, increases the risks of both heart attack and stroke substantially for all women, especially those over thirty-five years old. And, the combination of smoking, taking the pill, and being older than thirty-five greatly increases the risk of stroke and heart attack. For that reason, women over thirty-five who smoke should not use the pill as a means of birth control.

Can the Pill Decrease Your Fertility?

The pill has no long-term ill effects on future fertility. If a woman decides to stop taking the pill and tries to get pregnant, there may be a slight decrease in fertility in the first three months after stopping the pill as her body readjusts to being off the hormones. However, this adjustment is short-lived, and by the end of two years, more than 90 percent of former pill users will have been able to get pregnant. It is also important to note that the risk of miscarriage is no higher for women who have just stopped the pill in order to try to get pregnant, and there is no difference in the quality of eggs or the sex or health of the children born.

Who Should Not Take the Pill?

The pill is metabolized, or broken down, in the liver. Women with active liver disease such as hepatitis or cirrhosis should not take the pill unless their blood tests of the liver go back to normal. Women with a very rare form of liver disease called cholestatic liver disease should never take the pill because this is a chronic disease, and the liver never fully heals. Women with a history of blood clots or a known abnormality of blood clotting should not use the pill. Women who have had a heart attack or stroke should not take the pill, nor should women with severe systemic Lupus take the pill. Women with undiagnosed abnormal vaginal bleeding should wait until after they have had a gynecologic evaluation to determine the cause of bleeding. While the pill does not cause breast cancer, women with breast cancer should not take the pill because the dose of estrogen may stimulate cancer when it is already present.

Beth's Story

> Beth is a twenty-year-old woman who came in to the office to discuss birth control. She was hoping to get a prescription for birth control pills, but her mother had been diagnosed with breast cancer about five years ago, and Beth worried that this medical history would put her in the group of women for whom oral contraceptives was not recommended. Beth told us her mother, who was doing fine now, feared the pill's risk of increasing the chances of Beth also getting breast cancer. We sat down and reviewed the latest findings reported in the medical literature. Many studies have been done to see if the pill can increase a woman's risk of getting breast cancer, and they show that the answer is no.
>
> Beth told us that seeing the medical literature and taking a look at the conclusions gave her more peace of mind than she thought possible. "I got home and called my mother to tell her what I learned," Beth told us. "She immediately objected and repeated how fearful she was. I answered with a host of facts that I'd written down from my consultation with you. Those studies

convinced her. We're both comfortable with my being on the
pill now."

Does the Pill Increase Your Risk of Getting Cancer?

After much testing and follow-up on the pill regarding its potential to
cause cancer, to the best of science's ability we now know the following:

A few studies done many years ago suggested a slight increase in
the risk of breast cancer for young women who had taken very high-
dose pills for more than four years. Recent studies done on the low-dose
pills available today show no increased risk and, furthermore, no increased risk in women with a family history of breast cancer or women
with benign breast cysts.

The pill does not increase your risk for getting the conventional
kind of cervical cancer. However, an extremely rare form of cervical
cancer, called adenocarcinoma, does appear to be more common in
women who are taking the pill. However, the risk is very small. For
women not taking the pill, the actual risk of getting adenocarcinoma is
1 in 100,000. The risk is 2 in 100,000 for women taking the pill. Abnormal
cells can be detected with a Pap smear before they turn into cancer, so
it is important to get annual Pap smears when you are on the pill.

As noted before, *ovarian* cancer decreases by 50 percent for women
who take the pill for longer than five years, and decreases an additional
10 percent for every year the pill is taken thereafter. The risk of *uterine*
cancer developing in your lifetime will also decrease about 50 percent if
you take the pill longer than five years.

How Should You Take the Pill?

Most of the available pills are called Sunday start pills, meaning that the
first pill of the cycle should be taken on a Sunday. The reason for this is
convenience; if you start the first pill on a Sunday, your last active pill
will also be taken on a Sunday, and you should start to bleed in the next
day or two. Therefore, your period should never come on a weekend—
the time most women are more likely to be both physically and sexually
active. Also, if you start the pill on the first Sunday following the first day
of your period, and you do not miss any pills, the pill should be immediately effective on that very first cycle.

It does not matter if you take the pills during the day or at night,
with or without food. However, it is best to get in the habit of taking the
pills the same time every day. If you are late taking your pill by even a
few hours, you may experience spotting or bleeding. Missed pills may

also lead to irregular bleeding, which is usually light. If you miss a pill during a cycle and you have bleeding, this does not mean that the pill will not prevent pregnancy. If you miss one of the iron pills or placebo pills, then you do not have to make it up, and you can just pick up with the pill you are supposed to take that day.

What Should You Do If You Miss a Pill?

It is best not to miss any of the active, hormone-containing pills. However, sometimes you may slip and miss a pill, and you will need to make it up. If you miss any one of the first twenty-one pills in a package (the hormone-containing pills), then you should take the missed pill as soon as you can on the same day. If you cannot take it until the next day, then take two pills, the one you missed and the one you should take for that day. Some women may have mild nausea if they take two pills at once, but it usually will go away quickly. If you miss pills two days in a row, then take one of the missed pills with the scheduled pill for each of the next two days, then resume taking the pills correctly. If you miss more than two pills during a cycle, the pills may not be effective in preventing pregnancy. You should continue to take the pills, but should also use another form of contraception, such as foam or condoms, for the rest of that month for backup protection.

Merri's Story

Merri is a twenty-two-year-old woman who is getting married in two months. After the wedding, she and her husband plan to honeymoon in Hawaii. Merri is currently taking birth control pills and has very regular and predictable bleeding on the pill. However, she figured out that her period is due right when she plans to be having the time of her life at a resort on Maui. "I've spent the last eight months planning our wedding and honeymoon, and I can't bear to think of having a period during what's supposed to be the most romantic week of my life! What can I do?" She wanted to know if she could "postpone" her period for two weeks. It so happens she can. We told Merri to throw away the placebo pills from her next package of pills and to start the following package right away. Without a week off the active pills, no bleeding would occur. Once she was back in town, she could take the placebo pills at the end of the second package of pills and would get her period then. This would not harm her health or her future fertility. "Oh, you've really made my day with this news. I bet I'll even be thinking about you guys on my honeymoon because of this." We extended our best wishes on her impending marriage, but told her not to bother thinking about us until she was due for a checkup.

Can You Postpone Bleeding for an Event—Like a Wedding or Vacation?

Just as in the case of the new bride Merri in the anecdote above, some women find that they are scheduled to have bleeding at the end of a package of pills that falls at an inconvenient time, such as during a vacation. You can postpone bleeding by taking all the pills during a cycle except the seven placebo pills at the end of the package. Throw away the seven placebo pills and start a new package immediately after the first package is finished. You will postpone bleeding until you take the placebo pills at the end of the next cycle.

In fact, doctors have recently started to question the need to have monthly bleeding at all when you are on the pill. In times past, women were often pregnant or breast-feeding much of their lives, and it was rare for a woman to have periods every month. Avoiding monthly bleeding may prevent anemia by allowing your body to keep the blood it has manufactured over the course of the month. The extra blood may give you more energy. Some doctors now give the active birth control pills every day for three months followed by seven days of placebos, at which time bleeding will occur. It is also safe to take the active pills for an even longer period of time, say six months, before bleeding occurs. These new schedules have been shown to be entirely safe. New packaging on some pills will be designed just for this type of schedule.

Should You Stop the Pill Every Few Years "To Give Your Body a Rest"?

When the pill first became available, very little was known about it. One of the worries was that its continued use might impair fertility. As a result, doctors often suggested that women stop the pill every few years to "let their bodies rest" and recover normal menstrual function, which would, they thought, maintain fertility. However, it has been shown that even long-term use, twenty years or more, is not associated with any changes in fertility when the pill is stopped. Hormonal function and fertility return quickly, within a month or two. Therefore, you do not need to stop the pill for a "rest." In fact, women who do stop the pill for a brief period of time are more likely to get pregnant because they tend to use less effective birth control, or no birth control, during this rest period.

How Long Can You Take the Pill?

Low-dose pills can now be safely taken from adolescence until menopause. Most side effects occur in the first few months of taking the pill. Longer use is actually associated with decreased risk of problems. Again, if *you smoke*, then you MUST discontinue using the pill by the time you reach thirty-five years old. Obviously, it would be much better for your health if you stopped smoking. But the combination of being over thirty-five years of age, smoking, and taking the pill can significantly increase your risk of heart attack or stroke.

Sandy's Story

Sandy is a forty-seven-year-old woman who came to the office because she was having hot flashes and trouble sleeping. When asked, she also said she had been having longer menstrual cycles, now having a period about every forty-five days, for approximately the past six months. Sometimes she even missed an entire period. Because of her age, we knew these problems were caused by perimenopause, the transition time between normal predictable menstrual cycles and menopause, when all bleeding stops. During perimenopause, hormone levels fluctuate a great deal, resulting in levels both higher and lower than normal within the same month. The hormone fluctuations cause hot flashes, disturbance to sleep, and emotional swings. We suggested that Sandy try low-dose birth control pills to help with these symptoms. The pill works by shutting off the ovaries' supply of hormones and then supplying its own hormones on a daily basis. The level of hormones coming from the ovaries can vary on a daily basis, while those derived from the pill are exactly the same every day. Also, the hormone levels from the pill are high enough to stop the hot flashes and insomnia and effectively stop the emotional ups and downs of perimenopause. The pill also provided her with birth control, so she didn't have to fuss with putting her diaphragm in every time she and her husband decided to have sex. Sandy has been on the pill for one year now. "My husband and kids seem to like me better these days. Taking the pill is a lifesaver. I was even starting to dislike myself," Sandy told us. "I feel great."

Are There Benefits to Taking the Pill During Perimenopause?

Perimenopause is the time of hormonal transition from regular cycles to more irregular cycles. Perimenopause comes before menopause, the absence of cycles. This transition from perimenopause to menopause can take up to ten years, starting at age forty or so, with the average age of menopause at fifty-two. During perimenopause, hormonal levels produced by the ovary tend to be irregular and unpredictable. The changes in hormone levels can lead to mood swings, intermittent hot flashes, insomnia, and resulting fatigue. As noted on page 26, the birth control pill prevents pregnancy by shutting off the signals that lead to the development of an egg and, therefore, also shuts off the supply of estrogen and progesterone made by the developing egg.

If you take birth control pills during perimenopause, the pill shuts off the irregular supply of estrogen made by the ovary during this time and replaces it with the constant level of hormones contained in the pills. The constant level of hormones often eliminates most of the symptoms associated with perimenopause. Perimenopausal women on the pill tend to be free of hot flashes, sleep better, and have stability in their moods and energy. In addition, the contraception provided by the pill ensures they don't become pregnant.

If you choose to use the pill during perimenopause, you will have regular bleeding from the pill, and you will not know when menopause begins. So, as you approach your early fifties, your doctor can check your hormone level at the end of the week when you are taking the placebo pills. If the levels show that the ovary has stopped producing estrogen, you are in menopause and no longer need to take the pill. If you are menopausal, you should discuss with your doctor the benefits and risks of hormone replacement therapy in your particular situation.

What If You Have Irregular Bleeding on the Pill?

It is not uncommon to have some irregular bleeding when you start taking birth control pills. Not only is this bleeding not dangerous or worrisome, it is also not associated with an increased risk of getting pregnant. About 30 percent of women will have some irregular bleeding in the first month of taking the pill as the body gets used to the new hormones. By the third month, only 10 percent of women will have unexpected bleeding. If the bleeding persists past the third month, call your doctor.

In the past, gynecologists often recommended that you "double up" or take two pills every day for a few days. However, "doubling up" does not work and may make the bleeding worse. The doctor may recommend adding a small dose of estrogen for a week or so. If the bleeding persists, your doctor may want to see you for an evaluation.

What If You Don't Have Any Bleeding at the End of the Month?

The hormone progestin, one of the components of birth control pills, thins the uterine lining cells, so it is common to have lighter periods while you are on the pill. If the uterine lining gets very thin over time, there may not be enough lining to shed at the end of the cycle, and no bleeding may occur. Fewer than 5 percent of women miss their period while on the pill. The lack of bleeding poses no problems to a woman's health, future fertility, or the onset of menopause. Sometimes the absence of bleeding creates anxiety over whether you might be pregnant. As long as you have taken the pills properly, there is no increased risk of pregnancy. However, if the anxiety about a possible pregnancy gets to you, take an over-the-counter pregnancy test to confirm that you are not pregnant. If you miss periods frequently and that concerns you, you might switch to a higher-dose estrogen pill, or choose another method of contraception.

What If You Take the Pill Inadvertently When You Are Pregnant?

If you are on the pill, the risk of pregnancy is less than 3 percent per year. However, some women occasionally miss two or more pills during a cycle, and then the possibility of getting pregnant exists. If pregnancy occurs, the woman will usually not know it until after she has started the next package of pills. However, taking oral contraceptives during the first weeks of a pregnancy does not pose a risk to the health or well-being of the baby.

Molly's Story

> We got a frantic phone call from Molly, an eighteen-year-old woman who had been dating her boyfriend Josh for the past few months. Recently they decided to have an exclusive relationship and not date anyone else. Molly told us, "Once we made a commitment to each other, we started talking about *maybe* having sex. But last night, it just happened!' " Unfortunately, neither of

them was prepared. They hadn't used any contraception, and now Molly was filled with fear and remorse. She had heard about the "morning-after pill" and wanted to know if she could use "something like that" to make sure she and Josh had not conceived a child. Since it had been less than seventy-two hours since they had sex, we assured Molly that a "morning-after pill" should be effective, and we would call her pharmacist with a prescription for the new emergency contraceptive pills.

She feared getting terrible nausea and vomiting from this pill. "I just know if I start throwing up today my parents will suspect something, and then what would I say? I don't even want my best friend to know." We assured her that a serious reaction was uncommon. She sounded somewhat relieved and quickly got off the phone to go pick up the pills. When we saw her a few months later, she apologized for her panic, thanked us for our help, and informed us that the pills had indeed worked. "I was stupid about the whole thing, but at least I was smart enough to get help."

What Is Emergency Contraception?

We all make mistakes sometimes, but making a mistake regarding contraception can have major consequences. Some women have unprotected intercourse, or a condom breaks, or they take the diaphragm out too soon. In these situations, emergency contraceptive pills, taken within seventy-two hours following this unprotected intercourse, are fairly reliable in preventing pregnancy. Emergency contraception works by preventing or delaying ovulation. Two new pill packages, called Preven and Plan B, are now available specifically for this purpose. In some states emergency contraception is available over-the-counter without a prescription from a doctor. It is a good idea for all women who use barrier contraception to have on hand a supply of, or prescription for, emergency contraception.

Preven contains a higher dose of the same hormones that are present in the regular birth control pills. Plan B (the preferred choice) contains only the progesterone hormone (progestin). For each of these brands, one pill is taken as soon as possible following unprotected intercourse, and another pill is taken twelve hours after the first. Both of these brands have a success rate of 75 percent, so they are not as effective as most standard methods of contraception (hence the name Plan B). If 100 women have unprotected intercourse during the middle two weeks of their cycle, about 8 women will get pregnant. If emergency contraception is used, only 2 women will get pregnant. Emergency contraception is excellent for backup contraception, when needed.

Unfortunately, many women do not know about emergency contraception, and many unwanted pregnancies may occur as a result. If you are using a barrier method of contraception that you may occasionally forget to use, you should have a package of emergency contraception in your medicine cabinet to be safe.

What Are the Side Effects of Emergency Contraception?

Plan B, consisting of progesterone-only pills, has been found to be more effective than Preven and only rarely causes nausea. Therefore, this is the method of choice. The high dose of estrogen contained in the Preven pills frequently causes nausea, and some women will have vomiting as well.

What Is the Contraceptive Patch?

The ability to receive medications by absorption from a patch applied to the skin has recently been developed for contraception (see fig. 2.2). The patch contains both estrogen and progesterone and lasts for one week. It needs to be changed weekly for three weeks and then left off for one week to allow bleeding to occur. If used by 1,000 women for one year, about 10 will become pregnant. Pregnancy rates seem to be lower in women who weigh less than two hundred pounds. In early studies, women using the patch noted a bit more breast tenderness and menstrual cramps than women using contraceptive pills. The patch fell off about 2 percent of the time. More than 90 percent of the women who used the patch in these studies were happy enough to continue using it for contraception.

What Is the Contraceptive Ring?

Applying the technology developed for the estrogen vaginal ring now used by some postmenopausal women, the contraceptive vaginal ring has been recently introduced. Estrogen and progesterone are contained within the small silicon ring and are released over a three-week period (see fig. 2.3). After three weeks, the ring is easily removed and left out for one week so that bleeding can occur. Following this, another ring can be inserted into the vagina for the next cycle. The ring is comfortable to wear and cannot be felt during intercourse. If 1,000 women use the ring for one year, about 18 will get pregnant. About 70 percent of women who try the ring are happy enough with it to continue its use.

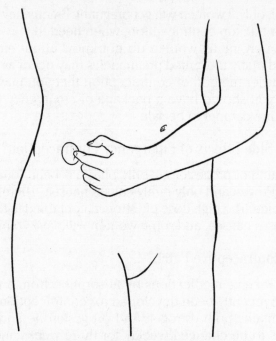

Fig. 2.2.   Contraceptive patch

What Is Implanon?

Implanon consists of one small progesterone-containing plastic rod that is implanted under the skin on the part of your arm that rests against your chest. This area is not visible, but you can feel the rod if you touch the skin in this area. The insertion is performed in the doctor's office under local anesthesia, with minimal discomfort and only takes a few minutes. A very low dose of progesterone is slowly released from the rod into the bloodstream and interferes with the hormonal signals that start the menstrual cycle. In addition, the progesterone makes the cervical mucus thicker, thus making it more difficult for sperm to pass through the cervix into the uterus. The progesterone lasts for five years. At that point, if you wish to continue with this method, the rod can be removed and a new one inserted. This method is very effective and requires no attention from the patient. The failure rate is very low. If 1,000 women use Implanon for one year, only 2 will become pregnant.

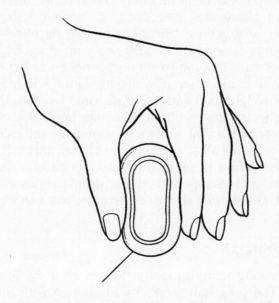

Fig. 2.3.   Contraceptive vaginal ring

What Are the Benefits of Implanon?

The most important benefit of using Implanon for contraception is the extremely high success rate of this method, due to both the effectiveness of the hormone and the fact that no care is needed to make it successful. The success rate equals that of permanent sterilization, since for every 1,000 women using Implanon for one year, only 2 will become pregnant. In addition, unlike sterilization, Implanon is reversible, so that you can regain fertility after the implant is removed. Because the method requires no attention from the patient, the success rate is predictably high in all users. Some women note a decrease in menstrual cramps with Implanon and some note a decrease in PMS.

What Are the Side Effects of Implanon?

Many women who use Implanon will initially experience some change in menstrual bleeding. Some women will have intermittent or continuous spotting, others may not bleed at all. Usually regular monthly bleeding returns after six months or so. If the bleeding is bothersome or persistent, low doses of estrogen can be given orally to control the bleeding.

Intermittent headaches can occur in women using Implanon. Over-the-counter headache medications should be effective in alleviating this problem. If not, you should see your doctor to make sure there is no other cause. Some women experience mood changes, depression, or loss of libido when they use Implanon and may request removal. Acne or weight gain can occur in some women. Despite these possible side effects, most women who use Implanon continue this method for longer than a year, and most women are still using Implanon at the end of five years. Most women who choose this method like the very reliable prevention of pregnancy and the ease of use. It usually takes a few months to resume normal menstrual periods after Implanon is discontinued. Once normal periods resume, you can expect normal fertility.

What Is Depo-Provera?

Depo-Provera is long-acting progestin that is given by injection every three months. The progestin works by interfering with the hormones that lead to the release of the egg. The success rate for Depo-Provera is very high; for every 1,000 women who use it for one year, only 1 will become pregnant.

What are the Benefits of Depo-Provera?

Depo-Provera is extremely effective for preventing pregnancy and is very easy to use. It is given by injection at your doctor's office every three months, and then you do not need to think about birth control until the next injection is due.

What are the Side Effects of Depo-Provera?

Almost all women who use Depo-Provera will initially experience irregular bleeding. This problem decreases in time. After one year of using Depo-Provera, about 50 percent of women have no menstrual bleeding at all. However, weight gain, loss of libido, and hair loss have been reported. About 30 percent of women will discontinue use of the Depo-Provera injections within a few years because of these side effects.

What is Lunelle?

Lunelle is also a form of contraception given by monthly injection; however, it contains both estrogen and progesterone. Lunelle is very effective. If 1,000 women use it for contraception for one year, only 1 will become pregnant. Because it contains the same hormones as the contraceptive pill, the side effects and risks are essentially the same, although Lunelle does appear to cause a slight weight gain. Most women using Lunelle are satisfied with it as a method of contraception.

What Is an Intrauterine Device (IUD)?

The history of the intrauterine device (IUD) dates back to ancient times when, as the story goes, nomadic people placed stones in the uteruses of their camels to prevent a pregnancy during long journeys. Now, the IUD is one of the most popular methods of contraception and is used by about 100 million women worldwide. Because of enormous negative publicity over the serious problems with infection with the Dalkon Shield (see p. 48) in the 1970s, IUDs are less popular in the United States than in other parts of the industrialized world. About one million American women have an IUD. The reputation of the IUD never recovered after the recall of the Dalkon Shield even though newer IUDs provide extremely high effectiveness with a very low infection rate.

The intrauterine device is a small plastic device placed inside the uterus in order to prevent pregnancy (see fig. 2.4). There are three IUDs now available in the United States, and a number of others are available around the world. The three available in the United States use a small (about one and a half inches) silicon rod shaped like a T. Two of the IUDs, one called Progestasert and the other called Mirena, contain progesterone and are called medicated IUDs. Progestasert needs to be replaced every year, and Mirena should be replaced every five years. The third IUD, called Paragard, has a small copper wire wound around the silicon rod and lasts ten years. Both the progesterone and the copper increase the effectiveness of the IUD.

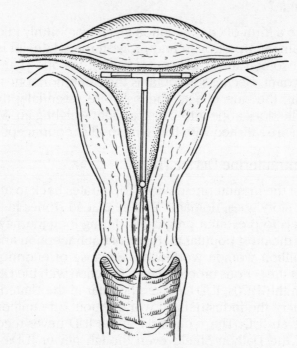

Fig. 2.4.   Intrauterine device

How Does the IUD Prevent Pregnancy?

The presence of the IUD within the uterus irritates the uterine lining cells without infecting them. The inflamed cells interfere with the movement of sperm and prevent the sperm from reaching the fallopian tubes where fertilization normally occurs. Once the IUD is removed, the inflammation goes away, and normal fertility is quickly restored.

The copper on the copper-containing IUD also causes the lining cells to produce a compound that kills sperm. The process is different with the progestin-containing IUDs. The progestin makes the cervical mucus thicker so that sperm have a harder time entering the uterus. When very sensitive pregnancy tests were done on women with progestin-containing IUDs, researchers learned that fertilization and pregnancy do not occur. Contrary to the belief of some people, the IUD does not work by causing the miscarriage of an early pregnancy.

Since the amount of copper wound around the IUD is extremely small, and no traces of copper are found in the bloodstream, there is no need to fear the effect of copper in the body. Likewise, the amount of progesterone in the medicated IUDs is very small and almost not measurable in the bloodstream.

Dory's Story

Dory is a twenty-eight-year-old mother of two young children. Recently she had heavier bleeding and cramping with her periods and came in to the office to make sure everything was all right. Her examination showed her to be perfectly normal, and we discussed some options for treating the bleeding and cramping. She had tried to take birth control pills in her early twenties, but she was nauseous for months and knew the pill was not a good solution for the bleeding and cramps. "I've had problem periods all my life," Dory said. "I've tried ibuprofen and all those painkillers; then I tried tolerating nausea with birth control pills. None of it helped. Now I have two kids, and I just can't stay in bed and moan all day like I used to." We discussed trying a progesterone-containing IUD because it makes contraception effortless, and it might solve the bleeding and cramping. During her next period, we inserted a Mirena IUD. After a few months with it, Dory had very little bleeding and almost no cramping with her periods. "Wow, I always thought IUDs were trouble, but this one is terrific for me. I've had problems during my period since I was a young teenager. I can't believe I'm free from all that."

How Effective Is the IUD?

IUDs are very effective for preventing pregnancy. For every 1,000 women using the copper-containing IUD for one year, less than 10 will get pregnant. The progesterone-containing IUDs are even more effective; they have a failure rate of fewer than 2 pregnancies per 1,000 women per year.

Are There Any Benefits to Using an IUD?

The IUD has some distinct advantages. Once inserted, it is immediately effective, and it does not require any care from the woman using it other than checking once a month to make sure that the string is present. In addition to preventing pregnancy, the IUD has other health benefits. The progesterone IUDs can decrease menstrual blood loss 40 to 50 percent and, therefore, will increase a woman's blood count over a few months and help avoid anemia. This is especially beneficial to women with heavy periods. The progesterone IUDs also decrease the amount of cramping you have with your period. As soon as you have an IUD removed, fertility is immediately restored, making this an extremely reversible form of contraception.

Does the IUD Increase the Risk of Uterine Infection?

Today's IUDs do not increase the risk of pelvic infection. Clinical studies provide some evidence that the copper-containing IUD may help to prevent pelvic infection. However, all IUDs still live under the negative cloud generated by the Dalkon Shield, an early version of the IUD. Many people still believe IUDs are dangerous and won't use them. All IUDs are attached to a string that comes through the cervix into the vagina and allows removal of the device. The Dalkon Shield had a woven string, and this design allowed bacteria to get in between the fibers and move up past the barrier of the cervical mucus and into the uterus. Once the bacteria reached the more fragile uterine lining cells, infection often followed. Some women got pelvic infections from this IUD, and the lawsuits that followed put the company that manufactured the Dalkon Shield into bankruptcy. The resulting publicity gave IUDs a permanent black eye, despite all the safer designs that followed.

The IUDs available today have a monofilament string (like fishing line) that does not allow bacteria to attach to the string or move up into the uterus. Therefore, the risk of infection is virtually never a problem. Unfortunately, the manufacturers of these IUDs still worry about possible lawsuits. They protect themselves by restricting the use of the IUD to women who are at an extremely low risk of getting an infection. Therefore, the IUD is only available for women who have completed their families, are in a monogamous relationship, and have never had a pelvic infection.

Nevertheless, there is a *very slight* risk of infection in the first three to four months after the IUD is inserted, presumably as a result of introducing bacteria from the vagina into the uterine cavity during insertion. About 3 women out of 1,000 may get an infection. This is true for all types of IUDs. Having recent negative tests for chlamydia and gonorrhea reduces that risk. Some doctors recommend that antibiotics be given to a woman at the time the IUD is inserted if she has any risk for infection.

What Is the Best Way to Prevent Both Pregnancy and Sexually Transmitted Infections (STIs)?

Choosing the best method of birth control depends on which method will be safe for you, which method you will be able to use consistently, and which method has the fewest side effects. However, only one method helps prevent STIs—condoms. Symptoms of STIs are fever, pelvic pain, or nausea and vomiting. Some infections are milder and can be treated with antibiotics at home, but more severe infections often require hospitalization for intravenous antibiotics. Other infections may be subtle, causing not much more than an upset stomach that will not lead to a doctor's visit. However, any of these infections can lead to scarring around the fallopian tubes or ovaries and may cause infertility. Therefore, prevention of STIs should be of great importance to women.

Condoms will protect the vagina from contact with both the skin of the penis and semen, both of which can carry infections. As a result, it is a good idea to use condoms in addition to other contraception. Once you are sure the relationship is mutually monogamous and both of you have been tested free of STIs, you may consider omitting condoms.

Who Should Not Use an IUD?

Again, the focus is on women who are at high risk for pelvic infection. Therefore, women who have previously had a pelvic infection should not use an IUD. Women with multiple sexual partners are at higher risk of developing an STI and should not use an IUD. Women who have conditions that increase the likelihood of getting infections, like leukemia, AIDS, or IV drug use should not use an IUD. Women who have abnormal vaginal bleeding should have appropriate testing done to determine its cause before using an IUD. Also, the IUD may not work properly in an abnormally shaped uterus, such as with fibroids, which could make pregnancy more likely.

What Are the Side Effects of the IUD?

The copper-containing IUD may cause a slight increase in the amount of menstrual bleeding and cramping. The progesterone IUD, because of the natural relaxing effect of the progesterone on the uterine muscle, often causes a decrease in the amount of bleeding and cramping. Most women experience some mild to moderate cramping at the time the IUD is inserted in the doctor's office. The cramping may last for a day or two and is easily treated with Advil or Aleve.

You need to check the IUD string monthly after your period, to make sure the IUD is still in place. In the unlikely event (less than 5 percent) that the IUD is expelled by your uterus, considerable cramping and bleeding can occur.

What If You Get Pregnant with an IUD?

Remember, pregnancy is very rare with the use of an IUD—less than 3 women per 1,000 users a year. However, if you do get pregnant with the IUD in place, there is about a 50 percent chance that you will have a miscarriage. Other than the risk of miscarriage, there is *no harm* to a developing baby from the IUD itself or from the copper or the progesterone. If a woman does get pregnant while using an IUD and wishes to continue with the pregnancy, a doctor can remove the IUD. If the IUD is removed, there is still a 30 percent chance of a miscarriage, but a 70 percent chance that the pregnancy will continue normally. As was true in nonpregnant women, the risk of infection during pregnancy with the Dalkon Shield in place was also higher. In fact, a few women died from severe infections while pregnant with the Dalkon Shield. However, with the newer IUDs, there is no increase in the risk of infection during pregnancy, and there have not been any deaths from infection with an IUD present during pregnancy since 1977.

If a pregnancy does occur with an IUD, as the uterus increases in size the IUD will be pulled up inside the uterus. If the IUD cannot be removed at the beginning of pregnancy there is an increased risk of labor starting before the end of pregnancy. While this risk of premature labor is low, it is four times higher than a pregnancy without an IUD in the uterus.

In addition, because the location of the IUD in the uterus makes it very good at preventing pregnancy in the uterus, it cannot prevent pregnancy in the fallopian tube. Accordingly, if you get pregnant with an IUD, it is very important that you see your doctor as soon as possible so a test can be performed to make sure the pregnancy is not in the fallopian tube.

What Are the Barrier Methods?

Barrier methods prevent pregnancy by preventing the sperm from reaching the cervix. Male condoms, female condoms, diaphragms, cervical caps, sponges, and spermicides all fit into this category of contraceptive. In general, barrier methods have a higher failure rate than the pill, IUD, or long-acting hormonal methods. However, barrier methods have the advantage of acting as a deterrent to infection as well as pregnancy and, thus, they decrease the rate of STIs.

What Is a Male Condom?

A male condom is a sheath used to cover the penis to prevent the passage of sperm into the vagina and cervix. Condoms are most often made of latex but can also be made from the processed intestines of animals, so-called natural condoms. Latex condoms have the advantage of preventing the passage of bacteria and viruses, while the natural membrane condoms have large pores that do not prevent the passage of these organisms. About 3 percent of condom users are sensitive to latex and will experience vaginal or penile irritation. Very rarely, people may have a severe allergic reaction, including hives or difficulty breathing.

What Is the Effectiveness Rate of the Male Condom?

If the condom is used every time you have intercourse, and it does not slip or break, the effectiveness is about 97 percent. However, in actual use, most studies show an effectiveness rate of about 84 percent. This means that for every 1,000 couples using condoms for contraception, about 160 will get pregnant every year. Semen may be ejaculated before a man can feel it, and semen may be left on the penis after ejaculation. Therefore, a condom should be put on right after the man has an erection and kept on until intercourse is finished. Putting the condom on after intercourse starts or removing the condom after ejaculation and then having intercourse again are not safe.

Jessie's Story

> Jessie is a twenty-year-old woman who is thinking about having sex with her boyfriend. She has heard so much about sexually transmitted diseases from her friends and wanted to use something that would protect her not only from pregnancy, but also from infections. We told her that the best protection from infection was the male condom and that we recommended this until she and her boyfriend agreed that they were only going to be with each other and both had tested negative for STIs. However, condoms are not the best protection against getting pregnant, so we also recommended that she take the pill for birth control. Jessie was agreeable to this idea since she wanted to be careful

about her health and her future fertility. Within a month, both she and her boyfriend tested negative to any STIs and clearly understood the risks should either stray from monogamy. Jessie also began taking the birth control pill and was confident about not having an unwanted pregnancy. "Talking about all this together and getting tested and all was really something for us as a couple," Jessie told us. "I feel like we both grew up a little during this process, and we both learned so much."

What Are the Advantages of Using a Male Condom?

Male condoms are easy to acquire, are easy for either a man or woman to carry, and are inexpensive. The male condom is also very effective at preventing the transmission of STIs—both from male to female and from female to male. Since the condom covers the skin of the penis, any bacteria or virus on the skin should not come in contact with the skin of the vagina, and transmission is unlikely to occur. Also, since the ejaculated semen does not come in contact with vaginal skin, infection in the semen should also be contained. This protection is not perfect. The condom may break or tear, or it may fall off prior to withdrawal. In addition, the condom only covers the penis, and any infection in other areas of the genitals will not be protected. Petroleum-based lubricants, baby oil, mineral oil, or vegetable oil should not be used with condoms because they can cause the latex to degrade and tear. Lubricants designed for use with condoms can be purchased at the pharmacy, as can prelubricated condoms. When used properly, latex condoms reduce the risk of sexually transmitted diseases by 99.9 percent.

What Are the Disadvantages of Using a Male Condom?

Male condoms have a number of disadvantages. First, they require the participation of men, who are not always willing to use them. The joke that condoms feel "like taking a shower with a raincoat" has been around for a long time. Some couples choose to have the condom applied by the woman as part of foreplay, but other couples find this embarrassing. Sensitivity during intercourse may be decreased for both partners, and some men find maintaining an erection more difficult with a condom. In addition, the condom must be used with every act of intercourse to be effective. While condoms rarely break if used correctly, it does occasionally happen. Testing the condom by filling it with air or water is not a good idea because the latex will stretch, and breaking the condom during intercourse will be even more likely.

How Does the Female Condom Work?

Invented in 1994, the female condom was designed to allow a woman the same protection from STIs and pregnancy as a male condom without having to rely on the man to use it. The female condom looks like a soft plastic tunnel, with one end open and one end closed. The closed end is inserted into the vagina against the cervix, and the open end stays outside the vagina. The female condom has a failure rate of 21 percent in actual use and is somewhat cumbersome to use. It is also expensive. So far, not many women choose to use it.

How Does the Diaphragm Work?

The diaphragm looks like a soft version of a hollow rubber ball cut in half. The rubber is very soft and flexible, and when inserted into the vagina, goes from the back of the vagina to just under the pubic bone, entirely covering the cervix (see fig. 2.5). If properly fitted, you should not be aware of the diaphragm at all. Prior to insertion, spermicidal jelly is placed inside the diaphragm, so that the diaphragm holds the jelly against the cervix. The barrier of the diaphragm prevents sperm from reaching the cervix, and the action of the spermicide kills any sperm that are able to get around the edges of the device. The diaphragm comes in different sizes and needs to be fitted by a health-care professional to ensure it will work effectively.

The diaphragm can be inserted as long as six hours prior to intercourse and needs to stay in the vagina for at least six hours after intercourse to make sure that all the sperm are dead. If you have repeated intercourse, an additional application of spermicide needs to be inserted each time. The diaphragm should not be left in longer than twenty-four hours, since this may slightly increase the risk of toxic shock syndrome, a dangerous infection.

Sara's Story

> Sara is a thirty-eight-year-old woman with two children. The life she and her husband lead is pretty hectic, and the only time they have to spend together is Saturday night. Even then, sometimes they fall asleep in bed reading and skip the "date" they intended to have. Although their sex lives are less active than when they were younger and childless, they still do enjoy a cozy Saturday night on occasion and find their physical relationship vital to

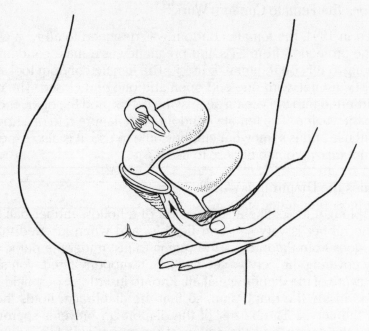

Fig. 2.5.   Diaphragm

their marriage. Sara came to the office wanting something for contraception that fit this situation, which she characterized as "married with children and almost no sex." We suggested a diaphragm because it was very safe and fairly easy to use. Plus she would only need to use it on Saturday night for her "date."

At her six-month checkup, Sara told us she was quite satisfied with the diaphragm. "It's not as messy as I expected it to be. I just pop it in when I brush my teeth before going to bed. My husband hasn't mentioned it at all—but that's what I expected. We're lucky some days if we say ten words to each other. But we still have our 'date,' so I'm not complaining."

How Effective Is the Diaphragm?

If the diaphragm is used absolutely every time you have intercourse, the failure rate is only 6 percent. However, in actual practice the failure rate is high, about 18 percent. Thus, for every 1,000 couples that use the diaphragm for one year, about 180 will get pregnant. Most likely this is because the diaphragm takes time and forethought, both of which may take some of the passion and spontaneity out of sex. This method is probably best suited for women who have a regular partner, so the when and where of having sex is predictable.

What Are the Advantages of Using the Diaphragm?

In that the diaphragm covers the cervix, it helps to prevent the passage of infectious organisms into the uterus. In addition, the spermicide used with the diaphragm kills many infectious organisms. Thus, the risk of acquiring pelvic infection from chlamydia and gonorrhea is reduced by about 50 percent. The diaphragm also prevents cervical infection with HPV, or human papillomavirus, which is responsible for causing most precancer and cancer of the cervix. The diaphragm also has the advantage of being inexpensive and independent of male participation.

What Are the Side Effects of Using the Diaphragm?

The spermicidal jelly used with the diaphragm may alter the normal bacteria present in the vagina and may increase the likelihood of getting a vaginal or bladder infection. This is not serious, but if you get recurrent infections, then consider choosing another method. If you are exposed to HIV while wearing a diaphragm, the spermicide used with the diaphragm may irritate the vagina and cause an increased susceptibility to the HIV infection. If a diaphragm is left in a woman's vagina for longer than twenty-four hours, the risk of toxic shock syndrome, a serious infection, may increase. This is a very rare event, however, with the incidence less than 2 in 100,000 women who use barrier methods per year developing toxic shock.

What Is the Cervical Cap?

The cervical cap is a rubber cup similar to the diaphragm, but it is smaller and seals directly around the entire cervix. Have the cervical cap carefully fitted by a health-care provider. The advantage of the cervical cap is that it can be safely left in place for forty-eight hours, and there is no need for additional spermicide with repeated intercourse during that time. However, the cervical cap is harder to insert, and some women cannot use it because it will not fit around their cervix properly. In addition, the failure rate is about 20 percent.

What Are Spermicides?

Spermicides are chemicals, usually nonoxynol-9, that kill sperm. Spermicides come in different forms including jellies, foams, creams, films, or suppositories that can be inserted into the vagina. They need to be inserted an hour before intercourse so they are at full strength when you have intercourse. Suppositories and films take about ten minutes to dissolve in the vagina before they are effective. If used alone, the failure rate is 26 percent for most women, mostly because the inconvenience of using the products leads to irregular use. If used reliably, the failure rate may be as low as 6 percent. As noted above, spermicides used with diaphragms and cervical caps increase their effectiveness.

What Are the Advantages to Using Spermicides?

Spermicides are available over-the-counter, are inexpensive, and their use is not dependent on participation by a man. Nonoxynol-9 has been shown to help protect against chlamydia and gonorrhea infections by killing the organisms. However, this protection is fair at best and cannot be counted on to protect you from infection. Although nonoxynol-9 kills HIV in the laboratory, the virus lives within white blood cells, which may shield it from the effects of the spermicide. In women who experience irritation from the spermicide, the risk of HIV may be higher due to the ability of the virus to get into the bloodstream through the irritated skin. Therefore, protection by spermicide against HIV in real life (as opposed to the lab) is uncertain.

What Are the Side Effects of Spermicides?

The active ingredient of all available spermicides is nonoxynol-9. Some women and men have sensitivities to this substance and develop rashes or irritations after using the spermicide. Sometimes switching to a product with a lower concentration of nonoxynol-9 or a product with a different type of cream may avoid this irritation.

What Is Natural Family Planning?

Women are fertile for only a portion of each menstrual cycle. Most women will ovulate fourteen days before they have a period, and if sperm are present at the time of ovulation, fertilization is likely to occur. At times further away from ovulation, fertilization is very unlikely. Women sometimes use their ability to detect fertile days to avoid intercourse on those days—this is called natural family planning. Some women prefer these methods because they require no medication, or devices, creams, or barriers inside their bodies. When used perfectly, these methods have a failure rate of less than 10 percent. Natural family planning requires very regular cycles, accurate and repeated monitoring of your own body's signals, and the ability to abstain from intercourse when required. For these reasons, this method is difficult to adhere to and has an actual failure rate of 25 percent. If 1,000 women use natural family planning for one year, 250 will get pregnant.

What Is the Rhythm Method?

This method uses a calendar to predict when ovulation will occur based on the fact that most women will ovulate fourteen days before they have a period. If you have very regular cycles, you can predict ovulation and avoid intercourse on the three days before and one day after the predicted date. Since sperm can survive in the fallopian tubes for up to five days and the egg can live for about twenty-four hours, this window of abstinence can avoid fertile times.

What Is the Ovulation Method?

Just prior to ovulation, most women have a change in their cervical mucus. The mucus becomes much thinner, clear, and slippery. This thinner mucus allows sperm to penetrate into the uterus more easily. By monitoring your cervical mucus every day, you can tell when ovulation is approaching and abstain at that time. To do this, you insert your fingers inside your vagina, touch your cervix, and withdraw some mucus to evaluate its consistency.

What Is the Basal Body Temperature Method?

Just prior to ovulation, the production of progesterone by the ovary causes an increase in body temperature of about half a degree (0.5). By monitoring your temperature every morning before you get out of bed, you can use this rise in temperature to signal ovulation. Since any activity will cause your temperature to rise, it is important to take your temperature before you do anything else every morning and record it on a chart.

What Is the Symptothermal Method?

This method combines the use of temperature changes and mucus changes, as described above, to improve your ability to detect fertile times.

What Are Home Ovulation Predictor Kits?

One day prior to ovulation, the pituitary gland sends out a hormonal signal that causes the release of the egg from the ovary. This chemical signal, called the luteinizing hormone (LH), can be detected in the urine by over-the-counter tests. While these tests were created to help women predict ovulation for women trying to get pregnant, they can just as easily be used to predict which days to avoid intercourse to not get pregnant. The disadvantage, however, is that these tests are expensive—about $50 per month.

What Is Female Surgical Sterilization?

Surgical procedures are available that block a woman's fallopian tubes, interrupting the passage of egg and sperm so that fertilization cannot occur. Sterilization is one of the most common forms of birth control in the United States. In a 1988 survey, about 17 percent of women using contraception used female sterilization. Although the procedure can be performed through a small bikini incision or an incision in the vagina, it is most commonly performed through the navel with the laparoscope. Usually performed under general anesthesia, laparoscopic tubal ligation takes about thirty minutes and has low, but not insignificant, risks such as bleeding and injury to other organs.

Sandra's Story

> Sandra is a thirty-nine-year-old mother of three who came to the office wanting to talk about contraception. She had been using a diaphragm for three years and had had her fill of the "fuss and bother." She was also certain that she did not want any more children. We discussed all the options, but the one that appealed to her the most was sterilization. She felt that if she did this, she would not have to think about birth control ever again. As we always do when we discuss sterilization with women, we suggested that Sandra consider some events that might be unpleasant to even talk about. What if something were to happen to her husband or to her marriage or to her kids? Would she want more children in any of those situations? Sandra decided to go home and talk this over with her husband. She called a few days later and said she decided to have the sterilization procedure. She told us, "This would be the best for me, and I know I

really would not want to get pregnant again, no matter what the circumstances." We scheduled the procedure for a few weeks later. A few years later, as we often do after a patient makes a significant medical decision, we asked Sandra whether she thought she had done the right thing. "Best thing I ever did," she said. "I don't have to think a minute about birth control, and we can be spontaneous about making love. I also like feeling absolutely sure I won't get pregnant again."

How Is Female Sterilization Performed?

Tubal ligation is most commonly performed with laparoscopic surgery. The procedure is usually done in the hospital under general anesthesia. Through a small incision made in the navel, a telescope is placed into the abdominal cavity. A second smaller incision just above the pubic hairline allows the entry of a small instrument. Each fallopian tube is grasped and blocked by either a clip or by electrical energy that scars the tube closed. (see fig. 2.6). The incisions are closed with self-dissolving sutures. Rest is required for the following day or two, and pain medication may be needed during this time. Strenuous activity and exercise should be avoided for about one week.

What Are the Advantages of Female Sterilization?

Female sterilization is extremely effective, with pregnancy rates of about 4 pregnancies per year for every 1,000 women who have the procedure performed. Once the procedure is completed, contraception is effective and no compliance issues exist. Although the procedure is expensive, when the cost is figured out over the entire time contraception is provided, sterilization becomes relatively inexpensive.

What Are the Disadvantages of Female Sterilization?

Sterilization is essentially permanent. Although surgical procedures can attempt to reverse the blockage of the tubes, they involve major surgery, are often not successful for returning fertility, and tubal reversal procedures are not covered by insurance companies. In addition, because scarring can occur in the tube after sterilization reversal surgery, scar tissue may block the path of the fertilized egg as it travels down the tube and result in a tubal pregnancy. Also, sterilization does not provide any protection from sexually transmitted diseases.

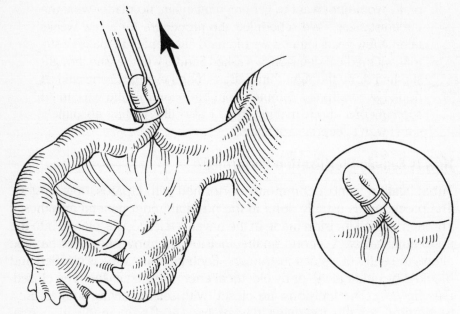

Fig. 2.6.   Tubal sterilization

What Is Male Surgical Sterilization?

Male sterilization, called vasectomy, interrupts the vas deferens, the tube that carries sperm into the fluid that makes up the semen. Ejaculation still occurs but no sperm are present. Unlike tubal ligation, which is most often performed in the hospital under anesthesia, vasectomy is usually performed in the urologist's office in about twenty minutes using local anesthesia. Thus, vasectomy is faster, safer, less expensive, and has a shorter recovery than female sterilization by tubal ligation.

What Are the Advantages of Male Sterilization?

Vasectomy is very effective as a means of contraception, even slightly more effective than female sterilization. Only one pregnancy will occur per year for the partners of every 1,000 men who have the procedure. It is safer, easier, faster, and less expensive than female sterilization. Once the procedure has been performed and semen analysis shows that no sperm are passing into the ejaculate, no further care or cost is needed. Vasectomy has been performed for many years, and no long-term side effects have been reported. Prior concerns about increased risks of autoimmune diseases, heart attacks, and prostate cancer following vasectomy have all been shown to be unfounded.

What Are the Disadvantages of Male Sterilization?

Because it is women who are at risk for pregnancy, male sterilization only protects each woman with one partner—the man who has been sterilized. Woman with more than one sexual partner will still need to have another form of contraception. The actual risks of the vasectomy procedure are very low. However, it is still a surgical procedure and can cause bleeding, infection, or postoperative swelling and pain. Although vasectomy can be reversed, a major surgical procedure would be required to do so. That procedure requires hospitalization and general anesthesia, is expensive, and is not covered by insurance. Also, reversal surgery fails to restore fertility in about 50 percent of men.

How is Male Sterilization Performed?

Vasectomy is performed in the doctor's office, most commonly by a urologist. Local anesthesia is injected into the skin of the scrotum directly over the vas deferens, the tube that carries sperm from where they are produced in the testicles into the ejaculate. A small incision is made in the scrotum, and a small loop of the vas deferens is identified and brought out through the skin. This tube is cut and cauterized with an electrical instrument, then placed back into the scrotum, and the skin is sutured closed. The procedure is then repeated for the other testicle. The procedure takes about twenty minutes. After surgery, ice is applied to the scrotum for a few hours to help prevent swelling. Normal daily activity can be resumed in two days, and strenuous activity or exercise can be resumed in about one week.

What About Male Hormonal Contraception?

Male hormonal contraception has been in development for a long time. The ability to stop all sperm production with minimal side effects has been more difficult than researchers originally thought. Monthly injections of the male hormone testosterone combined with progesterone have been tested with some success. However, it takes a few months for an adequate contraceptive effect to take place, and a small percentage of men continue to make sperm. More recent research focuses on the use of modified male hormones and synthetic progestins in either injectable or pill form. Longer-acting medications, given every three or four months, are also being tested. Researchers feel confident that these problems will be solved in the next few years and that male hormonal contraception will finally become a reality and a practical option for couples.

What Is Best for You?

As with most medical decisions, a lot has to do with what method of contraception suits you best. The one statement that applies to almost everyone is this: If you are in a new sexual relationship or a nonmonogamous relationship, you should use a condom in addition to another method of contraception. The male or female condom is the most effective means of avoiding STIs.

However, since the condom is not the best means of preventing pregnancy, an additional method for contraception is also advised. The diaphragm is a great method, but it won't work if you dislike using it so much that you often leave it in the drawer. Sterilization, either male or female, is very effective, but should be viewed as permanent so is not appropriate until you have completed your family. Hopefully, this chapter has provided enough information to help you make a reasonable choice. Ask your doctor or health-care provider for further information about your particular situation. It is important that you feel comfortable with your decision. After years of limited choices, recent advances have led to a number of new contraceptive methods now available. Other methods of contraception are in development and may be suited for you when they become available. New information about risks and benefits of current methods is regularly published and may influence your choice. This is an important decision and you should explore all your options.

REFERENCES

Ellerston, C., S. Ambardekar, A. Hedley, K. Coyaji, J. Trussell, and K. Blanchard. 2001. Emergency contraception: Randomized comparison of advanced provision and information only. *Obstetrics and Gynecology* 98:570–75.

Parsey, K., and A. Pong. 2000. An open-label, multicenter study to evaluate Yasmin, a low-dose combination oral contraceptive containing drospirenone, a new progestogen. *Contraception* 61:105–10.

Ronnerdag, M., and V. Odlind. 1999. Health effects of long-term use of the intrauterine levonorgestrel-releasing system. *Acta Obstetrics and Gynecology of Scandinavia* 78:716–21.

Smallwood, G., M. Meador, J. Lenihan, G. Shangold, A. Fisher, and G. Creasy. 2001. Efficacy and safety of a transdermal contraceptive system. *Obstetrics and Gynecology* 98:799–805.

Speroff, L., and P. Darney. 2001. *A Clinical Guide for Contraception*. Baltimore, Md.: Lippincott Williams and Wilkins.

3

PROBLEMS WITH YOUR PERIODS

Throughout history, menstruation has been associated with myth and superstition. Menstrual blood was felt to cure leprosy, warts, birthmarks, gout, worms, and epilepsy. It has been used to ward off demons and evil spirits. Menstruating women have been separated from their tribes to prevent a bad influence on the crops or the hunt. As recently as 1930, the cause of abnormal menstrual bleeding was felt to be an undue exposure to cold or wet just prior to the beginning of the period. "Excess" or "immoderate" sexual intercourse was felt to be the likely cause of profuse menstruation. Treatment for abnormal periods included avoiding thin shoes that exposed the feet to cold, taking warm baths, drinking a syrup made from cooked and mashed beets, and, not surprisingly, stopping intercourse altogether, or at least decreasing its frequency.

In modern times we have learned that menstruation is the end of the monthly cycle a woman's body goes through if conception has not occurred, allowing the uterine lining to start over again for the next cycle. We have made quantum leaps toward understanding the role menstruation plays in preparing a woman's body for reproduction. And we have learned a great deal about the treatment of many of the problems of abnormal periods. Science has thankfully dispelled the myths and superstitions that surrounded menstruation and sexuality, but the mystery and wonder of these processes stay with us still.

Since the days when I studied the female hormone system in medical school, new research has revealed an astonishingly complex system of hormones and nerve transmitter proteins that interplay to regulate the monthly menstrual cycle. The system is balanced, but in certain situations—such as times of stress, when body weight changes, or when taking medications—it is easily upset. Once the balance is upset, bleeding can occur that is outside the normal pattern. Also, cells that form abnormal growths within the uterine lining—polyps, hyperplasia, cancer—can cause bleeding as they develop. In the first part of this chapter, we will deal with the circumstances and solutions for problems with your periods. The second part of the chapter will deal with painful periods and the new ideas and treatments for this common, bothersome, and sometimes incapacitating problem.

What Kind of Period Is Normal?

The onset of menstrual periods occurs between the ages of nine and seventeen with the average age being thirteen. Adolescents tend to have periods that can vary from twenty to forty-five days for the first few years and then establish more regularity over the subsequent few years. Most young women have regular cycles by the sixth year after periods begin. Most adult women will have a menstrual cycle, measured from the first day of any bleeding to the next episode of bleeding, about every twenty-one to thirty-five days. Although women expect to bleed every twenty-eight days, only 15 percent of women actually have cycles that length. Bleeding usually lasts four to six days, with some women bleeding a few days longer or shorter. Most women lose about six teaspoons of blood each month. Interestingly, the number of days between periods changes over time, with periods becoming further apart as women reach their forties.

What Makes Your Cycle Regular?

The lining cells of the uterus go through a series of changes every month in response to the hormones made by your ovaries. These cells grow, they mature, they break down, and finally they are shed during your menstrual period. The changes these cells undergo are so predictable that a pathologist can determine how many days it has been since your last period just by looking at the size and shape of the lining cells under a microscope.

The first signal to start your monthly cycle comes from an area in the middle of your brain called the hypothalamus. The hypothalamus releases a hormone called GnRH (Gonadotropin-releasing hormone) that is transported to your pituitary gland at the base of the brain. If you touch your tongue to the roof of your mouth as far back as it will go, you will be touching directly below the site of the pituitary gland.

When GnRH reaches the pituitary gland, it provokes the release of another hormone, called follicle-stimulating hormone (FSH). This hormone causes the cells around an egg (the follicle) to develop. The follicular cells then begin to produce estrogen, the main female hormone. When estrogen reaches the uterus by way of the bloodstream, it stimulates the lining cells to grow.

Near the middle of your cycle, the pituitary gland produces another hormone called luteinizing hormone (LH). LH causes the cells surrounding the egg to break open and release the egg (ovulation). After ovulation, the ovary begins to produce progesterone in addition to estrogen. Progesterone causes the uterine lining cells to stop growing, and they begin to secrete nutrients that encourage the implantation of a fertilized egg.

If you don't become pregnant, the ovary stops making both estrogen and progesterone. Without these hormones, the uterine lining cells can't survive; they die and are shed as the menstrual flow, and the cycle starts all over again. This finely balanced symphony of hormonal events is crucial to controlling the normal pattern of bleeding that you expect.

Keep in mind that this whole system is designed to get you pregnant. Interestingly, at the time of ovulation the ovary increases its production of androgens, or male hormones. These hormones are known to increase libido, and it is probably no accident that they increase at the time a woman is fertile. The cycle is designed to increase your desire for sex at the time of the month in which you are most likely to conceive. The complex design inherent in this process is truly remarkable.

When Is Bleeding Abnormal?

Abnormal bleeding is said to occur if you have a period more often than every twenty-one days, less often than every thirty-five days, or if you have bleeding or spotting in between periods. Bleeding more than two ounces (twelve teaspoons) per month is abnormal and, if persistent, will lead to anemia. Very heavy bleeding—saturating a pad or tampon every hour or two for more than a few hours—is also abnormal. There are a number of causes of abnormal bleeding, and the good news is that almost all of them are benign and easily treatable. The most common causes are hormonal changes, ovarian cysts, uterine or cervical polyps, overgrowth of the uterine lining cells (hyperplasia), fibroids, and, rarely, precancer or cancer of the uterus. The following sections will explain each of these problems in detail.

HORMONAL PROBLEMS

Are Adolescents Prone to Abnormal Bleeding?

When you are an adolescent and begin having periods, it may take up to six years for the normal balance of hormones to be fully established. Most young women will not ovulate more than a few times during the first one or two years of their cycles, and periods can range from every twenty to forty-five days. The estrogen that is produced by the ovaries causes the lining of the uterus to grow, but without ovulation and the resulting production of progesterone, this growth is not controlled. These overgrown cells become fragile and start to bleed on their own. If the time between periods stretches out over a few months, the overgrown cells can accumulate, so that when bleeding finally does occur, it can be extremely heavy. It is, therefore, *common* for young women to have irregular and very unpredictable cycles until all the hormones come into balance, and ovulation occurs on a regular basis. If an adolescent has very heavy bleeding, she should contact her doctor. Treatment with the hormone progesterone can usually stop the bleeding within a day or two.

Kinesha's Heavy Bleeding

Kinesha is a fourteen-year-old whom I initially saw in the emergency room because she was having a very heavy menstrual period. She had not had her period for four months, and this period had started off fairly heavy. Now, four days later, she needed to change her menstrual pad every fifteen or twenty minutes. The examination showed that she was still bleeding. She was also starting to feel exhausted. Her blood count indicated that she had lost about one-third of her red blood cells. We began to give her high doses of progestin pills, and within two days the bleeding had stopped. We gave her the progestin for seven days during each of the next three months, and her periods returned to normal.

Unforunately, after a few more months of normal periods, her periods became irregular again. The next time I saw Kinesha, she was again bleeding very heavily and needed another treatment with progestin pills. Even though she was not sexually active, we discussed starting her on birth control pills to help regulate her periods. The pill contains high doses of progesterone and tends to thin out the lining cells of the uterus over time. The thinner the lining, the less severe the bleeding. Also, the pill supplies the body with steady levels of both estrogen and progesterone, rather than the irregular amounts Kinesha's ovaries had been making. Kinesha and her mother agreed she should start the pill, and within two months she was having regular and light periods. Her blood count returned to normal, and her strength and energy returned. She felt better than she had in a year. We stopped the pills after a year to see if her system had straightened out and found that she had begun to have regular periods of normal flow which have continued to this day.

Can Stress Interfere with Your Periods?

Today's scientists are only beginning to understand the relationship between stress and the functioning of the human body. We do conclusively know, however, that stress can affect the secretion of chemicals in the brain and the release of hormones from the pituitary gland. The sensitivity of the brain to stress is evidenced by the fact that about 20 percent of all female college freshmen will experience abnormal periods during that first year of academic and social pressure. The finely balanced symphony of events we referred to earlier, which is required for each menstrual cycle, can become upset due to stress.

Sara's Abnormal Periods

Sara, a twenty-four-year-old woman, came to the office because she had been experiencing spotting for the past few months in between her normally regular periods. While not excessive, the bleeding was becoming a nuisance. She had recently begun a new job and was preoccupied with her responsibilities. She was not sexually active, so she hadn't worried about pregnancy, but now she began to worry that something might be wrong.

The examination of her uterus, fallopian tubes, and ovaries was entirely normal. This was immediately reassuring to Sara, since she secretly suspected that something might be growing inside her. During our conversation, it became obvious that she was under a fair amount of stress at her new job. The demands of learning the job, getting along with the other employees, and pleasing her new boss were taking up a considerable amount of energy. Because of her young age, the possibility of cancer, polyps, or fibroids was small. With a normal examination, the most likely diagnosis was a hormonal imbalance as a result of her stress. Because these imbalances are almost always temporary, she and I discussed doing nothing for a while to see if the irregular bleeding would stop by itself. I asked her to call me if the bleeding became heavier or more frequent, or if the problem persisted after two months. Sara called three months later to say that the abnormal bleeding had resolved entirely, and she was feeling at home in her new job.

Can Your Weight Affect Your Periods?

The fat cells in your body take up hormones made by the adrenal gland and actually change the chemical structure of these hormones into estrogen. Women who are overweight have more fat cells and, therefore, change more adrenal hormone into more estrogen. Normally, your ovaries make lower levels of estrogen at the end of the menstrual cycle. These low levels act as a trigger to signal the brain to begin a new cycle. If the levels of estrogen never go down because of the extra estrogen from fat cells, then a new menstrual cycle won't begin. In this way, being overweight can interfere with the menstrual cycle.

Conversely, weight loss can also interfere with your menstrual cycles. It appears that women need a minimum percentage of body fat to maintain menstrual function. A loss of weight to 10 to 15 percent below the normal weight for your height may lead to loss of your menstrual periods. In one study of 170 women who had missed periods, 25 percent had lost weight prior to missing their periods.

While missed periods are not dangerous, avoiding the disruption of your hormones is one reason why slow and moderate weight loss is better for your body than rapid and drastic weight reduction. Slow, moderate weight loss allows your body to make the proper adjustments to keep your hormones normal. If you miss your period while on a diet, you should see your doctor just to be sure no other problem exists.

Can Changes in the Amount of Exercise You Do Cause Abnormal Bleeding?

Serious athletes who train vigorously sometimes will notice more irregularity to their cycles. Some even stop menstruating altogether. Abnormal periods occur in about 20 percent of women runners and 50 to 75 percent of women ballet dancers. The reason this happens is not totally understood, and a number of factors are felt to be at work.

Exercise and weight loss result in low levels of body fat. It appears that these low levels of body fat cause the body to change normal estrogen into another form of estrogen that is inactive. This inactive estrogen fails to give the proper signals to the brain, and menstrual function ceases. Strenuous athletic training associated with weight loss is also stressful to your body. It has been proposed that the body shuts down menstrual function during stressful times to prevent pregnancy at times of apprehension or turmoil.

Exercise also increases the levels of brain endorphins, the body's natural sedative. Interestingly, endorphins have about ten times the relaxant effect on the brain than does pure morphine. This may be the explanation for "runner's high," the feeling of relaxation and well-being that follows strenuous exercise. High levels of these endorphins can interfere with the production of your normal brain hormones and interfere with your menstrual cycle. One or all of these factors can be responsible for a decrease in estrogen production, the halting of ovulation, and the cessation of periods.

The lack of bleeding in and of itself is not dangerous. However, a low level of estrogen over a period of six months or longer can cause calcium to be lost from the bones and lead to the beginnings of osteoporosis. If very prolonged, this could lead to fractured bones, even in an otherwise healthy woman. Within a few months of ending high levels of exercise, weight loss, or stress, most women will return to normal cycles. If caught early, the beginnings of osteoporosis may be reversible with return to normal cycles. And happily, these women are also perfectly capable of getting pregnant once their normal cycles return.

Shawn Exercises Too Much

> Shawn is a thirty-four-year-old woman who recently decided to get back into the shape she was in when she was twenty. She began to run before work every morning. She was soon looking forward to this exercise and the "high" that she got after her run and morning shower. As the months went by, Shawn increased her run from the initial twenty minutes to an hour of vigorous, full-out running. Shawn was not only in the best shape of her life, but she was hooked on running. Each week she kept trying to in-

crease her time and distance. Soon, she noticed that her periods were becoming lighter, usually just spotting, and some months she missed them entirely. After missing two months in a row, she made an appointment to see what was wrong.

Shawn's examination was entirely normal. She was in superb condition and had lost twenty pounds since her appointment a year before. We discussed her exercise schedule and the fact that this amount of exercise can often lead to a decrease in the level of estrogen in the body, causing less growth of the uterine lining cells and less bleeding. Also, if her body continued to produce low levels of estrogen over a period of six months or longer, she was at high risk for osteoporosis.

We discussed two options. The first was for Shawn to decrease her exercise to a more moderate level that would allow her estrogen levels to rise back to normal and lead to a return of monthly periods. The second option was to continue her rigorous exercise schedule but to also take supplemental estrogen in pill form to replace what her body was not able to make. The idea of taking supplemental estrogen did not appeal to Shawn, so she chose to decrease her exercise to running only forty-five minutes four times a week. Within three months her periods returned to normal, and she has done very well since.

Can Anorexia Interfere with Your Periods?

Anorexia is a serious eating disorder that is associated with extreme weight loss. In addition, anorexia causes the cessation of menstrual periods. The majority of female sufferers are between the ages of ten and thirty. Anorexia appears to have deep psychological roots. It usually affects young women from achievement-oriented families who feel pressure to perform and be perfect. The initial loss of weight may be a way for the young woman to gain some sense of control in a life that may not be to her liking.

Our culture may also be contributing to the onset of this illness by placing a high value on young women being thin. Advertisements featuring women who in past decades would have been considered undernourished have set the contemporary standard of beauty. Many young women work very hard at achieving a thinness that may actually be detrimental to their health. Bulimia may also be a part of the disease of anorexia, involving cycles of binge eating followed by self-induced vomiting, which leads to further weight loss.

Because of the weight loss associated with anorexia, the brain shuts down the normal hormonal secretions associated with the control of the menstrual cycle. In effect, the brain returns to a prepubertal state. In an apparent effort by the body to conserve energy, other functions are also affected, resulting in low blood pressure, slow heart rate, constipation, and low body temperature. Anorexia is a serious and tragic disease with 5 to 15 percent of its sufferers virtually starving themselves to death. Psychiatric help is essential, and early intervention may prevent the problem from reaching its full extent. If you know someone with this problem, or if you think you suffer from it yourself, seeking help from a qualified psychiatrist is critical to defeating this disease. Under proper treatment, a return to normal eating habits is associated with return to normal weight and body functions.

Can Any Medications Interfere with the Menstrual Cycle?

Most medications used to treat medical illnesses do not interfere with menstrual function. However, sleeping pills, tranquilizers, and antidepressants can all change your cycle by affecting the area of your brain that regulates the flow of hormones. Taking these medications often results in missed periods, although frequent and irregular bleeding can occur. While these missed periods are not medically worrisome, missing periods may be emotionally worrisome, adding to the stress you already feel. Also, it may not be clear whether the source of your missed periods is the stress or the medication you are taking to help you cope with the stress. A discussion between your gynecologist and the doctor or therapist prescribing your medication can help clarify which medication might be best for you, and for how long it should be taken.

Can Drug or Narcotic Use Cause Abnormal Periods?

Drug use, particularly narcotics, affects the area of the brain that controls your menstrual cycle. This often leads to missed periods or more frequent bleeding. If you use drugs, you should inform your doctor. This information will be kept confidential but will be factored into your medical evaluation and treatment. Abnormalities of your period related to drug use should go away within a few months after stopping the drug.

Can Problems with Your Thyroid Gland Interfere with Your Periods?

For unknown reasons, thyroid problems are much more common in women than in men. The thyroid gland, found at the base of your neck, produces the hormone that controls the production of energy in all the cells in your body. Sometimes the symptoms of thyroid disease are obvious. An overactive thyroid can cause weight loss despite a normal or increased appetite. It may make you feel nervous or "hyper" and cause your heart to beat rapidly. You may feel warm at times when others around you are comfortable or even cold. An underactive thyroid can cause weight gain and make you feel sluggish or cold. However, subtle changes in thyroid function are fairly common and may not produce any unusual symptoms other than a change in your periods. These subtle changes may only be detectable by measuring thyroid hormone in your blood and should be checked by your doctor.

Abnormalities of the thyroid gland can cause abnormal bleeding, usually resulting in less frequent periods. Therefore, thyroid hormone blood tests will often be checked if your periods become less frequent. Problems with the thyroid gland are usually easy to treat with medication, and your periods should return to normal shortly after treatment.

Can Other Hormonal Problems Interfere with Your Periods?

Prolactin is another hormone that is produced in the pituitary gland. After childbirth, it is produced in large amounts and is responsible for stimulating your breasts to produce milk. For unknown reasons, and only in a small number of women, prolactin production may increase when a woman has not recently given birth. Higher than normal levels of this hormone can interfere with other female hormonal production, causing missed periods. The high level of prolactin may also lead to a little milky discharge from your breasts. After childbirth, breast-feeding maintains high levels of prolactin, which usually suppresses menstrual periods for at least a few months. Although unreliable, this is the reason nursing sometimes works as a form of birth control.

An elevated amount of prolactin can be detected by a simple blood test. An elevated level usually does not need to be treated and is not worrisome. Infrequently, the prolactin level can get extremely high, signifying a substantial but benign overgrowth of the cells that produce prolactin in the pituitary gland. Very rarely, this *benign* tumor can press on nearby areas of the brain and cause headaches or loss of peripheral vision. When the tumor causes these symptoms, it needs to be treated. A medication is available that can be effectively used to shrink the cells and relieve symptoms and restore menstrual function. In very rare cases, when the medication has been ineffective, surgery on the pituitary gland may be needed to remove the tumor.

Can Conditions That Interfere with Blood Clotting Cause Problems with Your Periods?

Your blood contains a group of proteins that are responsible for making your blood clot. The proper functioning of the clotting proteins is critical; otherwise, even a minor cut would lead to hemorrhage and death. The most well-known, but very uncommon, type of clotting abnormalities is hemophilia. However, a milder but much more common abnormality is called Von Willebrand disease, named after the doctor who first discovered it. This disease can be found in about 1 out of every 200 women. The first indication of a clotting problem may be at the time of the first period, when very heavy bleeding is noted. Especially if heavy bleeding continues with subsequent periods, it is a good idea to have your doctor check your blood for this condition. If Von Willebrand disease is found, treatment with medications or an infusion of clotting factors can be given if necessary.

Can Ovarian Cysts Cause Irregular Periods?

As an ovarian cyst develops, it often will interfere with the production of hormones from the normal ovarian tissue. As a result of this abnormal hormone production, the lining cells of the uterus start to break down and are shed irregularly, resulting in irregular bleeding. The cyst can lead to more frequent and lighter bleeding than normal, or it can be associated with missed periods later followed by heavy bleeding. Ovarian cysts and the problems associated with them are discussed fully in chapter 5.

Can Missing Periods Lead to Any Other Problems?

Missing periods over four to six months as a result of weight loss, stress, or too much exercise can be associated with a chronically low level of estrogen. Estrogen is needed to keep the calcium in your bones. Without estrogen, your bones start to lose calcium, and osteoporosis may result. While we know that exercise actually strengthens your bones, the benefit from exercise is totally negated by low levels of estrogen that result in decreased calcium absorption. Therefore, you can't rely on exercise to protect you from bone loss if you are not having periods. The amount of bone lost, about 1 to 2 percent per year, may not sound like very much, but over time it can add up. The overall effect of six or more missed periods in a row may be the start of the loss of bone strength. Osteoporosis resulting from missed periods can happen at any age!

What Is the Treatment for Abnormal Periods?

First, missing an occasional period is a common and not at all worrisome occurrence, and no treatment is necessary. Also, if you have an occasional irregular period, it is not uncommon for the amount of bleeding to also be irregular, either lighter or heavier than normal. However, if your periods are persistently abnormal, treatment should be considered. The first line of treatment for abnormal bleeding related to hormonal problems is the correction of the primary cause. Relief of stress, correction of weight gain or loss, changes in exercise patterns, or adjustments in medication use will often correct the abnormal bleeding. If a hormonal cause is fairly certain and these solutions fail, and if the bleeding is bothersome or persistent, then treatment with hormones can be undertaken.

If you are regularly missing periods, you should consider taking estrogen pills to prevent osteoporosis. Taking estrogen will prevent the loss of calcium from your bones and keep them from becoming brittle. In addition to estrogen, progesterone pills are also given to prevent overgrowth of the uterine lining cells. Also, it is important to take in about 1,500 milligrams of calcium a day. While better absorbed if taken as a part of your diet, calcium supplements can also be used. These supplements are best absorbed if taken a few times a day with food. Vitamin D is necessary for absorption of calcium. This vitamin is naturally and normally produced by the body in the fat layer below the skin when a person is exposed to sunlight. Calcium with vitamin D added, therefore, only needs to be taken if you live in an area with little sunlight, or if you don't often get outside, or if you regularly use sunscreen to protect your skin from the sun.

What Is the Treatment If Irregular Bleeding Is Due to Missed Ovulation?

For most women, the cause of infrequent but heavy bleeding will be a missed ovulation or two that results in a lack of progesterone. Therefore, progesterone tablets are usually given to correct the problem. Another alternative is to take birth control pills, which also contain progesterone and will cause you to have regular bleeding. While these treatments will correct your bleeding pattern during treatment, they obviously do not correct the original cause of bleeding. If the stress, exercise, or weight issues continue, the abnormal bleeding may return at a later time.

Are There Medications That Can Help with Heavy Bleeding?

If you have a problem with heavy bleeding, a number of medications exist that can help the problem. The most available of these medications are the group of anti-inflammatory medications called NSAIDs, nonsteroidal anti-inflammatory drugs. Advil (ibuprofen) and Aleve (naproxen) are well-known examples of these drugs. These drugs interfere with the production of biochemicals that dilate blood vessels. They therefore keep the blood vessels constricted and limit the amount of blood lost during the period. The best effect can be achieved if the medication is taken just before the period begins or as soon as bleeding is noted. If you wait until the bleeding is heavy, the biochemicals that dilate the blood vessels will already be present, and the medication will be much less effective.

Another group of medications, called antifibrinolytics, has also been shown to be effective in reducing heavy menstrual bleeding. These medications help blood clot more easily. One study showed a 40 percent reduction in bleeding when this medication was taken for the first four days of the menstrual cycle. These drugs are not yet available in the United States but have been available in much of the world for years.

Can Intrauterine Devices (IUDs) Be Used to Decrease Menstrual Bleeding?

In the past, IUDs have been known to cause an increase in menstrual bleeding. However, the use of newer progestin-containing IUDs is associated with greatly decreased menstrual blood loss. By releasing small quantities of progesterone directly to the uterine lining cells, the IUD makes the cells thinner. Thinner cells means less bleeding. The progestin IUD has been shown to decrease menstrual blood loss by *80 percent*. For most women, this is a significant change and will eliminate the need for any other treatment, surgical or nonsurgical.

Unfortunately, IUDs have a bad reputation in the United States as a result of serious infections associated with one IUD, called the Dalkon Shield, manufactured in the 1970s. A change in the design of the current IUDs makes pelvic infection extremely rare. Unfortunately, the benefits of the IUD have been lost in the confusion. Progestin-containing IUDs can have a significant impact on the quality of life of women who suffer from heavy bleeding.

When Is Dilatation and Curettage (D&C) Necessary for Abnormal Hormonal Bleeding?

If you are younger than thirty-five years old, abnormal bleeding is usually the result of irregular hormones, and hormonal treatment is nearly always effective. However, if the bleeding persists, or if it is very heavy (defined as bleeding through a tampon or pad every hour or two), then a D&C, which stands for dilatation (opening the cervix) and curettage (scraping the lining of the uterus) should be considered. The purpose of the D&C in this situation is twofold. First, the D&C removes the lining cells so that they can be examined under the microscope, and a precise diagnosis as to the cause of the bleeding can be made. The pathologist can sometimes tell what the hormonal abnormality appears to be, and then appropriate treatment can be started. Also, any other problem such as polyps, fibroids, or precancerous cells can be detected by the pathologist. Second, the D&C removes all the lining cells that are bleeding. This often will stop the abnormal bleeding and allow the uterus to form a new lining that is, hopefully, healthier. The D&C and other diagnostic tests are fully discussed below beginning on page 86.

Are There Homeopathic Remedies for Abnormal Bleeding Due to Hormonal Causes?

As with all homeopathic remedies, I feel it is important to make sure your examination is normal, and serious conditions have been eliminated. Homeopathics are prescribed by homeopathic practioners based on the type of abnormal bleeding in addition to other symptoms of exhaustion, discomfort, or irritability.

What Is Polycystic Ovarian Syndrome (PCOS)?

PCOS is a rare hormonal condition associated with infrequent periods and often with excess hair growth, oily skin and acne, and infertility. This condition has also been called Stein-Leventhal syndrome but is now more accurately referred to as persistent anovulation (lack of ovulation). The syndrome has been called polycystic ovarian syndrome because the ovaries are often filled with many small cysts, the remnants of eggs that failed to ovulate. The normal menstrual cycle depends on the proper balance and interplay of many hormones and other proteins within the body. There are many opportunities for this system to go awry, leading to a failure to ovulate, which in turn leads to hormonal imbalances that further inhibit ovulation, thus starting a continuing abnormal cycle. Persistent anovulation is not dangerous, and most of its symptoms are treatable. About one-third of women with persistent anovulation will have infrequent but heavy periods, and about 50 percent will stop their periods altogether.

Progesterone is not produced if ovulation does not take place, so it must be given to help bring about bleeding. Birth control pills (which contain progestins) or pure progestin pills are prescribed to help regulate the cycles. The lining cells are shed in the bleeding that results, thus preventing cell overgrowth. If no periods, or very few periods, occur over a number of years, the overgrown lining cells can develop into a precancerous condition called atypical hyperplasia. Progestin treatment or birth control pills, given on a monthly basis, can prevent the development of these abnormal cells.

Persistent anovulation also leads to an increase in male hormones, which are normally secreted in small amounts from a woman's ovaries. This increase in male hormone can lead to excess hair growth in about 70 percent of women with persistent anovulation. This problem also can usually be controlled by birth control pills, which decrease the production of male hormone. Stronger medications are also available if this regimen is unsuccessful. Laser hair removal is effective for the rare situation where medical therapy has not solved the problem.

Recently, an association between PCOS and a woman's inability to utilize insulin properly (diabetes) has been discovered. The exact details of how diabetes and PCOS are linked is still being worked out. However, treatment with a new class of drugs used for diabetes has been found to treat many of the problems associated with PCOS. Unfortunately, the medications can cause nausea and are not tolerated by some women. Weight loss has been shown to help correct some of the hormonal imbalances of PCOS and the resulting symptoms of anovulation, acne, and oily skin.

In some women, the infrequent and somewhat unpredictable ovulation associated with PCOS can lead to problems getting pregnant. For these women, other medications are available to help promote ovulation and fertility with excellent results.

What Is Premature Menopause?

The average age of a woman going through menopause, the time of her last menstrual period, is about fifty-one. Since this is an average, the actual age may range from the early forties to the late fifties. Very rarely, in fact in less than 1 percent of women, does menopause occur before the age of forty. Menopause before the age of forty is called premature menopause.

When you are born, your ovaries contain about two million eggs. However, the natural process of cell death decreases this number of eggs to about 300,000 by the time you have your first period. The number of eggs actually ovulated during your lifetime, about five hundred, is obviously only a small percentage of the original population of eggs. The rest regularly die off over time, even during the times you are pregnant or on birth control pills. In some women, the rate of egg death is very rapid and leads to premature menopause. One cause of this loss of eggs can be an autoimmune disease, a condition where the body makes antibodies that destroy its own tissue. Some rare genetic diseases may also lead to early menopause, as may exposure to radiation treatments or chemotherapy. Premature menopause is very rare, but if you start missing periods or having hot flashes at an early age, you should be evaluated by your doctor.

MENOPAUSAL BLEEDING

What Kind of Bleeding Problems May Develop During Menopause?

By definition, menopause is the date of your last menstrual period. The onset of menopause signifies that the eggs, and the cells surrounding the eggs that produce female hormones, are no longer present. Over the months or years preceding menopause, as your ovaries begin to run out of eggs, the ones that remain may not be quite as responsive to the hormonal signals sent from the pituitary gland. If a normal egg happens to be developing, your level of hormones will be normal. But, if a less responsive egg is developing, your level of hormones may be low for that month. This period of time, when your hormone levels vary, is called perimenopause. Because some, or even most, of your cycles are normal, it may not be clear that you are entering menopause. Symptoms such as hot flashes or vaginal dryness may be sporadically present or not present at all. In addition, hormonal tests can also fluctuate from month to month and may not reveal what is happening to your body.

The most common pattern of bleeding during perimenopause is lighter periods that are farther apart. If this pattern is accompanied by hot flashes, the approach of menopause may be recognized. However, in some women the diagnosis will not be certain until periods are missed, or blood tests clearly show the changes of menopause. Recent studies have shown that osteoporosis may start to develop during perimenopause as estrogen levels begin to decrease. Therefore, consideration should be given to taking hormonal therapy during this time. Taking estrogen and progesterone can prevent osteoporosis, as well as relieve the symptoms of menopause.

What Should Be Done If You Have Abnormal Bleeding During Perimenopause or After Menopause?

As menopause approaches, most women will experience lighter and less frequent periods. However, the likelihood of bleeding from other causes such as hyperplasia (lining overgrowth), polyps, or precancer or cancer of the uterus increases at this time of your life. Bleeding that is irregular, very heavy (requiring a pad change every hour or two), or prolonged (more than seven days) is abnormal, and it is important to establish the cause. The best way to accomplish this is with a sampling of the cells from the uterine lining. The diagnostic methods available, including hysteroscopy, endometrial biopsy, and D&C, are described beginning on page 86.

What If You Are Bleeding While You Are on Hormone Replacement Therapy for Menopause?

There are two basic regimens for taking hormone replacement therapy (see fig. 3.1). One regimen uses daily doses of estrogen, but uses progesterone taken *cyclically* for about half of each month (twelve days). With this regimen, some monthly bleeding is normal and occurs around the time that the progesterone tablets are finished. Bleeding at any other time of the month is not expected and should be reported to your doctor.

The other commonly used regimen calls for daily doses of both estrogen and progesterone, with no days off. This regimen works well to relieve the symptoms of menopause and is also felt to be effective in the protection from osteoporosis. During the first six months of this *continuous* therapy, as the uterus adjusts to the hormones, bleeding may be irregular and unpredictable. It is usually not heavy or persistent. After the first six months of therapy, 80 percent of women will have no bleeding at all for as long as they are on the hormones. If you are on continuous therapy, any bleeding after the first six months should be reported to your doctor. Also, heavy or persistent bleeding, even in the first six months, should be reported as well. For some women the lack of any bleeding with the continuous regimen is a plus, while other women prefer to have the monthly bleeding with the cyclic regimen. You should discuss the choice of regimens with your doctor. In either case, if bleeding occurs unexpectedly, let your doctor know.

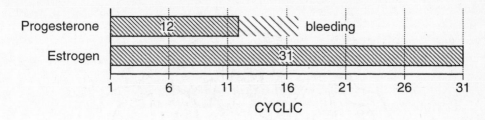

CYCLIC

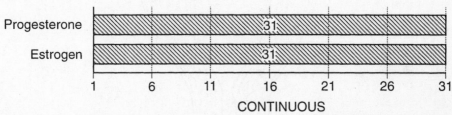

CONTINUOUS

Fig. 3.1. Hormone replacement therapy

POLYPS, FIBROIDS, HYPERPLASIA, AND CANCER

As the uterine lining grows, it normally appears smooth and regular. When menstrual bleeding occurs, the entire lining is shed over the course of a few days, again leaving an even surface. A number of things can grow within the uterus that disrupt the normal appearance and the bleeding patterns of the lining cells. Uterine polyps, fibroids, hyperplasia, and uterine cancer are the most common of these problems.

What Are Uterine Polyps?

Polyps are fingerlike overgrowths of lining cells that can occur in many areas of the body such as the nasal passages, the intestines, and also the lining of the uterus (see fig. 3.2). The cause of polyps is unknown, but in the uterus they are virtually always benign. As the cells of the polyp overgrow, they can become fragile and start to bleed. Polyps are now easy to diagnose in the gynecologist's office with a procedure called hysteroscopy. The hysteroscope is a very small telescope that allows us to see into the uterus and detect even small abnormalities that can cause abnormal bleeding (see page 86).

Can Polyps Be Cured?

Polyps are often loosely attached to the lining of the uterus. The hysteroscope is very helpful because it allows the doctor to see exactly where

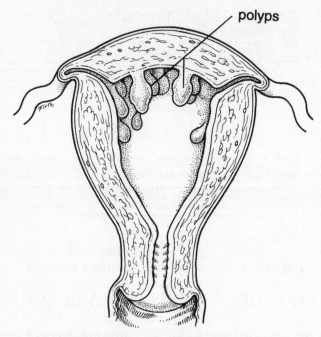

Fig. 3.2. Uterine polyps

the polyp is. Then the polyp can be easily removed by performing a D&C or by grasping the polyp with a small instrument. After removal, the hysteroscope can be reinserted to make sure that the polyp has been totally eliminated. In some cases the polyps may be very large or attached to the lining by thick stalks. In these rare instances, a resectoscope (see page 138) may be needed to cut the stalk of the polyp before it can be removed. This procedure is usually performed in the hospital under anesthesia.

Molly's Persistent Bleeding

Molly is a sixty-six-year-old woman who had been bleeding after menopause. She had already undergone three D&Cs and a variety of hormonal treatments, yet the bleeding persisted. Her examination was normal, but I suggested that we do a hysteroscopy in the office. This had never been done, and we really needed to see why the bleeding was not going away. She agreed, and we scheduled it for the next day. After using local anesthesia, the hysteroscope was inserted, and it was immediately apparent that a large polyp was inside the uterine cavity. Loosely attached to the uterine lining by a stalk, it flopped back and forth. Without the benefit of hysteroscopy to pinpoint the exact location of the polyp, the previous D&Cs had missed it entirely. The polyp was easy to remove with a polyp forceps. Another inspection of the uterine cavity with the hysteroscope now showed that the polyp was gone. Molly has not had abnormal bleeding again.

What Kind of Bleeding Problems Can Fibroids Cause?

Fibroids, benign overgrowths of the uterine muscle, can interfere with the ability of the uterus to stop the flow of blood once a period begins. As a result, the bleeding associated with fibroids is often heavy and prolonged. Fibroids and their associated problems are fully discussed in chapter 4.

What Is the Best Treatment If the Cause of Bleeding Is Fibroids?

While fibroids are a common cause of heavy bleeding, they often do not require treatment unless the bleeding is very heavy or persistent. Then, removal of the fibroids may be indicated. There are a number of ways to remove fibroids, including the standard treatment of abdominal surgery, as well as some newer developments. Removal of fibroids from within the cavity of the uterus can now be accomplished with a small instrument placed through the cervix, called the resectoscope. This procedure can be performed as an outpatient without any incisions. The recovery period is only one or two days, and the procedure is very effective for heavy bleeding associated with fibroids. A full discussion of this procedure can be found on page 138.

What Is Hyperplasia (Overgrowth) of the Uterine Lining?

The lining of the uterus grows in response to the hormones in your bloodstream. Estrogen causes these cells to grow, and constant, high levels of estrogen over a long period of time can cause an overgrowth of the cells called hyperplasia. As this overgrowth occurs, the cells can become fragile and start to bleed unpredictably.

One of the causes of hyperplasia is being overweight. All of the fat cells in your body normally take up the hormones produced by the adrenal glands and change them into estrogen. Therefore, if you are overweight, you have more fat cells to change the adrenal hormones into estrogen. This results in more estrogen floating around in your bloodstream, which can stimulate overgrowth of the uterine lining cells. And higher levels of estrogen can affect the brain hormones that regulate the menstrual cycle, leading to less frequent periods, less shedding of the lining, and eventually the accumulation of overgrown cells.

To diagnose hyperplasia, your doctor removes some of the lining cells with either a D&C or endometrial biopsy (see pages 86–87), and the cells are examined under a microscope. Simple hyperplasia is a benign condition. Because the underlying problem is too much estrogen (and not enough progesterone), progestin tablets are prescribed. Progestins will thin out the overgrown cells and help avoid further bleeding problems. If being overweight is the cause of the bleeding, then losing weight will usually correct the problem. Another condition, called *atypical* hyperplasia, also involves the overgrowth of uterine lining cells. These cells are different, however, in that they have the potential to develop into cancer. Atypical hyperplasia is discussed on page 305.

Can Abnormal Bleeding Be a Sign of Cancer?

Cancer of the uterus is a rare condition, occurring in about 2 out of every 1,000 postmenopausal patients and in many fewer younger women. The cause of uterine cancer is unknown but may be related to the presence of high levels of estrogen in the body over a very long period of time. The high levels of estrogen cause continued stimulation and overgrowth of the uterine lining cells, which may then become cancerous. As cancer cells develop and grow, they burrow into nearby normal cells and cause bleeding. While bleeding is often the first early sign of uterine cancer, most women who have abnormal bleeding will have a cause of bleeding other than cancer. The good news about uterine cancer is that, if it is discovered early, it is one of the most curable cancers in the body (see chapter 11). If you have abnormal bleeding, in all likelihood it is not uterine cancer. But to be sure, report any abnormal bleeding to your doctor.

How Do We Find Out What Is Causing Your Abnormal Bleeding?

The first thing that you should do if you have abnormal bleeding is let your doctor know. Depending on your age, the type of medications you take, and the amount and timing of the bleeding, your doctor will make some assessment as to what type of evaluation is needed. The first step is usually a pelvic examination. Your doctor will start by placing a speculum in your vagina and examining your cervix. Sometimes infections of the cervix can cause enough irritation to create bleeding, and this can be easily detected by looking at the cervix. Also, cervical polyps, which are benign fragile overgrowths of the cells that line the inside of the cervix, can be easily seen. These polyps can also cause bleeding.

Next, your doctor will examine your uterus by placing one hand on your abdomen and pushing the cervix and uterus up from inside the vagina. By feeling the uterus, fallopian tubes, and ovaries, your doctor can detect abnormal growths, like ovarian cysts or fibroids. If the uterus or ovaries are hard to feel, or if something feels abnormal, a sonogram may be helpful.

Julie Bleeds After Sex

Julie is a thirty-three-year-old woman who found bright red blood on her sheets right after she had sex. This had been going on for the past three months. Initially she was not alarmed because she just assumed it was a strange but passing thing and that it would go away by itself. Her periods were regular, and she had no pain, nausea, diarrhea, fever, or any other problems. When it didn't "just go away," she and her husband became concerned, and Julie came in for an examination. During her pelvic examination, a small polyp could be seen on her cervix (see fig. 3.3). When touched with a Q-tip, the polyp bled. The rest of the examination was totally normal. Her fallopian tubes, uterus, and ovaries were all the right size, and there was no tenderness or signs of infection. We were able to remove the polyp by grasping it with an instrument and twisting it off its stalk. This required no anesthesia, was painless, and took about two minutes. That put an end to Julie's bleeding.

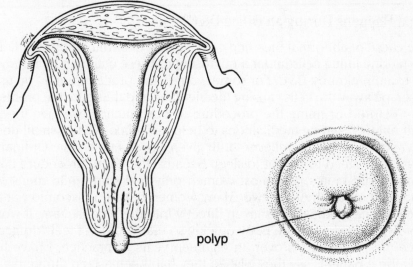

polyp

Fig. 3.3. Cervical polyp

When Are Further Tests Needed?

If your bleeding is very heavy or prolonged, or if it has not improved after treatment with progestins as described above, then other tests may be indicated to determine the cause of the bleeding and the appropriate treatment. Tests that may be performed include hysteroscopy, D&C, endometrial biopsy, sonogram, or saline-infusion sonogram. These tests are described below. As mentioned earlier, if you are approaching menopause or are postmenopausal and have abnormal bleeding, these tests are virtually always indicated to look for the presence of precancerous or cancerous cells.

What Is Hysteroscopy?

This test allows the doctor to look inside the uterus by placing the hysteroscope, a small telescope, through the vagina and into the opening in the cervix. Once inside the uterus, the lining cells can be inspected. Polyps, fibroids, hyperplasia, and cancer can all be seen with the hysteroscope. The procedure, called hysteroscopy, can be done in the office in about five minutes and usually does not require any anesthesia. The information the doctor can get from this procedure is invaluable. Because many problems can be clearly seen, the diagnosis is often certain. A number of studies have shown that the diagnosis made by hysteroscopy followed by scraping the visualized abnormal area of lining cells is more accurate than when a D&C is performed blindly without the hysteroscope.

What Happens During an Office D&C?

The cause of abnormal bleeding can often be determined by examining the uterine lining cells under a microscope. These cells can be removed for examination by D&C. For some women the procedure may be used to scrape away the cells causing the bleeding and thus cure the problem.

Before beginning the procedure in our practice, we give the patient mildly sedating medications to help her relax. We use small doses of Valium plus a pain reliever, both given slowly into a vein. Ordinarily, you do not need to be put to sleep because the entire procedure takes about five minutes, and most women only feel some mild menstrual cramping for a minute or two. Many women have no discomfort at all. Because the medication is given directly into the bloodstream, it works rapidly. It also leaves the body quickly so that you don't feel "drugged" once the procedure is over. In eighteen years of practice, I have had only three patients say they wished they had been asleep during the office D&C. The anticipation is usually much worse than the reality.

After you are relaxed from the medication, a local anesthetic is injected near the cervix to numb it. Then the cervix is held with an instrument and gently dilated so that the hysteroscope can pass easily through the cervix. Once through the cervix, the uterine cavity can be seen and inspected for polyps, fibroids, overgrowth, or cancer. If any abnormalities are seen within, the doctor then knows exactly where to scrape to remove these cells. After the hysteroscope is removed, a small metal instrument called a curette is inserted into the uterine cavity, and the lining cells are scraped out. If any polyps are present, a grasping instrument can be placed into the cavity to remove them.

To be sure that all the cells are removed and collected, a tubular plastic instrument is inserted into the uterus, and a suction is attached to vacuum any remaining cells into a container. All of these cells are sent to the laboratory so that a pathologist can examine them. Cancer, precancer, polyps, and hyperplasia (overgrowth of the lining cells) can all be detected by the pathologist. The pathologist may also be able to see evidence in the cells of any hormonal imbalance that may have caused your abnormal bleeding.

Between the information that the doctor obtains by viewing the uterine cavity with the hysteroscope and the information the pathologist gets from looking at the lining cells with the microscope, the cause of your bleeding can be determined and the treatment appropriately chosen.

What Is an Endometrial Biopsy?

While an office D&C is a far cry from major surgery, it often requires some form of medication—usually mild sedation and local anesthesia. It also involves a fair amount of time, expertise, and equipment. In an effort to get information about the lining cells of the uterus with a simpler procedure, a smaller biopsy of the lining, called an endometrial biopsy, has been used for years. An endometrial biopsy is performed by placing a small plastic tube, about the diameter of spaghetti, through the cervix and into the uterus. As the tube is removed, it scrapes some cells from the uterine lining. Because this only samples a small area of the lining, it is not quite as accurate as a hysteroscopy and complete D&C. But recently, a number of small suction-type instruments have been developed to improve the accuracy of the procedure. The results show that, in most cases, these newer instruments work fairly well. I find an endometrial biopsy most helpful when I am *not* very suspicious that cancer is the cause of the bleeding. But if the results of this test are not 100 percent normal, I think a full office hysteroscopy and D&C are required to make sure that everything is okay.

Also, if the bleeding is persistent or heavy, or if a sonogram shows increased thickness of the lining cells (see below) that suggests that precancer or cancer is possible, then I always recommend that a hysteroscopy and office D&C be done, since this is the most accurate test we have.

Janet Bleeds on Hormone Replacement Therapy

Janet is a fifty-five-year-old woman who was experiencing irregular bleeding while taking her estrogen and progesterone therapy for menopausal symptoms. One year earlier, Janet had a similar problem while living in another city. Her gynecologist there had performed a D&C and hysteroscopy, with lab results showing her to be entirely normal. Because the D&C had been done within the recent past, another one did not seem warranted. However, we decided some evaluation was necessary to be sure that nothing new was developing. Therefore, I recommended that Janet have a sonogram of her uterus. We were easily able to see that the uterine lining cells were not thickened, as might be seen with precancer or cancer. In fact, the sonogram showed that the lining cells were too thin and not getting enough estrogen, and we just needed to adjust her hormone dose.

Can a Sonogram Be Used to Diagnose the Cause of Abnormal Bleeding?

In the past few years the equipment and techniques used for sonography have improved enormously. Patterned after a ship's sonar, the sonogram machine bounces harmless sound waves off the organs inside your body. The reflected sound waves are picked up and recorded in the form of a black-and-white picture on a screen. Photographs can then be made to record the images. The newest technique, called transvaginal sonography, makes images using a small wand placed within your vagina. This allows the end of the instrument to get very close to the uterus, fallopian tubes, and ovaries. Because it is so close, it is able to sense very small detail, including the thickness and regularity of the lining of your uterus. A thick uterine lining may be associated with hyperplasia, precancer, or cancer. Polyps can show up as irregular structures within the cavity, and fibroids appear as enlarged round areas of tissue growing within the uterine wall. If you have irregular bleeding and the lining appears very thin on the sonogram, you are probably fine. Cancer almost never appears that way. Recently, a new technique has been developed to improve the detail the doctor can get from a routine sonogram. Normally, the inside of the uterine cavity is collapsed; the wall on one side touches the wall on the other side. As a result, some of the detail on the walls is hard to see. Small polyps or fibroids may blend into the opposite side and go undetected. If a small amount of fluid, in this case sterile salt water (saline) is gently pushed into the cavity to hold it open, the picture on the sonogram will be much clearer, and we can see fine detail. In addition, the fluid appears black on the sonogram so that there is a sharp contrast to the lining cells that appear white. This technique is called saline-infusion sonography. Polyps, fibroids, and thickening of the uterine lining cells can be seen clearly with this technique. However, all of this technology is still being developed, and I do not rely solely on sonography to make a diagnosis. Currently, the only way to make a *diagnosis* is by examining the lining cells under the microscope. Perhaps in the future, sonography may be accurate enough to use alone to diagnose the cause of bleeding problems.

What Is the Best Treatment If the Bleeding Does Not Go Away?

For some women, the bleeding may persist even after hormonal treatments and the removal of the lining cells by the D&C. In these women, the cause of the continued bleeding may be subtle hormonal changes or changes in the uterine lining or muscle wall itself. Once precancerous or cancerous cells have been ruled out by a D&C, one option is to do nothing. From a medical perspective, as long as the bleeding does not make you anemic, it is not dangerous. And if the bleeding is not very bothersome, you may choose to live with it. On the other hand, if the bleeding causes severe anemia or is bothersome because it is extremely heavy or continuous, a new treatment called endometrial ablation may interest you. This procedure is only appropriate if you do not want to have children. Endometrial ablation is described below.

What Is Endometrial Ablation?

Endometrial ablation is an outpatient surgical procedure used to stop or decrease bleeding from the uterus. The traditional method of performing endometrial ablation uses electrical energy passed into the uterus at the end of a telescope to burn and destroy the lining of the uterus (see figs. 3.4a–b). The uterus is filled with fluid, and the doctor is able to look through the telescope and watch to make sure the entire lining is destroyed. This technique is very effective, but does require special training and skill on the part of the doctor. As a result, many doctors never learned how to perform endometrial ablation and do not offer the procedure to their patients as an alternative to hysterectomy.

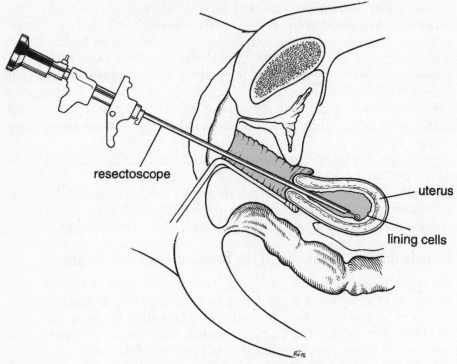

resectoscope

uterus

lining cells

Fig. 3.4a.   Endometrial ablation

Newer methods of ablation have recently been developed that should allow most gynecologists to perform the procedure without involved special training. Some of these devices may even be able to be used in a doctor's office, avoiding anesthesia and the added costs of a hospital. In addition, many of the new methods do not use fluid to hold the uterus open during surgery and thus avoid the extremely rare chance that extra fluid might get absorbed into the bloodstream and cause complications. One of these methods uses an expandable metal device that is inserted into the uterus like an IUD. Once the device is expanded inside the uterus, a gentle suction pulls the uterine lining close to the instrument and an electrical current burns the lining cells. This procedure only takes ninety seconds, and the results have been excellent. Another device circulates hot water inside the uterus to burn the lining cells. This device has been specially engineered to keep the water at a low pressure so that it cannot escape through the fallopian tubes. If the device senses a leak, it automatically shuts off. Because the water circulates freely throughout the entire uterine cavity, the shape of the cavity will not affect the results. As a result, the device is very effective for women with fibroids, or enlarged or abnormally shaped uterine cavities. This procedure takes about ten minutes, and results have been comparable to the other methods. Other devices are in development, and, hopefully, endometrial ablation will become more available to women as an alternative to hysterectomy for heavy bleeding.

How Well Does Endometrial Ablation Work?

After endometrial ablation, the ovaries continue to make normal amounts of hormone, but without lining cells, bleeding cannot occur. In 50 percent of patients, all the lining cells have been destroyed, and these women never have another menstrual period again. In an additional 40 percent of women, a few lining cells have been left behind, and these women will experience a light flow for a few days each month. For 10 percent of women, no improvement is noted. Still, 90 percent of the women who have this procedure are extremely happy not to have to tolerate the severe and debilitating monthly bleeding they previously had. Women who have had an endometrial ablation are among the most satisfied patients in my practice. After surgery, they are

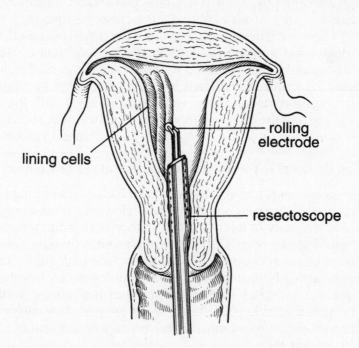

Fig. 3.4b. Uterine lining cells destroyed

able to return to normal activity and life unencumbered by the fatigue and inconvenience associated with heavy bleeding.

Endometrial ablation may only be performed on women who do not wish to have children. Once the lining cells of the uterus are destroyed by the procedure, there is no place for a developing fetus to attach within the uterus. Despite this, it is best to use some form of contraception after the procedure. If some cells remain following endometrial ablation, there exists the rare possibility of pregnancy. In the few cases where pregnancy has occurred, termination of the pregnancy has been recommended. Doctors have been concerned that without adequate cells lining the inside of the uterus, the placenta would grow abnormally, directly into the muscle wall of the uterus, and take hold like the roots of a tree. As a result, the placenta would not be able to separate at the time of delivery, and hemorrhage could occur.

When Is a Hysterectomy Necessary for Abnormal Bleeding?

Hysterectomy should be performed for bleeding only as a last resort. After appropriate evaluation of the problem, hormonal treatment or D&C will often stop abnormal bleeding. If this fails, you should consider endometrial ablation or, if you have fibroids, resectoscope myomectomy (see page 138). However, if these treatments have been tried but failed, or if you or your doctor feel they are not appropriate for you, then hysterectomy may be a reasonable option. Recently, the Maine Women's Health Study (see page 348) found that women who tried but failed to control their bleeding with nonsurgical means were quite satisfied with the relief of their symptoms and the quality of their lives after they went ahead and had a hysterectomy. The subject of hysterectomy is discussed in chapter 12.

What Can Be Done If You Have Uterine Precancer or Cancer?

If uterine precancer is found, treatment with high doses of progestin may effectively change the cells back to normal. However, often hysterectomy is suggested as a way of removing the abnormal cells to prevent cancer from developing (see page 328). If cancer is present, hysterectomy will almost always be the recommended treatment (see page 319). Only if the cancer appears to be fast-growing (the pathologist can see this under the microscope), or has spread deep within the muscle wall of the uterus, or spread outside your uterus, will more extensive surgery and/or radiation therapy be required. Uterine precancer and cancer are discussed in chapter 11.

BLEEDING PROBLEMS AND PREGNANCY

What If You Are Pregnant and Have Bleeding?

About 20 percent of pregnant women with totally normal healthy pregnancies will have some bleeding in the first three months. As the placenta burrows into the lining of the uterus seeking blood to supply the fetus, blood vessels may be disrupted, and bleeding may result. Therefore, most women with light bleeding early in pregnancy should not be concerned. If the bleeding becomes heavy or if it is associated with bad cramping, then the possibility of miscarriage should be considered. At this point, your doctor will likely perform an examination and, possibly, a sonogram to help determine whether a miscarriage is occurring. The small fluid-filled sac surrounding the developing fetus should be visible on the sonogram after about five weeks from your last normal menstrual period. If this sac is collapsing, then a miscarriage may be inevitable. Also, if no fetus is seen within the sac by the sixth week of pregnancy, a miscarriage may be likely.

In addition to the sonogram, the blood test measurement of HCG, the main hormone of pregnancy made by the placenta, can help make the diagnosis. If the pregnancy is continuing normally, the level of this hormone continues to rise in early pregnancy. If the pregnancy is destined to end in a miscarriage, then the HCG level starts to drop. Again, most bleeding in early pregnancy is normal and does not indicate a problem with the baby.

What Should Be Done If You Are Miscarrying?

Miscarriage is the body's way of expelling a pregnancy that is not developing properly. This is fairly common, occurring in about 15 percent of all pregnancies. Often miscarriage results from *nonhereditary* chromosomal abnormalities that occur by chance before or during fertilization of the egg. As a miscarriage proceeds, the uterus begins to contract and pushes the pregnancy tissue out through the cervix, causing cramping and bleeding. If you are pregnant and begin to bleed and cramp, then you should be examined by your doctor. The first thing the doctor will do is look at your cervix. If your cervix has dilated, then miscarriage is inevitable. Over the next hours or days, the uterus will continue to contract to expel the tissue. On occasion, this process may be uncomfortable or associated with heavy bleeding. Sometimes, the uterus may not fully empty, and a D&C may be necessary to completely remove any remaining tissue. Some women may choose to have a

D&C as soon as the diagnosis of miscarriage is made to avoid prolonging the bleeding and cramping and to ensure that all the tissue
is gone.

If your cervix is not dilated, then the diagnosis may not be certain.
As described above, doing a sonogram or testing pregnancy hormone
levels in the blood can often establish whether this is a normal pregnancy, a miscarriage, or an ectopic pregnancy (see below). Again, if the
diagnosis of miscarriage is established, you may wish to have a D&C to
avoid the inevitable bleeding and cramping associated with expelling
of the pregnancy tissue.

While the physical effects of a miscarriage may cause some discomfort, the emotional effects usually cause more distress and suffering.
The loss of a pregnancy is often accompanied by sadness and even depression. Having your partner, family, and close friends to talk to and cry
with is important. Also, it is helpful to remember that having a miscarriage does not make it any less likely that you will be able to go on to
have a healthy pregnancy.

Can Bleeding Mean You Have an Ectopic Pregnancy?

Normally, the fertilized egg implants itself inside the uterine cavity. In
some women, however, the fertilized egg may not reach the uterus, and
it starts to develop within the fallopian tube (see fig. 3.5). The uterus has
the remarkable ability to expand enormously with the growing fetus,
but the fallopian tube can only grow to about the diameter of your
thumb before it begins to tear. As time goes on, this causes pain on the
side where the tube is located. The fallopian tube is also not able to supply the placenta with adequate amounts of blood, and the placenta fails
to develop properly. Without the support of the normal hormones of
pregnancy from the placenta, the lining cells of the uterus break down,
and bleeding results. If you think you are pregnant, and have bleeding
and pain, you should see your doctor.

What Causes an Ectopic Pregnancy?

After the egg is released from the ovary (ovulation), it passes into the fallopian tube, where, if sperm are present, the egg may be fertilized. The
fertilized egg then travels down the rest of the tube over the next two
days. A few days later, when the egg is ready to implant (attach), it is
normally in the uterus. It then burrows into the uterine lining and continues to develop. If anything blocks the travel of the fertilized egg, the
egg may still be in the tube at the time it is ready to implant. Scar tissue

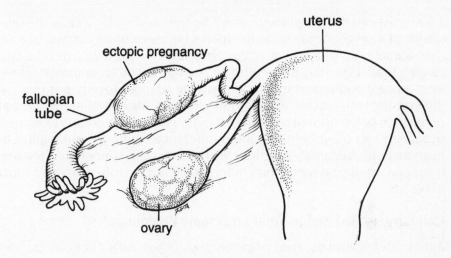

Fig. 3.5.   Ectopic pregnancy

from a previous pelvic infection or endometriosis can block the tube. Other factors, not yet well understood, can slow the movement of the egg down a normal tube. Then, at the time the egg is ready to implant, it is still in the tube and begins to grow there. The end result is an ectopic pregnancy.

How Can the Doctor Tell If You Have an Ectopic Pregnancy?

Enormous advances have been made in the ability to diagnose an ectopic pregnancy early before it tears the tube and causes serious bleeding inside the body. Ten years ago, the diagnosis of an ectopic pregnancy was usually made only if a woman had a swollen, tender abdomen that had filled with blood as the pregnancy tore open the tube. With good medical care, that situation is now, fortunately, a very rare occurrence. We are now able to detect an ectopic pregnancy with blood tests and sonograms very early, and before it tears the tube.

As a normal pregnancy develops, the placenta makes increasing levels of the hormone HCG. If the level of pregnancy hormone does not continue to increase as expected, suspicion of either a miscarriage or ectopic pregnancy is raised.

Five to six weeks after your last period, the amount of pregnancy hormone should be about 1,500 units or greater (this number may vary from lab to lab). At this point, the pregnancy can be seen as a fluid-filled sac within the uterus. If the level of hormone in the blood is greater than

1,500 units and the pregnancy cannot be seen within the uterus, the possibility of a pregnancy outside the uterus becomes more certain.

Sometimes, the growth of the pregnancy in the fallopian tube will cause a tender swelling in the tube that can be felt on examination. However, since the fallopian tube and ovary lie so close together, it may be difficult for your doctor to tell whether this tender swelling is a tubal pregnancy or the normal ovarian cyst of pregnancy, the corpus luteum. A sonogram can often help to tell the difference. Using a combination of examination, pregnancy hormone blood tests, and sonogram, the diagnosis can usually be made long before the fallopian tube tears and starts to bleed.

Can Surgery Be Used to Treat an Ectopic Pregnancy?

Again, advances in the field of gynecology have totally changed the way we treat ectopic pregnancy. Ten years ago, the only way to treat this problem was with major surgery and often removal of the entire fallopian tube along with the pregnancy it contained. A woman who had this type of surgery spent four or five days in the hospital and took six weeks to recover before she went back to normal activity.

One of the first applications of laparoscopic surgery, however, was the removal of a tubal pregnancy. By placing the laparoscope in the abdominal cavity, the enlarged fallopian tube can be seen. Using a small scissors or a laser, the fallopian tube can be cut open, and the pregnancy tissue removed. The open fallopian tube will go on to heal by itself. The advantage of laparoscopic surgery is that women with ectopic pregnancies can usually go home a few hours after surgery and can go back to normal activity within a week or so. Blood tests for HCG are performed following surgery to ensure that all of the pregnancy tissue has been removed.

What Is the Current Treatment of Early Ectopic Pregnancy?

In the past few years, an attempt has been made to treat ectopic pregnancies with medication only, instead of surgery. A drug called methotrexate has been very successfully used for the past twenty years to treat a rare cancer of placental tissue called gestational trophoblastic disease. The drug was so successful that it changed the survival rate from this cancer from about 10 percent in 1965 to almost 100 percent today. Most of the tissue that develops in the fallopian tube during an ectopic pregnancy is placenta, so researchers felt that perhaps this tissue could be destroyed by methotrexate as well. The drug was tried originally in women who had surgery for an ectopic pregnancy and were later found to have a positive pregnancy test, signaling that not all the pregnancy tissue had been removed. As they had hoped, after treatment with methotrexate, the remaining placental tissue was destroyed, and the pregnancy hormone levels went down to zero. Methotrexate is now commonly used to treat early ectopic pregnancies detected by sonogram and blood tests and allows most women with an ectopic pregnancy to avoid surgery.

Methotrexate is given by injection as soon as the ectopic pregnancy is diagnosed. If the pregnancy is too far along or too large as measured by ultrasound, the medication may not work and surgery will be necessary. Usually, only one injection of the medication is needed. Following the injection, blood tests are performed every few days to ensure that the levels of pregnancy hormone decrease appropriately. Side effects from this medication are very rare, with less than 1 percent of women experiencing some nausea. Ninety percent of women with early ectopic pregnancies can be successfully treated with methotrexate. If pregnancy hormone levels do not decrease appropriately, or if there are early signs of bleeding from the tube inside the abdomen, laparoscopic surgery can be used to remove the pregnancy tissue from the tube. Fertility rates after methotrexate are even slightly higher than women treated with surgery alone.

Lee's Story

Lee is a twenty-eight-year-old woman who had been trying to get pregnant for about five months. When her period was a week late, she went to the pharmacy and bought a home pregnancy test. Much to her dismay, the test came out negative. She felt fine and decided to wait and repeat the test in another week. Within a few days, she noted some light spotting and figured her period was about to start. The bleeding was unusual for her, though, because the spotting went on for a few days and never really turned into her normal flow. At this point she went to see her doctor.

Other than the fact that she was bleeding, Lee's examination was normal. A blood test for pregnancy hormone was performed, and it was positive, but at a fairly low level—1,200 units. Lee's doctor explained that she was pregnant, but that the low level of hormone might just mean that the pregnancy was earlier than they thought. She also mentioned the possibility of either a miscarriage or a tubal pregnancy, although there was no evidence for either. Lee was instructed to call her doctor if she developed any heavier bleeding or pain in the pelvic or abdominal areas. She was also scheduled to come back to the doctor's office in two days for a repeat test of the level of pregnancy hormone. Lee was happy about being pregnant but anxious at the same time.

Normally, the levels of pregnancy hormone just about double every forty-eight hours. A smaller rise or any fall in the level signifies either a miscarriage or an ectopic pregnancy. In two days, Lee's blood test came back as 1,700 units. While it was higher than before, it was not as high as it should be, and her doctor ordered a sonogram. Although no pregnancy could be seen in the tube, none was seen in the uterus either. Because at this level of pregnancy hormone, a normal pregnancy should be visible in the uterus, her doctor suspected an ectopic pregnancy. Lee still felt fine and was shocked and upset that anything was wrong.

Because of the likelihood of a tubal pregnancy, her doctor discussed with Lee the possibility of using methotrexate to treat her. She was unhappy about the outcome of her pregnancy, but relieved to know that she would probably not need surgery. Her doctor gave Lee the injection that day and had her return three days later to check her pregnancy hormone level. It had not gone down, which is common right after the medication is given, but it had not gone up either, which was encouraging. Her subsequent levels showed a fairly quick fall in the pregnancy hormone and within three weeks it was no longer present. She had no side effects from the medication and was relieved that the treatment had gone so well. Lee is nervous about getting pregnant again, but her doctor assured her that she would be monitored closely and, hopefully, all would go well.

PAINFUL PERIODS

How Common Are Painful Periods (Dysmenorrhea)?

Nearly 50 percent of all women have some degree of pain associated with their periods. About 10 percent of adult women are unable to perform their normal activities because of this pain, and 50 percent of young women miss school for this reason. Painful periods, called dysmenorrhea, can occur at any age. Painful periods are uncommon in the first six months after the onset of menstrual periods and relatively uncommon in the years prior to menopause. The most common ages for this problem to occur are in the late teens or early twenties.

What Symptoms Can Occur with Painful Periods?

Dysmenorrhea is cyclic, with pain most often occurring just before or during the first few days of each period. Women with dysmenorrhea often feel sharp, crampy pain below the pubic area, but some may also have pain in the back or down the thighs. Although rare, some women have such intense pain that they feel weak and may even feel close to passing out. And some women may also have nausea, vomiting, or diarrhea associated with their painful periods.

What Are the Causes of Painful Periods (Dysmenorrhea)?

Dysmenorrhea refers only to the pain accompanying a period. While sometimes associated with premenstrual syndrome (PMS—the cyclic change in *mood* associated with a period), the two conditions are not necessarily connected. While the symptoms may occur together, some women have painful periods without mood changes, and other women have mood changes unassociated with painful periods.

Most menstruating women have uterine contractions of moderate strength that each last for less than thirty seconds and occur about every three to five minutes. However, women who experience severe dysmenorrhea have cramps that last up to ninety seconds with only a few seconds of rest in between. And the strength of the contraction may be up to five times greater than normal.

We now know that dysmenorrhea results from the release of a chemical substance, called prostaglandin, from the lining cells of the uterus at the time of the menstrual period. The prostaglandin causes contractions of the muscle wall of the uterus that are called menstrual cramps. In fact, if you give prostaglandin to a woman by injection, severe menstrual cramps result. Prostaglandin is now used to help start the contractions of labor in women who, for medical reasons, need to deliver their babies promptly.

Women who have dysmenorrhea have been found to produce more prostaglandin in the lining cells of the uterus than woman who do not have cramps. And, when the increased amount of prostaglandin is released at the time of the period, stronger uterine contractions are the result. As we will discuss later, new medications are now available that prevent the formation of prostaglandins in the uterus and thus can prevent or decrease menstrual cramps.

How Is the Diagnosis of Dysmenorrhea Made?

Because menstrual cramps are the result of an increased amount of a chemical (prostaglandin), there is nothing abnormal for your doctor to feel on your examination. Therefore, the diagnosis of dysmenorrhea can be made by the history of cramping in the presence of a normal pelvic examination. If the pain is severe, it is a good idea to have an examination to be sure that other causes of pelvic pain, such as endometriosis (see page 215) or adenomyosis (see page 148) are not present. And unless another condition is suspected, other tests such as a sonogram, CT scan, MRI, or blood tests are unnecessary.

What Is the Best Treatment for Painful Periods?

Medications called the nonsteroidal anti-inflammatory drugs (NSAIDs) work exremely well, controlling cramps in about 75 percent of women with dysmenorrhea. The medications work by preventing the formation of prostaglandins in the uterine lining cells. Therefore, they are more effective if taken *before* the prostaglandins are formed and before the onset of cramps. The pills should be taken *every* six to eight hours (depending on the type of medication) starting the day before you anticipate the cramps to start, or the day before your period is expected to begin. The pills should be continued until the day after your cramps would normally disappear. If you cannot tell when your period is about to begin, the medication should be started the moment bleeding starts. If you wait until you have cramps, the prostaglandins have already been formed, and the medication may be less helpful.

If you do not get relief from one type of the many NSAIDs available, switching to another may provide relief. Most of these medications are now available over-the-counter in the form of Advil, Aleve, ibuprofen, etc. You should discuss the proper dose and schedule of taking these pills with your doctor.

Birth control pills are another effective way to decrease or even prevent dysmenorrhea. As noted above, prostaglandin is produced in the uterine lining cells and released when the cells begin to disintegrate prior to the menstrual period. The synthetic hormone progestin, present in all birth control pills, acts to make the uterine lining cells thinner. As a result, many women on the pill note that their periods are lighter and shorter. But because the cells are thinner, they also produce less prostaglandin. And less prostaglandin means less dysmenorrhea. Accordingly, if you take birth control pills, you may find a dramatic decrease in menstrual cramps. For some women with severe dysmenorrhea, a combination of birth control pills and NSAIDs may be very helpful in controlling the pain of the menstrual period.

Leslie's Painful Periods

Leslie is a twenty-two-year-old woman who had been bothered by painful periods for as long as she could remember. When she was in high school, she had tried over-the-counter remedies for menstrual cramps, but none had been helpful. Over the past few years, she had used increasingly stronger pain medications and now was fairly dependent on narcotic drugs to get her through those few days every month. She was not happy to be taking these medications but couldn't make it out of her house without them during her periods.

When I saw Leslie, her pelvic examination was totally normal. I was concerned about her need for narcotics and the potential for addiction and discussed other possible medical treatments for dysmenorrhea with her. Leslie had never taken birth control pills for the cramps, and because she was not sexually active, she was embarrassed and a little reluctant to start taking them now. Therefore, I recommended that Leslie stop using the narcotics and begin to take four Advil (800 milligrams) every six hours, starting the day before her period. I recommended she try this for two months and then call to tell me how she was doing. She agreed.

When she called two months later, she said that she got some relief from the Advil, but was still having a lot of discomfort from her periods and still needed to stay in bed for a few days each month. I suggested that she again consider taking birth control pills to help with the pain, and she agreed. After two months of taking the pill, Leslie noted a marked decrease in her pain, but not complete relief. Finally, we had her continue to take the pill, with the addition of Advil for the first few days of her period. She now has almost no cramping and has tolerable periods for the first time in her life. She is able to work and take part in all of her regular activities every day of the month and has never needed to take narcotics again for pain relief.

Another way to decrease painful periods is to have the progestin-containing IUD inserted into the uterus. As noted on page 46, this type of IUD gives off small amounts of progestin continuously and directly to the lining cells that produce prostaglandins. The progestin interferes with the production of these prostaglandins and results in less discomfort. Studies show a significant decrease in the amount of pain associated with periods in women using a progesterone-containing IUD.

Can Heat Be Used to Treat Painful Periods?

A recent study found that heat, applied to the lower abdominal area, can be very effective treatment for menstrual cramps. Hot water bottles have a long history of use for cramps, but had never been studied to see if the treatment worked. This study showed that a specially designed heat patch, placed in the underwear overlying the abdomen for twelve hours a day for two days, was just as effective as ibuprofen for menstrual pain relief. If both heat and ibuprofen were used together, the onset of pain relief was faster, although the amount of relief was not better than if either treatment was used alone. The way the heat works is unclear, but it may have something to do with changing the ability of the brain to sense pain.

Can Homeopathic and Herbal Therapies Be Used for Period Pain?

A number of homeopathic and herbal therapies have been used to treat dysmenorrhea. Tea made from chamomilla may be effective, as may pulsatilla. Herbs such as cramp bark, rosemary, black haw, and lobelia used in combination may also bring relief. The type of homeopathic or herbal therapy prescribed depends on the symptoms experienced and your general health. Eight hundred milligrams of calcium, the amount found in three cups of milk or yogurt, and magnesium, found in whole grains, tofu, and vegetables, may also be used to relieve cramps.

Can Acupuncture Be Used to Treat Painful Periods?

Acupuncture has been shown to reduce menstrual pain. After using acupuncture twice a week for six weeks, pain relief may last as long as six months. Your doctor may be able to recommend an experienced practitioner.

Can Surgery Help Period Pain?

For women who experience severe menstrual pain that is not relieved by medication, interrupting the nerves that "feel" pain from the uterus can be attempted. This can be accomplished with a surgical procedure called a presacral neurectomy. A gynecologist performs this procedure, usually through an abdominal incision, although laparoscopic techniques have recently been developed. Fortunately, cutting these nerves does not interfere with any other function of the uterus, fallopian tubes, or ovaries, including sexual response, the ability to get pregnant, go into labor, or have a normal delivery. However, some women do note constipation following presacral neurectomy. This procedure will not mask the pain from other sources such as appendicitis or other serious conditions for which pain is a warning signal. Not all nerves travel in exactly the same path in all women, and some nerves may not be severed. For this reason, some women do not get relief from this procedure. In addition, some women notice return of pain months or years following presacral neurectomy. Since surgery entails risk, time, and expense, it should be considered rarely and only for those women who have not had relief from other methods of treatment.

What If Your Pain Occurs in the Middle of the Cycle?

Around the middle of the menstrual cycle, ovulation occurs, and an egg is released from the ovary into the fallopian tube. The fluid that normally surrounds the egg as it develops is also released at this time. If a large amount of fluid has formed, its release may irritate the inside lining cells of the body, causing pain. This pain has been called *mittelschmerz*, which in German means "pain in the middle" (of the cycle).

The irritation from the fluid may even lead to a low fever (100° F) and nausea. The body usually reabsorbs the fluid quickly, and the pain and other symptoms should resolve over a few hours or a day. The key to making this diagnosis is the description of sudden onset of pain in the middle of your cycle along with the findings of a slightly tender but otherwise normal pelvic exam. If the diagnosis is uncertain, a sonogram may confirm that fluid is present behind the uterus. Rest and mild analgesics should get you through until the pain goes away. Resting in bed will stop the fluid from moving around inside you and reduce the irritation.

REFERENCES

Akin, M., K. Weingand, D. Hengehold, M. Goodale, R. Hinkle, and R. Smith. 2001. "Continuous low-level topical heat in the treatment of dysmenorrhea." *Obstetrics and Gynecology* 97:343–49.

Barnhart, K., M. Esposito, and C. Coutifaris. 2000. "An update on the medical treatment of ectopic pregnancy." *Obstetrics and Gynecology Clinics of North America* 27:653–67.

Cumming, D., C. Cumming, and D. Kieren. 1991. Menstrual mythology and sources of information about menstruation. *American Journal of Obstetrics and Gynecology* 164:472–6.

Duffy, J. 1979. *The Healers: A History of American Medicine.* Chicago: University of Illinois Press.

Ehrenreich, B., and D. English. 1978. *For Her Own Good—150 Years of the Expert's Advice to Women.* Garden City, N.Y: Anchor Press.

Falk, R. Ovarian malfunction: When is it exercise induced? 1994. *Contemporary Obstetrics and Gynecology* October:187–93.

Munro, M. 1999. Abnormal uterine bleeding in the reproductive years. Part I: Pathogenesis and clinical investigation. *Journal of the American Association of Gynecologic Laparoscopists* 6:393–416.

Munro, M. 2000. Abnormal uterine bleeding in the reproductive years. Part II: Medical management. *Journal of the American Association of Gynecologic Laparoscopists* 7:19–32.

Munro, M. 2000. Abnormal uterine bleeding in the reproductive years. Part III: Surgical management. *Journal of the American Association of Gynecologic Laparoscopists* 8:18–48.

Neistein, L. 1985. Menstrual dysfunction in pathophysiologic states. *Western Journal of Medicine* 143:476–84.

Shangold, M. 1985. Factors affecting menstrual flow. *Contemporary Obstetrics and Gynecology* April:73–81.

4

IF YOU HAVE FIBROIDS

What Are Fibroids?

Fibroids are noncancerous (benign) growths of the muscle wall of the uterus. They are probably responsible for more unnecessary gynecologic surgery than any other condition. Every year a staggering *600,000* American women have a hysterectomy. And about 30 percent of those hysterectomies, 180,000 in all, are performed because of fibroids. For many years gynecologists have surgically removed these growths, often because of fear of the problems they might cause in the future. And those problems are often overstated. Fibroids are extremely common. More than 75 percent of women can be found to have small fibroids, using MRI, a very sensitive imaging technique. However, only about 30 percent of all women will have fibroids large enough to be noted during a pelvic exam, and the vast majority of even these women, more then 80 percent, will *never* have symptoms and will *never* require treatment. And for the rare patient who does have problems, there are a number of sound and effective options available. Hysterectomy should be the solution of last resort.

What Causes Fibroids?

While there is much we don't know about fibroids, we do know that each individual fibroid starts from a single cell growing the wrong way.

But, despite ongoing research, the reason why this one cell grows to cause a fibroid remains a mystery. Recently, gene mutations have been discovered in fibroid cells that alter the cell's growth. It is very likely that the cause of fibroids relates to genes, but the entire mechanism has not yet been worked out. There may also be environmental causes that stimulate fibroid growth. We simply do not know. It is important to realize that there is no evidence that fibroids turn into cancer. Fibroids are benign from the beginning and remain benign.

We do know that the female hormones estrogen and progesterone are necessary for fibroids to grow. We know this because fibroids do not occur before puberty when estrogen and progesterone production begins, and once a woman has a fibroid, it will shrink after menopause when hormone production ceases. It appears that fibroids may start from a single cell mutation, but growth of the fibroid requires the complex interaction of estrogen, progesterone, and cell growth factors. Studies are now under way to try to determine how fibroids arise and what influences their growth. We hope this research will lead to new, noninvasive ways to stop fibroids before they grow and cause symptoms.

Surprisingly, even though the body greatly increases estrogen and progesterone production at puberty, fibroids usually do not develop until much later, generally between ages twenty-five and thirty-five. You might expect that women with fibroids are making too much estrogen or progesterone, which causes the fibroids to grow. However, if we measure hormone levels in the blood, these women have *absolutely normal* amounts. It appears that the muscle cells in the uterus undergo a change that causes these cells to use up, or metabolize, more of the estrogen and progesterone in the blood than usual. As a result, the cells are stimulated to overgrow, causing a round swelling of the uterine muscular wall. Importantly, this change in metabolism does not appear to affect any other area of the body. Women with fibroids are not more prone to fibrocystic changes in the breast, a totally different and unrelated condition. And they are *not* more prone to develop any other benign or cancerous conditions.

Do Birth Control Pills Cause Fibroids?

At one time, birth control pills were felt to be responsible for an increased risk of developing fibroids. Since the pills contain estrogen and progesterone, it made some sense that they might cause this problem. However, recent studies have convincingly shown that women who take birth control pills are no more likely to develop fibroids than women who have never taken the pill. And another study found that most women who already have fibroids may take the pill without any increased growth of the fibroids. There are rare women who are noted to have some growth of fibroids on the pill. If you have fibroids, you may certainly take the pill, but it is a good idea to be checked by your gynecologist within a few months to make sure no fibroid growth has occurred.

What Are the Different Types of Fibroids?

All fibroids begin as a growth somewhere within the uterine muscular wall. The symptoms caused by fibroids depend on where they grow in the wall (see fig. 4.1). Fibroids that grow and bulge toward the outside of the uterus, called *subserosal* fibroids, can press on the organs surrounding the uterus such as the bladder or rectum. Sometimes, they may grow large enough to push outward and cause a noticeable swelling in the abdomen.

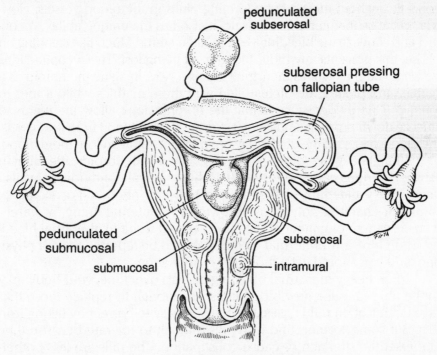

Fig. 4.1. Types of fibroids

Fibroids that grow and bulge toward the inside of the uterus are called *submucosal* fibroids. These grow directly below the lining cells of the uterus and may interfere with the cells that are shed during the menstrual period. As a result, submucosal fibroids may lead to heavy or irregular bleeding. Fibroids that stay mostly embedded within the middle of the wall of the uterus are called *intramural* fibroids. If they grow closer to the outside of the uterus, they can cause pressure, and if they grow closer to the inside, they can cause bleeding. Some fibroids may form on stalks that connect them to the uterus. These are called *pedunculated* fibroids and can be either submucosal or subserosal in location.

Can Fibroids Cause Bleeding Problems?

It is not uncommon for fibroids to cause an increase in the amount of menstrual bleeding. There are a number of theories as to why this happens. At the time of the menstrual period, when the uterine lining is shed, the inside of the uterus is raw and bleeding. The uterus has two basic ways to stop itself from bleeding. The first is the normal blood-clotting mechanism that works throughout the body by forming plugs in the blood vessels. However, because the uterus is a muscle, it also has the unique ability to contract and squeeze the bleeding vessels of the uterus. Much like stepping on a hose, this prevents any more blood from being lost. These contractions are what you may feel as menstrual cramps. Now imagine the fibroid as a marble, and picture the uterus filled with these marbles while it tries to contract. One theory suggests that the fibroids don't allow the uterus to squeeze down properly, and it can't stop the flow of blood from the vessels. The blood vessels in the uterus stay open longer, and you lose more blood.

While heavy bleeding is often associated with fibroids, bleeding in between periods can also result. But other medical conditions may also cause heavy bleeding or bleeding in between periods. For example, hormonal changes, polyps, overgrowth of the uterine lining, or, rarely, even precancer or cancer of the uterus can all result in abnormal bleeding. Therefore, any abnormal bleeding should be reported to your physician, and you should get a thorough examination.

When heavy menstrual bleeding persists over time, your body may not be able to make new blood cells fast enough to replace those that have been lost. In mild cases, this may be easy to correct by taking iron pills. But some women find iron pills difficult to tolerate because they can upset the stomach or cause constipation. The pills are less bothersome if they are taken with food. And an increase in fluids and vegetables in the diet will alleviate the constipation. Some women with fibroids find that the bleeding is so severe that even iron pills cannot correct the problem, and anemia develops. Anemia results in weakness, fatigue, and, if severe, light-headedness. Women with significant anemia sometimes notice that they may not be thinking clearly, likely the result of less blood to bring oxygen to the brain. If you have any of these symptoms, treatment beyond iron pills should be considered.

Emily's Abnormal Bleeding and Myomectomy

One afternoon last spring, Emily, a new patient to my practice, came bounding angrily into my office. Her regular gynecologist had recommended a hysterectomy for fibroids, but Emily was resistant to that idea. As far as she was concerned, her fibroids had taken too much time out of her life already. She was hoping for another solution and would only consider major surgery as a last resort. After she explained her circumstances to me, I understood more why she didn't want to lose any more time. Emily, a forty-five-year-old mother of two grown children, was injured in an automobile accident seven years before. The accident had been quite serious, and Emily had to endure many months of pain and treatment. As part of her rehabilitation, she began to lift weights. She had never been the least bit athletic or even interested in fitness prior to this time. Much to her delight and to the shock of her family, Emily loved weight lifting and began to crave her daily workout. She found she loved to sweat and just loved the way this sport made her feel. From the original emphasis on rehabilitating her injured body, Emily began to train seriously. The "cuts" of her muscles became an enormous new source of pride and self-esteem to this full-time mother and homemaker. In her second year of bodybuilding, Emily started competing at bodybuilding events.

For a year she had been having heavy and irregular bleeding. By the time she saw her gynecologist, she was changing menstrual pads every hour for four of the seven days of her period. The bleeding was sapping her strength; she was often exhausted. When her gynecologist diagnosed fibroids, he recommended a hysterectomy. Although she realized that a hysterectomy would provide a permanent solution to her problem, having to stop training for two months while recovering from major surgery wasn't acceptable. She came to my office seeking a second opinion.

After examining her, I noted that she had small fibroids, altogether about the size of a lemon. Although she came to me requesting a laparoscopic hysterectomy (a hysterectomy done through small incisions with the aid of a small telescope), I also discussed other procedures that might alleviate her symptoms with even less risk and less time for recovery.

First, a simple procedure called hysteroscopy was performed in the office and revealed a small fibroid protruding into the cavity of the uterus. Based on this information and Emily's desire for a rapid recovery, I recommended a procedure called hysteroscopic myomectomy and endometrial ablation (see pages 89 and 132). This procedure was performed as an outpatient in the hospital without any incisions. A small telescope was inserted through the vagina into the uterus, and the fibroid was removed. I also removed the lining cells of the uterus so that her periods would decrease or stop altogether. Emily spent less than four hours in the hospital. She was back lifting weights in two days and was able to successfully compete in her next bodybuilding competition. It is now six years later, and Emily never had another period. When she went through menopause, she chose to take hormones and has never had any bleeding. She is thrilled that she avoided the hysterectomy she had been told was inevitable.

Can Fibroids Cause Pain or Pressure?

Your uterus lies below the pubic bone, well down in the pelvis (see fig. 1.1, page 3). It is just under the bladder, just above the rectum, and surrounded by the intestines. Since it is so near to these other organs, growth of the uterus from fibroids may cause pressure or, rarely, pain in the pelvis. The uterus is normally about the size of a small pear and weighs less than one-quarter of a pound. But with fibroids, the uterus may enlarge to the size of a small watermelon and weigh one or two pounds or more. Just the change in the size and weight of the uterus can cause an awareness of fullness or pressure that was previously not apparent. If the fibroids grow toward your back, pressure on the rectum can cause constipation (see fig. 4.2). You may also feel pressure or pain in the lower back or discomfort with activity or intercourse.

If the uterus grows as large as a cantaloupe, it may be seen as a noticeable swelling in the lower abdomen, perhaps even making a woman appear pregnant. While not dangerous, the enlarged uterus may cause enough discomfort or enough visible change to warrant treatment.

Sybil's Abdominal Pressure

Sybil is a forty-two-year-old woman who has been coming to my office for routine gynecologic care for about ten years. She had no health problems until two years ago when I noted that her uterus

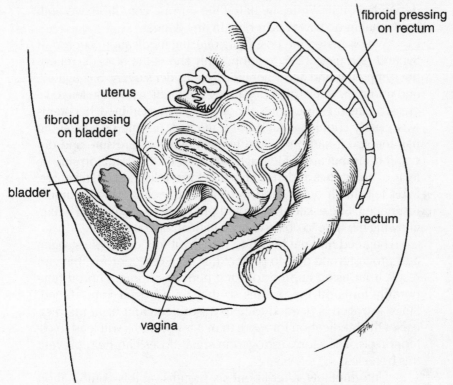

Fig. 4.2.   Fibroids may cause pressure

was beginning to enlarge from fibroids. The enlargement was
only of a moderate degree; her uterus was then the size of a large
lemon. Since she was feeling well, no treatment was needed, and I
examined her every four months to keep track of the fibroids.

Sybil's fibroids continued to slowly enlarge, which is unusual and not at all what we had hoped for. Sybil assumed she
was just putting on weight and had to switch to long overblouses
and pants with elastic waists. At the time of her next scheduled
exam, she looked about five months' pregnant. The fibroid could
be felt reaching up to her navel. She was increasingly uncomfortable from the pressure of the fibroids on her bladder and back.

The combination of discomfort, change in her appearance,
and fear about just how big these fibroids were getting galva-
nized Sybil's desire to begin some kind of treatment. But she
was reluctant to have surgery. Sybil was fearful of anesthesia and
had long ago promised herself to have surgery only if her life

depended on it. While she hated her current condition, we both knew that in no way was her life in any danger.

We discussed the possibility of using medication, Lupron or Synarel (see page 123), to temporarily shrink the fibroids, relieve her symptoms, and allow her time to consider surgery. She agreed, and about six weeks after beginning the medication, she felt a decrease in the pressure in her abdomen. When examined, her uterus was clearly shrinking. After three months, her uterus was about half the size it had been, and her symptoms of pressure and discomfort disappeared. Although bothered by the common side effects of hot flashes and insomnia that the medication often causes, Sybil felt much better, and her negative feelings about surgery resurfaced. She asked if we could put off her surgery for a while, allowing her time to come to grips with an operation.

I agreed and we began to give Sybil low doses of estrogen and progesterone pills to protect her from osteoporosis that can result from using Lupron for long periods of time. Lupron temporarily turns off the ovaries so that no estrogen is produced. Since estrogen is needed to help absorb calcium from the diet, use of the medication for more than a few months will lead to osteoporosis. Therefore, estrogen in small doses can help prevent this bone loss.

Unfortunately, after about six months on this combination of medication and estrogen, her uterus began to grow again. At this point, we had tried the simple solutions and had failed. She now wanted to have surgery. We planned to perform a myomectomy, removing just the fibroid.

Sybil was worried because she had been told by another doctor that a hysterectomy might be necessary. I told her that I had only once performed a hysterectomy for a woman who wanted to preserve her uterus, and I did not think she would be the second. We also spent a great deal of time talking about anesthesia, which had been so frightening to her. We arranged for her to meet her anesthesiologist prior to surgery, who reassured her about the minimal risks and her likelihood of a safe surgery.

At the time of the operation, we found a single large subserosal fibroid. We were able to remove the fibroid and easily reconstruct her uterus. In the recovery room, Sybil smiled in relief; her fibroid was gone, and her worst fears had not come true. At her six-week postoperative visit, the pressure, discomfort, and "pregnant" appearance were gone, and she felt like herself again.

Can Fibroids Cause Sudden Pain?

Fibroids are living tissue, and need blood and oxygen to survive. If a fibroid grows quickly, blood vessels feeding the fibroid may not be able to grow fast enough to supply the new tissue with enough blood and oxygen to keep it alive. If this happens, the fibroid undergoes a process called degeneration, or cell death. As the cells in the fibroid die, chemical substances are released that cause pain and swelling in the uterus. This pain may be severe but is not usually associated with any serious problems. If these chemical substances from a degenerating fibroid reach the bloodstream, they may cause a low fever. As some of the fibroid dies, the blood supply to the rest of the fibroid will be enough to keep it alive and healthy. At this point, the pain will go away. When pain develops in a woman with fibroids, examination by a physician is important to help figure out the source of the problem. If you have a degenerating fibroid, a heating pad on your abdomen will be comforting, and pain medication should provide relief for a few days until the pain naturally begins to subside.

In rare instances, a fibroid on a stalk, or *pedunculated fibroid,* can twist around on the stalk so that *no* blood can get through the stalk to the fibroid. If that happens, the *entire* fibroid begins to die, and the pain becomes very severe. Then, surgery is usually necessary to remove the dying fibroid.

Can Fibroids Cause Urinary Problems?

The uterus lies directly beneath the bladder, and the uterus and bladder are partially attached at one point. If a fibroid begins to grow forward, it may squeeze the bladder so that it cannot fill properly with urine (see fig. 4.2). Then you may notice that your bladder often feels full, and you need to urinate more often. Also, when you laugh, cough, or sneeze, the fibroid may push against the bladder and cause you to lose urine. This is called *stress incontinence.* While this may only be a minor inconvenience for some women with fibroids, others may be so bothered by the incontinence that they limit their activity to avoid embarrassment. There are also other causes of incontinence, so you should get a careful examination (see chapter 8). There are now a number of treatments available other than surgery for many of the causes of incontinence. Stress incontinence is not something you "just have to live with."

Denise's Frequent Urination

Denise is a forty-year-old woman who had a myomectomy three years before being seen in our office. New fibroids had recently grown, and she noticed that she needed to urinate all the time. She had been advised to have a hysterectomy and came requesting a second opinion. Denise could no longer sit through a two-hour movie and sometimes had to leave the theater twice to go to the bathroom. At work, she was frequently getting up from her desk and felt that these trips to the bathroom were breaking her concentration and making her less productive.

A pelvic examination revealed a four-inch fibroid on the outside of the uterus (subserosal), pushing right against the bladder. We discussed her options, which included follow-up with frequent exams, myomectomy, or hysterectomy as a last resort. After a full discussion of all her options, she chose to be followed closely with frequent pelvic exams. Denise also began to see a homeopathic doctor and started taking homeopathic remedies for her fibroids.

The fibroid remained unchanged for one and a half years, but then on her routine exam it was noted to have grown to about five inches, and a new three-inch fibroid was also felt. She was beginning to feel more unhappy about the frequent trips to the bathroom, feeling that they were part of the reason why she was passed over for a promotion at work. Her homeopathic physician could offer nothing new. Denise was glad she had given homeopathy a chance, but at this point, frustrated with her symptoms, she requested surgery.

We discussed all her options including myomectomy, hysterectomy, and embolization. Denise was interested in a quick recovery so that she could get back to work, where she was needed, and she asked if laparoscopic removal of the fibroids was possible. I thought that laparoscopic myomectomy was possible, and she decided to have that procedure performed. Surgery went very well, and we were able to remove both fibroids with minimal blood loss. Denise went home the same day, and when I saw her two weeks later, she was back to almost all of her normal activities, including work. The only activity she was not doing was making those frequent trips to the bathroom that had caused her so much distress.

Can Fibroids Cause Infertility?

Fibroids are *not* usually a cause of infertility. A recent scientific article reviewed the published studies on fertility and fibroids. This careful analysis found no relationship of subserosal or intramural fibroids to infertility. Fertility only decreased in women who had submucosal fibroids, those bulging into the uterine cavity. Therefore, if you have fibroids, surgery will rarely be necessary to help promote fertility. And if you have submucosal fibroids that interfere with fertility, treatment can now be easily performed with resectoscope myomectomy, as an outpatient, without incisions and with a very short recovery (see page 138).

Can Fibroids Cause Miscarriage?

Fibroids may rarely cause repeated miscarriages. The fertilized egg comes down the fallopian tube and takes hold in the lining of the uterus. If a submucosal fibroid happens to be nearby, it often thins out the lining and decreases the blood supply to the developing embryo. The fibroid may also cause some inflammation in the lining directly above it. The fetus cannot develop properly, and miscarriage may result. However, with the next pregnancy, it is very unlikely that the egg will settle in exactly the same location, and pregnancy may proceed without problems. However, if you do have a miscarriage and a fibroid is found bulging into the uterine cavity, it is advisable to have it removed. Studies do show a notably higher pregnancy rate in women who have submucosal fibroids removed.

Sara's Miscarriages

Sara is a thirty-two-year-old woman who had been trying to have a baby but had two miscarriages in the past year. She also realized that her periods were getting heavier. Her gynecologist had performed a number of tests and had been reassuring, but a recent ultrasound had shown a small fibroid. I recommended that a hysteroscopy be performed to see if the fibroid was in the uterine cavity and perhaps responsible for her problems. The hysteroscopy did reveal a small submucosal fibroid that was bulging into the uterine cavity. Because of her history of repeated miscarriages and abnormal bleeding, removal of the fibroid seemed indicated. Sara was admitted to the hospital, and a hysteroscopic resection of the fibroid (see page 138) was performed without any difficulty.

She left the hospital a few hours later and was back to work in two days. The outcome was excellent; Sara got pregnant four months after surgery and went on to have a healthy baby boy.

Can Fibroids Cause Problems During Pregnancy?

The vast majority of women who are pregnant and have fibroids encounter no problems. They go on to have full-term, healthy babies without difficulty. Although many women will have fibroids during their lifetime, the fibroids most often occur in women in their late thirties and forties, a time in life many women have already completed their families. Therefore, fibroids are only present in about 3 percent of all pregnancies.

During pregnancy, the placenta makes large amounts of estrogen. These high levels of estrogen often will cause any fibroids already present to grow larger. If the fibroids grow too quickly, the blood vessels supplying them may not be able to get enough oxygen to the tissue. As mentioned earlier, death of the fibroid cells can then occur. Just as it does in non-pregnant women, this process of degeneration usually resolves in a few days without treatment and without harm to the baby. Some women may have mild contractions during this time, but it is extremely rare for premature labor to actually begin. However, it is crucial that a pregnant woman with fibroids see her physician if she experiences pain or contractions. Bed rest, heat, and pain medication will usually be prescribed, and medications to inhibit premature labor may sometimes be needed.

Do Fibroids Mean You Need a Cesarean Section?

Rarely, a fibroid may grow during pregnancy in the lowest portion of the uterus, near the cervix. It is then possible for the fibroid to get in the way and prevent the baby from coming through the birth canal. This problem is not dangerous for the baby and can often be diagnosed by a sonogram before labor begins. Sometimes we discover this problem during labor because the baby does not come down the birth canal. A cesarean section is performed, and the fibroid is seen in the birth canal when the baby is delivered. Because of the large amount of blood supplying the pregnant uterus, removal of a fibroid at the time of cesarean section is associated with excessive blood loss and is not recommended. What I have just described is actually unusual. Most women with fibroids deliver their babies without any problems.

Do Growing Fibroids Mean Cancer?

Fibroids, by definition, are *benign* uterine growths. However, a *leiomyo-sarcoma*, an extremely rare form of malignant tumor of the uterine muscle, also causes enlargement of the uterus. But only 1 out of every 1,000 women admitted to the hospital for surgery because of fibroids will be found to have a sarcoma. And since 80 percent of women with fibroids are never admitted to a hospital for surgery, the incidence of sarcoma in all women with fibroids is extraordinarily low. The average age of women who develop fibroids is thirty-eight. And although sarcoma can rarely occur in young women, the average age of a woman who develops a sarcoma is fifty-eight. So, if you have fibroids, there is not much reason to worry about sarcoma.

Most gynecologic textbooks teach physicians that if a woman has a rapidly growing uterus, she should have surgery to see if she has a uterine sarcoma. Surgery would be needed to remove tissue for microscopic analysis since no other available tests could make the diagnosis of sarcoma. However, during the course of my training and years in practice, I have never seen a "rapidly growing fibroid" actually turn out to be a sarcoma. And when I review all the medical information available on this subject, it appears that while this statement about rapid growth and sarcoma is often made, there is no evidence to support it.

Although often presented as fact, the science and art of medicine includes both carefully studied principles and other assumptions based on unstudied observation. Unfortunately, the enormous amount of information absorbed during medical education often blurs the lines between fact and assumption. This appeared to have been the case with sarcomas. Gynecologists have assumed that rapid growth means sarcoma, but that fact has never been proved.

To look into this assumption, I began a clinical study at the two hospitals where I practice. I reviewed the charts of 1,330 women admitted for surgery because of uterine fibroids. Interestingly, only three women (0.2 percent) were found to have a sarcoma. In addition, of the 370 patients admitted because of rapidly growing fibroids, only one (0.2 percent) had a sarcoma. This study showed that the risk of developing a sarcoma is extremely low, even if your fibroids are rapidly growing.

If you have a growing fibroid, it is perfectly reasonable to be followed by having a pelvic examination every one to three months. If the fibroid begins to cause bothersome symptoms, then surgery may be considered. If the fibroid continues to grow very rapidly, doubling in size in a few weeks or months, then surgery may be indicated. However, because of the rarity of sarcomas (especially in women younger than fifty), we found no justification for assuming that growth in a fibroid means that cancer is developing. And, as stated before, there is no evidence to suggest that fibroids turn into cancer. Therefore, surgery is not usually indicated.

If you are a woman in her fifties or sixties, the issue of growth of fibroids is a little different. Published reports show that sarcomas most often occur in women in their fifties and sixties. If you are *postmenopausal* and *not* on estrogen replacement therapy, your body will lack the estrogen and progesterone that fibroids need for growth. Therefore, any growth in your uterus is cause for concern. Since there are no tests at the present time that can diagnose sarcoma, surgery is needed to remove the growing fibroid. A pathologist performs an examination of the tissue under a microscope to conclusively show if cancer is present.

Interestingly, in our study, we found that in the small number of postmenopausal women who were taking estrogen and were noted to have growing fibroids, none was found to have a sarcoma. Therefore, a reasonable option for these women would be to discontinue the estrogen and see if the uterus shrinks back to its previous size. If the fibroid does shrink (because the estrogen is no longer present), then you would need to consider the following options. You could stay off estrogen and avoid surgery. Or, if estrogen is necessary for bothersome menopausal symptoms or because of your risk for osteoporosis, you can restart the estrogen with the knowledge that surgery will probably be necessary if the fibroids grow again. If you stop taking estrogen and your uterus does not shrink, or especially if it continues to grow, then surgery should be performed because of the possibility of uterine sarcoma.

Laura's Fibroids Grow Rapidly

Laura is a twenty-four-year-old single woman who saw her gynecologist because of a feeling of pressure and discomfort in her lower abdomen. Her mother had been assuring her that her symptoms were "just gas" and were caused by her fast-food diet. Laura tried changing her eating habits, but the symptoms remained. She fearfully realized that what she was feeling in no way resembled the sensation of gas, and it was time to see her family doctor.

On examination she was noted to have a very enlarged uterus, the size of a large grapefruit. This concerned her doctor because her uterus had felt normal during her last examination one year ago. The doctor questioned whether this rapid growth might represent cancer of the uterine muscle, called sarcoma, and suggested that immediate exploratory surgery was necessary. Laura was referred to me by her family physician, and at the time she was very anxious about the rapid change in her body and the possibility of cancer. Laura's mother accompanied her to the office, feeling extremely anxious and guilty about the advice she had given her daughter.

After the examination, we discussed the *extremely rare* possibility of Laura's having cancer. Most patients with a rapidly growing uterus have benign fibroids, and most patients with sarcoma are sixty to seventy years old. I felt Laura had two options; close observation or surgery. Observation would require frequent pelvic examinations, perhaps every month, until we were certain there was no further growth. Following that, exams every three months would be recommended to monitor any change in symptoms or growth of the uterus. If further growth were noted, we would reconsider surgery.

However, Laura was so worried she requested immediate surgery. The goal of surgery would be the removal of the fibroid (myomectomy) and repair of the uterus. Only if obvious cancer were found, would a hysterectomy be performed. At surgery, a bikini incision was made, and we found what appeared to be a benign fibroid. We removed the fibroid and repaired the uterus without difficulty. The next day the pathology report came back disclosing a benign fibroid and no evidence of cancer. Laura was very relieved and then recovered without problems. She and her mother came for her follow-up visit feeling very grateful for Laura's good health.

What If You Have Large Fibroids?

Gynecologists are often taught that a uterus enlarged because of bulky fibroids should always be removed. However, as discussed below, this is not true. Doctors measure the size of a uterus containing fibroids by comparing it to the size of a pregnant uterus, according to the number of weeks of pregnancy. We often also express uterine size by comparing it to common items such as fruits. Talking about fibroids in relation to lemons and grapefruits, while not exactly precise or scientific, helps us all to visualize their size more easily.

Doctors have been taught that if a woman walks around with large fibroids, about the size of a large grapefruit (or a twelve-week pregnant uterus), she would be at risk for other health problems; even if she felt perfectly fine, eventually she would begin to feel discomfort because of her large fibroids. This reason—the future possibility of problems—simply does not make sense to me. If you have a large fibroid and you are feeling fine, I can't see the need for you to undergo surgery. It is actually likely that your large fibroid will never go on to cause you any bothersome symptoms.

Doctors also feel that large fibroids make it very difficult to perform a thorough pelvic examination. In chapter 1, it was noted that a pelvic exam is done so that the doctor can feel for the size, texture, and presence of any abnormalities of the ovaries, fallopian tubes, and uterus. A large fibroid can get in the way, and doctors fear that a less than optimum pelvic examination can result in missing an early diagnosis of ovarian cancer.

Unfortunately, ovarian cancer is extremely difficult to diagnose in the early stages, with or without fibroids, even with the most sophisticated and expensive testing (see chapter 10). This is a frustrating and difficult reality for us all. Usually, by the time a gynecologist can feel an abnormality of the ovary during the pelvic exam, the disease has already spread. It is also common for gynecologists to not be able to feel every patient's ovaries because of the size of the ovaries, the position of the ovaries, or the weight of the patient. It would make no sense to recommend a hysterectomy to every women whose ovaries were unable to be felt by her gynecologist. And no study has ever shown that removal of a uterus enlarged with fibroids will make any difference in the early detection of ovarian cancer.

Another argument proposed for the aggressive removal of a fibroid uterus states that the ability to detect leiomyosarcoma, a rare cancer of the muscle wall of the uterus (see page 117), is difficult if the uterus is too large. The risk of sarcoma among patients with fibroids is extremely low (0.23 percent), and, therefore, justifying surgery for everyone on this basis doesn't make any sense.

Another argument for aggressive surgery relates to the belief that the risks and complications of surgery are greater if the surgery is delayed and the uterus grows larger. Based on my fifteen years of performing these surgeries and discussions with my colleagues, it is my observation that the risks and complications for a woman with a large uterus who has a hysterectomy are not greater. As shown in a recent study by Dr. Robert Reiter of the University of Iowa College of Medicine, the complication rate for women who have hysterectomies for large fibroids is no different from that for women with small fibroids. Also, as noted on page 131, a myomectomy may also be safely performed on a woman with large fibroids.

Therefore, surgery is only reasonable if you have symptoms that truly warrant the risk, time, stress, and money that an operation entails. Remember, *most patients with uterine fibroids need no treatment*. If you have fibroids, the odds are you will not need to do anything about them.

Can My Fibroids Just Be Watched?

Although 30 percent of all women will have fibroids during their lifetime, only a small number of them will ever need treatment. The vast majority of women with fibroids are unaware of them until their doctor feels them at the time of a routine exam. Some women have very minor symptoms, which are not bothersome at all. If that is the case for you, then no treatment is necessary. I consider careful observation to be the primary treatment option.

The cause of the growth of fibroids is not well understood, and the rate of growth is unpredictable. Most fibroids never grow; others grow gradually over the course of many years; and some seem to go through growth spurts and then may stop growing entirely. The only way to know what is happening is to have a pelvic examination on a regular basis. I usually examine women with fibroids every three to six months. If the fibroid grows during that time period, the growth will be discovered early, and a number of options, short of hysterectomy, should still be available. If the fibroid seems to be growing, I usually do exams more frequently, generally every month, until the growth stops. Ultrasonography, a simple test that uses sound waves to make a picture, may also be used to determine the size of the fibroids. This is an accurate way to measure both the number and the size of the fibroids present and is sometimes necessary to give your doctor more information about the fibroids and your uterus.

On the other hand, fibroids may sometimes grow large enough to cause constant discomfort, pressure, and even pain (see page 118). And, while not dangerous, the discomfort may lead you to choose surgery as treatment for fibroids. One added note: Very large fibroids may partially block blood flowing from the legs back to the heart. This can lead to swelling of the legs and some discomfort. Very rarely, it can also lead to formation of blood clots in the legs that can be dangerous. If you have very large fibroids, it is important that you not sit for prolonged periods of time so that clots have less chance to form.

TREATMENT FOR UTERINE FIBROIDS ▰▰▰▰▰▰▰

What Are the Treatment Options for Fibroids?

If you do need treatment for fibroids, there are a number of options available to you. The choices regarding treatment of uterine fibroids are guided by the medical problems the fibroids are causing, your desire to have children, and your feelings and thoughts about surgery. I think it is helpful for you to know all the options available. At the time of the consultation, I usually begin with an overview of all the treatment options. Even if some treatments do not apply at the current time, your condition or symptoms may change. If you understand the potential for future symptoms and problems, as well as the alternative means of treatment available, much of the mystery of fibroids will disappear. Once the unknown is discussed, some of your anxiety will diminish. For the vast majority of women, there is plenty of time for careful thought and planning.

Can You Take Medication for Fibroids?

A variety of medications have been used in an attempt to treat the symptoms of fibroids. Unfortunately, there are no medications currently available that are able to *prevent* the formation of fibroids or *permanently* shrink them once they are present. Medicines are often used to buy time or reduce symptoms. For some women, a reduction in discomfort is enough to indefinitely postpone surgery. For others, medication allows a more relaxed time period to prepare emotionally and physically for an inevitable surgery. Medications may also temporarily reduce the size of the fibroids enough to allow for a less invasive surgery with a quicker recovery. For some women who are approaching menopause, the "bought time" may lead them right into menopause, when the natural loss of estrogen and progesterone shrinks the fibroids. Once again, hysterectomy is the choice of last resort.

Are There Any Medicines Used to Treat Fibroids?

About twenty years ago a number of new medications were developed based on the hormone that regulates the menstrual cycle. The hormone, produced in the brain, is called GnRH, short for Gonadotropin-Releasing Hormone. By slightly altering parts of this hormone and by changing the length of time it could last in the bloodstream, scientists were able to completely change the effect of the hormone on the menstrual cycle. Normally, the release of this hormone in the brain causes the cyclic release of estrogen and progesterone from the ovaries. These cyclic hormonal changes then lead to the monthly menstrual period. But the new medications work by *temporarily* shutting off the ovaries' ability to make estrogen and progesterone, and menstrual periods temporarily cease. Since estrogen and probably progesterone are also necessary for fibroids to grow, the lack of hormones causes fibroids to shrink.

Lupron and Synarel are two of the GnRH-based medications most often used to shrink fibroids. Because these medications are destroyed by digestive fluids in the stomach, they must be given in a nonpill form. Lupron is given by injection, and Synarel is administered by nasal spray. The nasal spray, used twice a day, coats the thin nasal tissue with medication and is absorbed directly by the blood vessels. The advantage of the nasal spray is that the patient can give herself the medication and avoid the extra trips to the doctor for injections. Lupron's advantage is that it is usually administered only once a month, or in a shot that will last three months. The effectiveness of Lupron and Synarel is virtually identical, so the choice of medication should be up to the patient.

These medications take about two weeks to begin shrinking the fibroids, and the full effect is seen after three months. At that time, most fibroids will decrease in size by about 50 percent of their volume. The shrinking effect is maintained for as long as you use the medication, but there is rarely any further shrinkage after the third month of treatment. Unfortunately, if the medication is stopped, the ovaries begin to produce hormones again, and the fibroids return to their original size within three months. Therefore, the medication has no permanent effect and is primarily used to reduce symptoms and allow time to correct anemia and plan surgery. In addition, long-term use of these medications is limited by their side effects.

What Are the Side Effects of Lupron and Synarel?

Like most medications, Lupron and Synarel cause side effects. Your brain needs estrogen to regulate your body temperature. Since the medications stop the ovaries' production of estrogen, minor temperature changes can occur that are felt as hot flashes, which may be bothersome during the day and may disturb your sleep. The lack of restful sleep can lead to irritability or mood changes. One patient told me that the Lupron affected her husband as much as it did her; her restless nights kept him sleep deprived as well. Progestin pills, given at the same time, have been found to help the hot flashes and allow more restful sleep. However, their use during the first three months of therapy prevents the shrinkage of the fibroids. If you are planning to be on Lupron or Synarel for longer than three months, low doses of estrogen and progesterone can be added after the fibroids have shrunk without any increase in fibroid growth. Another medication, Bellergal, may also relieve hot flashes. It has a mild sedative effect on some women, but if used before bedtime, it often helps you get a good night's sleep.

The lack of estrogen caused by the treatment may also cause a decrease in normal vaginal secretions, leading to vaginal dryness and discomfort during intercourse. About 20 percent of women experience headaches when using these medications. Some women using Synarel, the nasal spray, have reported nasal irritation, which may cause them to discontinue the medication. You may experience an initial episode of menstrual bleeding two weeks after starting the medication. Following that, periods should cease until after the medication is stopped. And when the medication is discontinued, periods resume within a few weeks. These medications have absolutely no effect on a woman's fertility. In fact, they are also used in some infertility patients to make fertility drugs more effective.

The maximum benefit from Synarel or Lupron occurs after three months' use, and surgery is usually scheduled at that time. If these medications are used alone for longer than six months, the resulting low levels of estrogen may prevent your body from absorbing calcium from the foods you eat. So prolonged use may put you at risk for developing osteoporosis or thinning of the bones.

Osteoporosis can be a serious problem, and research efforts are under way to prevent the side effects that may result from prolonged use of these medications. Recent studies have shown that after the initial shrinking of the fibroids, you may take small doses of estrogen and progesterone while you continue to use Lupron or Synarel. Remember, these medications stop the normal supply of estrogen from the ovaries, which is necessary for fibroids to grow. But a small dose of estrogen, the same dose used for postmenopausal women, seems to be too low to allow the fibroids to flourish. And these small doses of estrogen are enough to prevent osteoporosis from developing over limited periods of time. Perhaps there will come a time when a medication is developed that permanently, not just temporarily, shrinks fibroids.

In addition to being temporary and often causing hot flashes, another disadvantage to using these medications is cost: Lupron or Synarrel are expensive, nearly $550 per month. If you are worried about what to expect when taking these medications, most of the women I have treated with either Lupron or Synarel report the following: hot flashes that can disrupt sleep; moderate bleeding within a few weeks after beginning the medication, but generally not heavy and lasting less than a week; cessation of menstrual periods; fibroid shrinkage of 50 percent at the end of three months. Fortunately, the medication only needs to be given for a few months, so most women can tolerate the side effects fairly well during this relatively short period of time.

When Should Lupron or Synarel Be Used?

Lupron or Synarel are most often used prior to anticipated surgery when anemia is present. For women who have experienced heavy bleeding because of fibroids, cessation of the bleeding that results from the medication is a major benefit. This allows you to rebuild your blood supply and regain energy and strength prior to surgery. When the blood count returns to normal, surgery can be planned.

After shrinking the fibroids, it may sometimes be feasible to remove them by laparoscopic surgery, with a few small incisions (see page 129). Also, a few studies have shown that blood loss from surgery is decreased after the use of these medications. However, the need for blood transfusions is no lower in women treated with Lupron or Synarel, so the decrease in blood loss may not be significant.

What Is Tibolone?

A new medication called Tibolone, now available in Europe, may change the medical treatment of fibroids. Tibolone is a synthetic steroid that shares some properties of estrogen, progesterone, and testosterone. It may be possible to decrease or eliminate many of Lupron's long-term side effects if it is given in combination with Tibolone. One study showed that a group of women taking Tibolone and Lupron had a 50 percent reduction in the size of their fibroids, no loss of bone, and only rare hot flashes. Importantly, at the end of six months, none of these women required surgery as opposed to the almost 70 percent of women on Lupron and placebo who did require surgery. Hopefully, further studies will show that Tibolone may allow women to safely use Lupron for prolonged medical treatment of fibroids and avoid surgery altogether.

Can Lupron Be Used for Women Approaching Menopause?

A woman with fibroids who is approaching menopause can use Lupron or Synarel until menopause begins. Then the natural supply of estrogen will cease, and the fibroids will remain small without any medication.

However, because the exact age of natural menopause is unpredictable, this can turn into an expensive proposition—$2,000 per year—and is usually not covered by medical insurance. But, for some women, this treatment plan may be useful.

Can Progesterone Be Used to Treat Fibroids?

Progesterone was one of the first medications used to treat women who developed symptoms from fibroids. In certain areas of the body, progesterone has the opposite effect of estrogen. Since estrogen makes fibroids grow, it only seemed reasonable that progesterone would make fibroids shrink. Unfortunately, this does not happen, and recent studies have found that progesterone increases the growth of fibroids. In fact, ongoing research on the antiprogesterone drug mifepristone has shown some promise for its use to help shrink fibroids.

In addition, progesterone has a number of bothersome side effects. It can cause emotional changes or even depression, which abate after the medication is stopped. Mild water retention is another side effect that resolves after the medication is finished. Although not effective for shrinking fibroids, the thinning effect of progesterone on the lining cells of the uterus may decrease vaginal bleeding. However, because of the possible detrimental effect of progesterone on fibroids, I do not prescribe it.

Are There Any Promising Medications on the Horizon?

Pirfenidone is a new, not yet available, medication that blocks the growth of existing fibroids and may stop the formation of new fibroids. Although the exact mechanism of action is not known, pirfenidone affects the production of collagen, a major component of fibroids. Other effects of pirfenidone on cell growth factors may also be important. Studies are now under way to evaluate how fibroids respond to this new drug and to evaluate its side effects. In the future, women with small fibroids may be able to take pirfenidone, or a medication like it, to prevent fibroid growth and avoid any other need for treatment.

Are Holistic Remedies Effective for Treating Fibroids?

After practicing medicine for many years, it is apparent to me that Western medicine does not have all the answers. A number of my patients have tried holistic therapy for fibroids while under my observation. However, my overall impression has been that these remedies have not been effective. The growth of fibroids is unpredictable, often ceasing even when no treatment has been given. Therefore, claims that holistic remedies have been successful may be no more than coincidence. The only way we have of assessing the value of a treatment is to give a large number of women one treatment and another large group no treatment and compare the results. If the group of people given the treatment do better, then the therapy is felt to have some value. Unfortunately, holistic practitioners have not performed scientific studies to determine the effectiveness of their therapy.

On the other hand, what really matters is how *you* feel after treatment. Therefore, I am comfortable with patients seeking alternative remedies for fibroids. A number of my patients have tried vegetarian diets, eliminating meat that might contain estrogen used in animal feed. Others have tried various vitamin supplements or acupuncture. Although none of these remedies or diets has been shown to be effective, I have never seen a patient harmed by these treatments. I do feel it's important for a woman exploring holistic alternatives to be closely monitored by a physician, so that any change in the fibroids or symptoms can be evaluated.

Do You Need Surgery for Fibroids?

There are three main indications that require surgery for fibroids: uncontrollable bleeding, a concern that the fibroids may be causing kidney damage, or a concern that cancer might be present.

What If You Have Uncontrollable Bleeding?

Surgery is indicated if you experience heavy bleeding that is persistent and leads to severe anemia. Anemia can lead to chronic exhaustion and light-headedness and will eventually lower your body's resistance. We can measure the amount of blood that you have in your body by two tests; the hemoglobin and hematocrit. The *hemoglobin* is a measure of the weight of the number of molecules present in the blood that carry oxygen. Normal amounts are about 12 to 14 grams per liter (quart) of blood. The blood is made up of many components, but the two largest components are the fluid that carries the blood cells, the *plasma*, and the red blood cells that carry oxygen. The normal percentage of red blood cells in the blood is about 40 percent; 60 percent of the blood is plasma. The *hematocrit* measures the percentage of the blood that is red blood cells, and higher numbers are better.

If your fibroids cause heavy bleeding and if your hemoglobin is less than 10 grams (or your hematocrit is less than 30 percent), you have a fairly significant anemia and probably will need treatment. Resectoscope myomectomy and/or endometrial ablation are very effective for most patients with this problem (see pages 89 and 138). Uterine artery embolization works well to decrease bleeding from fibroids. Other women may choose to have a myomectomy (see page 129), and others with severe or unrelenting symptoms may choose to have a hysterectomy.

What If You Are at Risk for Kidney Damage?

Another indication for surgery relates to your kidneys. The ureters are thin tubes that connect the kidneys (which are below the shoulder blades) to the bladder, which is in front of the uterus. In the pelvis, the ureters are about one-half inch away from the uterus. In some women, the fibroids may grow sideways and press against the ureters, slowing or stopping the flow of urine out of the kidney. If urine cannot flow freely from the kidney, pressure builds up in the kidney. This pressure damages the cells that clean the blood of impurities and can be dangerous. This process is slow and usually produces no symptoms. It is also *extremely rare*. If you are being closely followed by a physician, it is very unlikely that any damage will occur to the kidneys. On examination, a doctor can feel if the fibroids are too near the ureters. Some action would then be advised, before the slow process of damage to the kidneys begins.

Blockage of the ureter can be detected by an X-ray called an *intravenous pyelogram (IVP)* or by a CAT scan. During these X-rays, a special iodine dye is injected into a vein of the arm. The dye then collects in the kidneys and flows down the ureters. The X-rays show the path of the dye, and abnormalities of the kidneys or ureters can be detected. In my many years of practice, I have never seen a woman suffer kidney damage from fibroids. If IVP or CAT scan shows a risk to the kidneys, then surgery is indicated. Either myomectomy or hysterectomy can reestablish the normal flow of urine and prevent permanent damage to a vital organ.

What If There Is Concern That the Fibroids Might Be Cancer?

As discussed on page 117, surgery is often performed when a woman is found to have rapidly growing fibroids because of the fear of cancer. However, uterine sarcoma, a cancer of the uterine muscle, is extremely rare, occurring in less than 1 patient per 1,000 who have surgery for fibroids. And since 80 percent of women with fibroids never even have surgery, the incidence of this cancer is extraordinarily low. Also, most patients determined to have sarcomas are postmenopausal women in their sixties or seventies, whereas most patients with fibroids are in their thirties and forties. Virtually all premenopausal women with growing fibroids have benign uterine fibroids. Therefore, most patients with rapidly growing fibroids may be followed with frequent pelvic examinations. However, if you are postmenopausal and not on estrogen, any growth of the uterus is an indication for surgery.

TYPES OF SURGERY FOR FIBROIDS

What Is a Myomectomy?

Myomectomy means the surgical removal of just the fibroid, with reconstruction and repair of the uterus. There are now a number of techniques used to perform myomectomy: through an abdominal incision, vaginal excision, with a laparoscope, or with a hysteroscope. These procedures are described in the following sections. General considerations regarding surgery are discussed in chapter 13.

What Is an Abdominal Myomectomy?

First performed about ninety years ago, abdominal myomectomy is excellent for women who wish to maintain their ability to have children, or who just prefer to avoid removal of the uterus. The standard method of performing a myomectomy is by *laparotomy*, making a four- to six-inch "bikini" incision on the abdomen just below the pubic hairline. After the incision is made, the intestines and bladder are held out of the way so that the uterus can be seen in the pelvic cavity.

After inspecting the uterus to determine the number and position of the fibroids, the uterus is injected with pitressin, a solution that slows bleeding during the surgery. Then the covering of the uterus overlying the fibroid is cut, and the fibroids are separated from the normal uterine muscle (see figs. 4.3a–c). The remaining normal uterine muscle is then sewn back together. This procedure takes about one to two hours, depending on the number and position of the fibroids. The intestines often take a few days to recover from the pushing and irritation; eating too soon after surgery sometimes can lead to nausea and vomiting. For this reason, and because of the moderate discomfort associated with the incision, a woman having an abdominal myomectomy may need to stay in the hospital for two to three days.

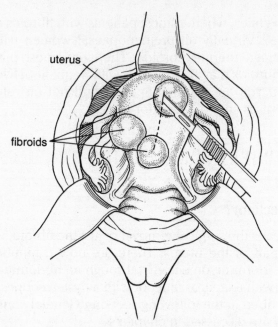

Fig. 4.3a.   Abdominal myomectomy: incision in the uterus

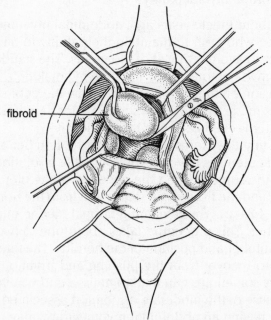

Fig. 4.3b.   Removing the fibroids

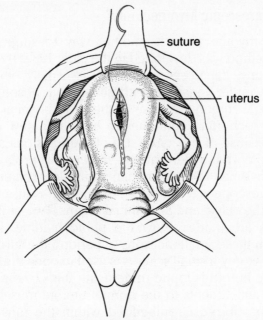

suture

uterus

Fig. 4.3c.   Repairing the uterus

Are Some Fibroids Too Big for a Myomectomy?

The short answer is no. Some doctors and some managed-care organizations have policies stating that a myomectomy cannot be attempted if the uterus is bigger than a certain size—hysterectomy is the only option that they will offer. However, skilled gynecologic surgeons can perform a myomectomy on just about any size uterus. One of the risks of a myomectomy is bleeding from the uterus during surgery. However, there are a number of techniques that can be used to reduce bleeding. A medication can be injected into the uterus that causes the blood vessels in the muscle to constrict, and less blood will seep out of the incisions in the uterine wall. Or the doctors can place an elastic tourniquet around the lower portion of the uterus to decrease the blood flow to the uterus. For very large fibroids, some doctors use a machine called a cell-saver during surgery. Blood that pools around the uterine incisions is removed, filtered by the cell-saver and replaced back into the patient's circulation through a vein. Thus, the patient receives an immediate transfusion of her own blood, and there is no risk of HIV infection or mismatched blood. Many gynecologic surgeons don't have training in these techniques and so don't offer them. Ask your doctor and get some clarification on this issue.

What Is a Laparoscopic Myomectomy?

Laparoscopic myomectomy is another way to surgically remove fibroids. This method was developed in the early 1980s by Dr. Kurt Semm, in Kiel, Germany. Laparoscopic surgery is usually performed as outpatient surgery under general anesthesia and has absolutely revolutionized gynecologic surgery because of the short hospital stay and quick recovery. The technique continues to evolve as new instruments are developed. Because of the small size of the incisions and the level of skill needed to correctly perform the surgery, this procedure is actually harder for a physician to perform than abdominal surgery.

The laparoscope is a slender telescope that is inserted through the navel to view the pelvic and abdominal organs. Two or three small, half-inch incisions are made below the pubic hairline. Instruments are passed through these small incisions to perform the surgery. For laparoscopic myomectomy, a small scissors is used to open the thin covering of the uterus. The fibroid is found underneath this covering, grasped, and freed from its attachments to the normal uterine muscle (see fig. 4.4). The deeper the fibroid is embedded within the muscle wall of the uterus, the more difficult the procedure.

After the fibroid is removed from the uterus, it must be brought out of abdominal cavity. The fibroid is cut into small pieces (*morcellation*), which are removed through the small incision. New morcellating devices allow the easy removal of even large fibroids in a few minutes. The openings in the uterus are then sutured closed with the use of specially designed laparoscopic suture holders and grasping instruments. The procedure can take one to three hours, depending on the number, size, and depth of the fibroids within the muscle wall.

Following laparoscopic myomectomy, many women are able to leave the hospital the same day as surgery. For more extensive surgery, a one-day stay may be necessary. Because the incisions are small, recuperation is usually associated with minimal discomfort. Since the abdominal cavity is not opened, bacteria are less likely to reach the area of surgery, and the risk of infection is low. The intestines are not exposed to the drying effect of air, or the irritating effects of the sterile gauze sponges used to hold the bowel out of the way during abdominal surgery. As a result, the intestines usually begin to work normally again immediately after laparoscopic surgery. This avoids the one- or two-day delay before a person is able to eat following regular abdominal surgery. After laparoscopic myomectomy, women usually return to normal activity, work, and exercise within two weeks (see page 377).

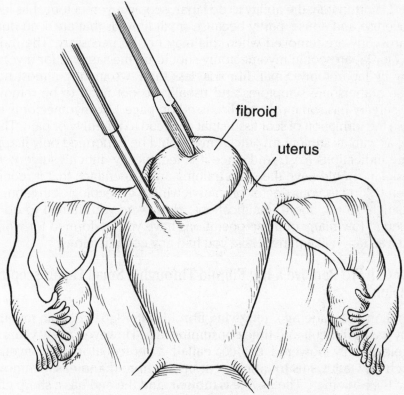

Fig. 4.4. Laparoscopic myomectomy

The use of laparoscopic myomectomy for women who desire to have children is controversial. The concern is how well the uterus will be able to withstand the stress of labor after having been cut and repaired with laparoscopic techniques. Fewer women have gone through labor and delivery after having a laparoscopic myomectomy than the numbers of women going on to have children after a nonlaparoscopic myomectomy. The uterine scar, however, appears to heal as securely with a laparoscopic myomectomy as with myomectomy done by laparotomy. While many women have gotten pregnant and delivered safely, some physicians may recommend cesarean section for delivery to avoid the stress of labor on the uterus. There are now a number of studies showing the safety and success of laparoscopic myomectomy for women who wish to get pregnant. However, a study comparing laparoscopic myomectomy and standard myomectomy with regard to fertility, labor, and delivery has not yet been performed by the research community.

Unfortunately, the ability to do laparoscopic myomectomy has led to its overuse and abuse, partly because small fibroids that are seen during laparoscopy are removed when this may not be necessary. The indications for laparoscopic myomectomy should be the same as for myomectomy by laparotomy. Small fibroids, less than two inches, almost never cause bothersome symptoms and usually do not need to be removed. Any surgery has some risk. As discussed on page 136, myomectomy may cause the formation of scar tissue that can lead to infertility or pain. Therefore, as with all surgery, myomectomy should be performed only if appropriate indications exist. And since it is technically difficult surgery, your physician should have the extra training and experience that it requires. When talking to your doctor or interviewing a gynecologic surgeon, it is your right to ask about qualifications: How were you trained to do this surgery? How many of these operations have you performed for women with a situation like mine? Have you had any complications?

How Can We Remove a Big Fibroid Through a Small Laparoscopic Incision?

Less than a decade ago, removing fibroids after laparoscopic myomectomy was a difficult and time-consuming task. However, a few years ago an electrically powered device, called a morcellator, was invented, which now allows us to quickly cut up the fibroid and easily remove it from the abdomen. The device is tubular, and the end has a sharp circular blade that rotates quickly and takes small slices off the fibroid in a few seconds. A very large fibroid can now be removed in about fifteen minutes. Therefore, we are now able to operate on women with larger fibroids without prolonging surgery and anesthesia. This device has allowed a major advance in our laparoscopic technique.

Karen's Large Fibroid

Karen is a twenty-five-year-old student who came for her first visit to our office for a bladder infection. When I performed her pelvic examination, I felt a large mass behind her uterus, about the size of a very large grapefruit. Her previous doctors had never mentioned this to her, so we assumed this was a new growth. I was a bit concerned, but luckily an ultrasound showed that this was a fibroid coming off the back of her uterus. After some discussion, Karen realized that the fibroid was causing her recent abdominal discomfort. Karen asked if it could be removed. Because of the way the fibroid felt on examination, I thought it might be attached to the uterus by a stalk and, therefore, surgery might be possible with laparoscopic techniques. Karen was excited about this possibility and the quick return to work it might allow her.

I suggested Karen get an MRI to show us more detail about the attachment of the fibroid to the uterus. When I reviewed the MRI with the radiologist, it was clear that the fibroid was indeed attached by a thin stalk. During the scheduled laparoscopic surgery, we were able to cut the stalk attaching the fibroid to the uterus, and the small amount of bleeding was easily stopped. Using the morcellator, we removed the fibroid in pieces. The entire operation took about one hour, and Karen went home the same day. That was four years ago, and Karen has never had another problem.

Can Lasers or Ultrasonic Instruments Be Used for Myomectomy?

Lasers have been used to perform gynecologic surgery since 1982. By concentrating very high-energy light in a very small area, lasers are able to cut through tissue quickly and accurately. Traditionally, surgery has been performed using a scalpel or electrosurgical instruments that create heat that cuts through tissue. Lasers were originally thought to cause less damage to the tissue during surgery. However, recent studies have not found a significant difference between the results of surgery performed with a laser versus that done by electrosurgery or with a scalpel.

Some studies have reported that the use of the laser decreases the amount of blood lost during surgery by a small amount, but there is not enough difference to make this an important advantage. In fact, the transfusion rate is the same whether a laser, electrosurgery, or a scalpel is used. Lasers cost a medical facility approximately $100,000, and the use of a laser during a surgical procedure adds about $800 to the hospital bill. Also, a surgeon requires a substantial amount of specialized training and experience before he or she is truly competent to use a laser.

More recently, ultrasonic surgical instruments have been designed with metal tips that vibrate 30,000 times per second. This rapid motion creates enough heat to boil the water found inside a cell. When the water boils, the cell explodes. When cell after cell explodes, the tissue is cut following the path of the instrument. This phenomenon has been successfully applied to surgery. The advantage of ultrasonic instruments is that they cause very little damage to surrounding tissue and, therefore, may be slightly safer to use. They also create water vapor that disappears quickly from the surgical area, rather than smoke that needs to be suctioned away every few minutes.

Since scientific studies have not shown the results of surgery to be dependent on the type of instrument used, your physician should use whatever instrument he or she is most comfortable with. Don't be fooled because an instrument or technique is new—it may not be any better or safer.

Laparoscopic myomectomy can be performed with either electrosurgery, laser surgery, or ultrasonic instruments. All are equally effective and safe. My own preference for laparoscopic myomectomy are the ultrasonic shears, available at the hospitals where I operate. This instrument performs both cutting and coagulation (stops bleeding) quickly and safely. However, new electric instruments are also safe and provide similar accuracy with less expense.

Can Myomectomy Lead to Scar Tissue?

Any surgery can cause scar tissue to form. Your body makes new tissue as part of the healing process to help paste things back together. This new tissue is called scar tissue or adhesions. The inside of your body can scar from what it perceives to be an injury just as the skin on your knee forms a scar after a bad cut. Unfortunately, this natural defense can work against us when it occurs internally after surgery, because scar tissue may stick to the normal tissue around it, pulling on it and causing pain. Myomectomy performed by either laparotomy or laparoscopy may lead to the formation of scar tissue near the uterus, fallopian tubes, or ovaries. This new tissue is sometimes thin and flimsy, but can be thick and inelastic. Scar tissue near the fallopian tubes or ovaries may decrease fertility by making it difficult for the egg to travel to the fallopian tube.

One of the major benefits of laparoscopic surgery is the principle that it causes fewer adhesions than laparotomy. A group of Italian doctors recently performed laparoscopy on a group of women a few months after they had fibroids removed by either laparoscopy or traditional abdominal surgery. The number of women studied was small (thirty-two women), but the doctors found fewer and thinner adhesions in the women who had laparoscopic surgery. Further studies need to be performed, but this information is encouraging for women wishing laparoscopic surgery.

Can Adhesion Barriers Prevent Scar Tissue?

Another new advance in surgery has been the use of special substances, called adhesion barriers, that help prevent the formation of scar tissue after surgery. Scar tissue forms after virtually all types of surgery, but after pelvic surgery it may lead to scarring of the fallopian tubes and problems with fertility. Therefore, to lessen the chances of adhesion formation, two forms of adhesion barriers have been developed: in the first, small sheets of clothlike material can be wrapped around the areas raw from surgery; or a gel can be poured into the pelvis to bathe and surround the organs after surgery. Both materials prevent nearby tissue, such as the intestines, from sticking to the surgery sites. After a few weeks, the materials dissolve, leaving the newly healed surgery sites fairly free of adhesions. While the barriers are not perfect, they have been shown to help reduce the formation of adhesions.

What Is Vaginal Myomectomy?

In rare instances, a fibroid growing within the uterus on a stalk is pushed, by contractions of the uterus, out through the cervix. This process is usually associated with crampy pain and vaginal bleeding. When a speculum is placed in the vagina, the fibroid can be seen coming out, or prolapsing, through the cervix. Because of the bleeding and discomfort, removal of the fibroid is necessary.

Vaginal myomectomy is performed as an outpatient procedure. The doctor places a speculum in the vagina, cuts the stalk of the fibroid, and removes the entire fibroid. To see if any other fibroids are inside the cavity, the doctor views the inside of the uterus with a telescope (hysteroscopy). If the fibroids are small and appear easy to remove, a small wire attachment to the telescope, called a resectoscope, can cut through the fibroids and remove them (see page 138). If the fibroids are large, they may need to be removed at a later time after shrinking them with a medication such as Lupron.

What Is Myolysis?

Myolysis is a surgical procedure developed to shrink fibroids without removing them. The procedure is performed through the laparoscope and uses either a laser or electrical needle that is passed directly into the fibroid. When the instrument is activated, it delivers high-temperature energy to the tissue and destroys both the fibroid tissue and the blood vessels feeding it. The procedure takes less time than either abdominal or laparoscopic myomectomy because no tissue needs to be removed, and no suturing of the uterus is necessary. At the present time, myolysis is not being recommended for women who wish to have children. Two potential problems exist. First, in some women, scar tissue has formed around the uterus after myolysis, and this might impair future fertility. Second, the effect of myolysis on the strength of the uterine wall is not known. Because of this potential risk of the uterus tearing during labor, we advise that women do not attempt to get pregnant after they have had myolysis.

Although myolysis has been performed on thousands of women throughout the world with very good results, it is still too early to know what its long-term results will be. In our practice, the results have been very good to date.

What Is a Resectoscope Myomectomy?

Resectoscope myomectomy (or hysteroscopic myomectomy) is a technique that can be performed only if the fibroids causing the symptoms are within the uterine cavity (*submucosal*). This procedure is performed as outpatient surgery without any incisions (see fig. 4.5). Anesthesia is needed because the surgery may take one to two hours and would otherwise be uncomfortable. A small telescope, the resectoscope, is passed through the cervix, and the internal uterine cavity is seen. A small camera is attached to the telescope, and the view is projected on a video monitor. This magnifies the picture and also allows your physician to perform the surgery while sitting in a comfortable position. The surgery can then proceed more rapidly.

Electricity passes through the thin wire attachment of the telescope, allowing the instrument to cut through the fibroid like a hot knife through butter. As the fibroid is shaved from within the uterine cavity, the heat from the instrument sears blood vessels so that the blood loss is usually minimal. Patients go home the same day, and recovery is remarkably fast, with most patients able to go back to normal activity in one or two days.

When fibroids are the cause of infertility, pregnancy rates following resectoscope myomectomy have been about 50 percent. And when performed for heavy bleeding, nearly 90 percent of patients return to normal menstrual flow. Only a few years ago, treatment for fibroids in the cavity of the uterus involved major surgery—an abdominal incision and either cutting open the entire uterus to remove the fibroid or performing a hysterectomy. Resectoscope myomectomy has been a major advance in the treatment of women who have submucus fibroids.

What Is Endometrial Ablation?

Endometrial ablation is an outpatient procedure used to stop or decrease bleeding from the uterus. It is described in detail on page 89. En-

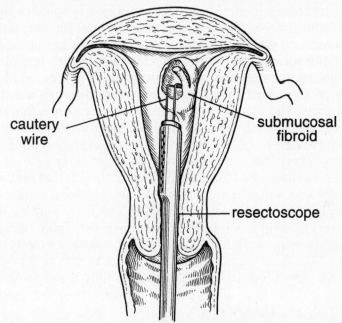

cautery
wire

submucosal
fibroid

resectoscope

Fig. 4.5.   Myoma resection

dometrial ablation can be very effective in treating women who experience bleeding from fibroid and who do not wish to have children. The
procedure may be performed at the same time as a resectoscope myomectomy. In women who have a fibroid uterus larger than a fourteen-
week pregnancy, endometrial ablation has not been as successful.
However, recent advances in the methods used for endometrial ablation make it likely that the procedure will be able to be performed for
women with large fibroids.

Do I Need a Hysterectomy for Fibroids?

I believe hysterectomy for uterine fibroids should be performed as a last
resort. The issues concerning hysterectomy are fully discussed in chapter 12. Hysterectomy is a major operation and carries with it risks of infection, injury to other organs, anesthesia complications, and blood loss
that can sometimes result in the need for transfusion. While complications are uncommon, they should not be taken lightly. Recovery from
abdominal hysterectomy takes four to six weeks, recovery from vaginal
hysterectomy takes about three to four weeks, and recovery from laparoscopic hysterectomy takes about two weeks. The cost of surgery is

expensive, including doctors' fees, anesthesia fees, hospital charges, and operating room charges. It's preferable to avoid major surgery if possible.

Hysterectomy has two positive attributes as treatment for fibroids. One is that the surgery has been shown to cause slightly less blood loss than abdominal myomectomy. Yet, with today's sophisticated testing of blood donors (see page 364), the risk of infection from a transfusion is extremely small. The second advantage of hysterectomy is that since the entire uterus is removed, the possibility of new fibroids growing back is eliminated. However, the likelihood of requiring surgery for fibroids a second time is very low and gets lower as you get older.

For the woman who has symptoms from fibroids that *require* her to have surgery and who does not wish to have children, removal of the uterus may be discussed as one option. Hysterectomy may be appropriate for a woman who has multiple fibroids, or very large fibroids, and who does not want to take a chance that another surgery may be needed for fibroids at a later time. Hysterectomy can be an option for women who have fibroids, but only when fertility is not an issue, only when other options have been tried, only when they are emotionally prepared, only as a last resort.

It is important to remember that hysterectomy means removal of the uterus only, not including the ovaries and tubes. The medical word for removal of the ovaries and tubes is *salpingo-oophorectomy*. The issues regarding whether your ovaries should or should not be removed are also discussed in chapter 12.

Can Focused Ultrasound Be Used to Treat Fibroids?

Ultrasound is a form of energy, and when used at high intensity and focused on an object, the energy can be used to destroy that object. This principle has recently been used in experiments for the treatment of fibroids. The ultrasound energy is generated outside the body but focused on a fibroid in the uterus. The procedure presently takes a few hours to treat each fibroid. The size of the fibroid that can be successfully treated is limited to about a one-inch diameter. This procedure is in its early development. We hope these techniques can be refined so that the procedure time will be shorter, and the size of the treated fibroid can be larger.

What Is Uterine Fibroid Embolization?

Uterine fibroid embolization (UFE) is a nonsurgical technique that shrinks fibroids without removing them. The procedure is performed by an interventional radiologist, an M.D. with basic certification in radiology and special education and certification in interventional radiology. The interventional radiologist guides a long thin catheter (tube) into the blood vessels that supply the uterus while monitoring the process under X-ray. Small plastic particles are pushed through the catheter until they form a blockade to the blood flowing to the uterus. Fibroids have a limited supply of blood vessels, and with the blood flow blocked, the fibroid cells start to die off. The surrounding normal uterine muscle has a better blood supply and is able to survive. Deprived of blood, nutrition, and oxygen, fibroids shrink like prunes for the three to six months following embolization, and the symptoms from the fibroids often lessen as well.

Embolization has been used in medicine for many years and has been used in gynecology since 1972 to stop heavy bleeding from cervical cancer or heavy bleeding from the uterus that rarely occurs after childbirth. Embolization has been very effective in these cases, with success rates of 85 to 100 percent. Embolization was first used to treat fibroids by the French physician Dr. Jaques Ravina in 1995. Interestingly, his idea was to stop the vaginal bleeding caused by large fibroids prior to performing an abdominal myomectomy. To his surprise, many of the women who were scheduled to come back for surgery after embolization canceled surgery because most of their symptoms had disappeared as a result of the embolization. It became clear to Dr. Ravina that embolization might be more than a preparation for surgery; it might be the only treatment needed. Shortly after Dr. Ravina published his findings, uterine artery embolization became available in many countries around the world. It has now been performed in about 20,000 women in the United States and another 5,000 women worldwide.

How Is UFE Performed?

An interventional radiologist performs UFE in a specially designed hospital procedure room. The patient lies down on a flat table, and an overhead X-ray machine takes moving pictures during the procedure. You do not need to be put to sleep, but sedating medications are given in the vein to help you relax during the one to two hours the procedure takes. A small (one-inch) incision is made in the groin directly over the artery carrying blood to the leg. The catheter, about the diameter of a piece of thick spaghetti, is threaded up this artery into the main artery of the body, called the aorta, and then threaded back down one side into the main blood vessel that supplies the uterus, called the uterine artery (see fig. 4.6).

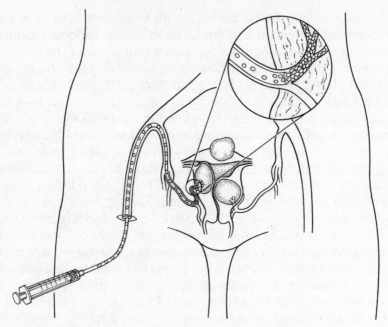

Fig. 4.6.   Uterine fibroid embolization

The radiologist can tell the position of the catheter by injecting a special liquid through the catheter that shows up on the X-ray. Once the catheter is in position, tiny particles the size of fine sand are injected through the catheter and into the uterine artery. There are presently two types of particles used: polyvinyl chloride (PVC) particles made of plastic, and embospheres made of acrylic and gelatin. The particles build up until they block off the uterine artery and stop the blood flow to the uterus. However, there are two smaller blood vessels that supply blood to the uterus, one branch from the artery supplying the ovary and one from the artery supplying the vagina. These braches allow some blood to reach the uterus even though the main blood supply is stopped. After one side is treated, the catheter is redirected into the corresponding artery on the other side of the uterus, and the procedure is repeated. After the procedure is completed, the patient is transferred to a hospital room for recovery and pain medication.

What Is Recovery Like After UFE?

After embolization blocks the blood supply to the fibroids, the cells of the fibroid start to die off immediately. The dying cells release toxins that irritate the surrounding tissue and cause pain and inflammation. Almost all women have moderate to severe pain for the first day or so after uterine artery embolization. All women are kept in the hospital for one day so that they can be given intravenous narcotic pain medication. Anti-inflammatory medications, like Anaprox or ibuprofen, are also given to keep the inflammation down in the uterus. Tylenol is given for the fever that commonly follows the procedure. However, most women are able to go home the next morning and only need to take oral pain and anti-inflammatory medications for the next few days. As with all medical procedures, the recovery varies from woman to woman. Many women feel back to normal within a few days and return to regular activity within a week or so. Other women have pain or discomfort for weeks and may not get back to normal activity for a few weeks or, rarely, even months.

How Effective and Safe Is UFE?

Many women will notice a relief of fibroid symptoms within six weeks after the procedure. However, it takes a few months for the fibroids to fully shrink and the full effect of the procedure to be evident. Three to six months following UFE, the uterus and fibroids will have decreased about 40 percent in size. About 90 percent of women who were bothered by symptoms related to the size of their fibroids will have a significant improvement and be satisfied with the results. Likewise, about 85 percent of women who had heavy bleeding from their fibroids will have lighter and shorter periods and be satisfied with the results. About 10 to 15 percent of women who have UFE will continue to have bothersome symptoms and usually require other treatment. Many of the initial women who had UFE have now been followed for three years and are still symptom free. Because the procedure has only been widely available since 1997, we do not have longer follow-up on these women yet.

About 25,000 women worldwide have had UFE performed for uterine fibroids. To date, the procedure has been extremely safe. The Society of Interventional Radiology reports only four deaths from this procedure or 1 out of every 6,000 women who have had UFE. For comparison, the risk of dying from surgery or anesthesia for a hysterectomy is about 2 out of 6,000 women. Risks for an individual are related to your medical condition, your age, and the disease for which you are being treated. Comparing risks of UFE to hysterectomy for women of similar age and condition with fibroids, it appears that the serious risks may be slightly lower with UFE.

Are You a Good Candidate for Embolization?

Embolization is still a relatively new procedure, and selecting the appropriate women who will clearly benefit from UFE is still a work in progress. There remains some difference of opinion among interventional radiologists, and even more differences between gynecologists and interventional radiologists, as to which women should have the procedure. Obviously, the first criteria for treatment would be the presence of fibroid symptoms bothersome enough to require that something be done. As is true for fibroid treatment in general, the option of doing nothing exists unless the fibroids are causing significant anemia or the fibroids are blocking the ureters and threatening harm to the kidneys.

UFE works well for women who have large fibroids that are causing discomfort or pain because of their size. If shrinking the fibroids to a little more than half their present size would relieve your symptoms, then UFE may be right for you. However, UFE may not be very helpful for women with extremely large fibroids because they may not shrink enough to make a difference in the symptoms.

Women with fibroids on a stalk outside the uterus, called pedunculated fibroids, should not have UFE. Embolization can cause the stalk to deteriorate and allow the fibroid to float around the abdominal cavity. The dead tissue causes an inflammation inside the abdomen resulting in pain and fever. Surgery may be required to remove the degenerating fibroid. Fibroids that mostly bulge inside the uterine cavity, submucus fibroids, may also detach and float inside the uterine cavity after embolization. The uterus will then cramp and contract to expel the fibroid. Discharge and blood may accompany this process, and sometimes infection develops. If the fibroid is not expelled, surgery may be needed to remove it.

If your fibroids are small, endometrial ablation (see page 138) may alleviate heavy bleeding. This outpatient procedure also allows you to avoid hysterectomy and is painless, inexpensive, fast, and has a one-day recovery period. However, ablation may not be technically possible if your fibroids are very large. Embolization works very well for women with bleeding and large fibroids.

What Is Postembolization Syndrome?

Following UFE, some women may develop fever, increasing rather than decreasing pelvic pain, and a vaginal discharge. This combination of symptoms is called postembolization syndrome. Many of these women will also experience nausea and exhaustion. The symptoms may last for days or even weeks and cause concern because of the possibility that serious infection is present in the uterus. If the symptoms get worse over time, rather than better as would be expected, then an examination and evaluation for infection is important. Postembolization syndrome will resolve over time, even if it takes a few weeks. However, if infection is present in the uterus, hysterectomy is usually necessary to prevent the spread of a very serious infection throughout the body. This infection, called sepsis, has led to the deaths of 2 women (out of 25,000) following UFE. Good communication between the gynecologist and interventional radiologist will be helpful to differentiate between postembolization syndrome and infection.

What Are the Long-Term Risks of UFE?

Uterine fibroid embolization was first performed to shrink fibroids in 1995 and has only been widely available since 1997. For that reason, there is presently no long-term follow-up information. However, since embolization has been used for a long time for other reasons, we do know that it is very safe. There have not been any allergic reactions to the particles. Also, there is no evidence, or even any reason to believe, that embolization could cause cancer of the uterus.

Some women worry that the particles will travel to other parts of the body during the procedure or at a later time. Misembolization, particles traveling during the procedure, is discussed below. After the procedure, the particles become embedded into the vessel wall by scar tissue and do not travel in the bloodstream. After about six weeks, the blood vessels open back up and start supplying blood to the uterus again. Since the fibroids have already died off, they do not grow back again.

Childbirth after embolization is now viewed with caution. We know that women who have had embolization of the uterus for hemorrhage following childbirth have been able to safely have more children. However, those women have not had embolization for fibroids, a somewhat different situation. Fibroids are an integral part of the uterine wall, and embolization destroys them. Therefore, the strength of the remaining tissue is uncertain. Hopefully, further study will clarify whether childbirth is safe after UFE.

What Is Misembolization?

The particles that are used for embolization are very small, about the size of a grain of sand. In a few instances, the particles have been noted to travel through blood vessels to areas other than where they were intended to go. We call particles ending up in the wrong place nontarget embolization, or misembolization. In one patient reported in the medical literature, the particles went to the wrong blood vessel and caused the breakdown of her buttocks. Some women have noted a loss of clitoral sensation following embolization that is presumed to be the result of particles blocking the artery that supplies the clitoris. We do not know how often this happens, but it appears to be uncommon. In an attempt to avoid these complications, many interventional radiologists are paying close attention to the pattern of the blood vessels in the pelvis for every patient, noting that the path of the vessels can be different from woman to woman. An attempt is made to avoid vessels going anywhere other than the uterus. However, the vessels supplying one area may interconnect with the vessels of another area. If this is the case, it may be difficult to completely avoid particles going to other areas. In over 25,000 women having UFE to date, serious misembolization has only been reported in a very few. Less dangerous but still concerning misembolization, such as to the clitoral or cervical vessels, may often not be reported, so we do not really know how often this occurs.

Can UFE Affect Fertility?

The answer is maybe. Misembolization, or particles traveling to unintended areas as described above, may rarely block off blood flow to the ovaries and interfere with the function of the ovaries. In addition, in about 10 percent of women, the main blood vessels supplying the ovaries start as a branch from the uterine artery. If the uterine artery is blocked, the blood supply to the ovaries is also blocked, and the ovaries cease functioning. Following embolization, in about 5 percent of women, the ovaries stop functioning, and early menopause follows. While this is never a good thing at any age, it is devastating for a twenty-five-year-old woman who wishes to have children.

Another unanswered question is whether the age of menopause will be affected in women who have UFE. If misembolization allows particles to block blood flow to some eggs, those eggs may die. The ovaries have many eggs, and the surviving eggs may continue to produce some hormone even if lots of other eggs have been destroyed. Hormone tests during this time may appear normal. However, if fewer eggs than normal remain in the ovaries, both eggs and the hormones they produce may be depleted before normal menopause is expected, around age fifty-two. We do not know whether any women who have had UFEs are destined to enter earlier menopause. This question will take many years to answer.

The problem of early menopause has been seen after hysterectomy in some women. If the blood vessels supplying the uterus also have a branch as the main supply to the ovaries, then suturing the uter-ine arteries during the hysterectomy will destroy the ovaries. Myomec-tomy, which does not disturb the uterine or ovarian blood vessels, has not been found to cause this problem.

Pregnancies and healthy babies have been born to women who have had UFE. However, we do not know how many women tried to get pregnant and were unsuccessful. We do not know how many had a mis-carriage. To date, no cases of rupture of the uterus during pregnancy or labor have been reported following UFE. However, since the number of women getting pregnant after UFE is very small, we do not know what the risk really is. As a result of all this uncertainty, most interventional ra-diologists recommend that women who wish to have children not use UFE as treatment for their fibroids.

Are There Surgical Techniques That Mimic UFE?

As mentioned earlier, there has been a bit of discord between some gynecologists and interventional radiologists over UFE as treatment for fibroids. Some of this disagreement is medical—an honest debate about which women will benefit most from UFE instead of myomec-tomy or hysterectomy—and some of the disagreement is self-interest and economics.

Gynecologists recently created a surgical technique to tie off the uter-ine arteries (rather than block them with particles) using the laparoscope. So far, the first two years of results in a small number of women have been as good as those achieved with UFE. There may be advantages to the sur-gical approach, called laparoscopic uterine artery ligation, and there are some clear disadvantages. The current surgical approach requires an anes-thetic and is an invasive procedure with the risks of any laparoscopy. How-ever, the surgical approach only ties off the uterine artery, and since no particles are used, there is no risk of misembolization to other areas. La-paroscopic uterine artery ligation may, theoretically, decrease the small risk of premature menopause that accompanies UFE. If, however, some women have a branch of the uterine artery as the only blood supply to the ovaries, then surgical ligation of the uterine artery will cut off blood supply to the ovaries, and the result will be early menopause for these women. A variation of this surgical technique that is being developed blocks the uter-ine artery though a small vaginal incision and does not require general anesthesia, and thus avoids some risk. It is still too early to tell whether there will be any long-term differences between these techniques, so you will need to ask your doctor about new results as they are published.

How Do You Find a Doctor to Perform UFE?

Interventional radiologists, M.D. subspecialists in the field of radiology, perform uterine artery embolization. Interventional radiologists are not only trained to interpret X-rays, but they take three years of special training and are certified to place catheters into blood vessels to deliver medications or, in these cases, particles to block blood flow. As is true for gynecologists and gynecologic surgery, some interventional radiologists have more experience with UFE than others. You need to ask the same questions you would ask of your surgeon: How many of these procedures have you performed? How many in cases similar to mine? How many complications have you had, and what was the extent of those complications?

The other important issue to consider is whether UFE is right for you in the first place. Unfortunately, interventional radiologists are not trained in gynecology, and there may be other less invasive treatments available to treat your symptoms. It might be best to get a second opinion from a gynecologist in addition to an opinion from an interventional radiologist before choosing treatment. UFE has been performed on women who were not appropriate candidates for the procedure and who would have been better off with another type of treatment.

Hopefully, in the future, more gynecologists and interventional radiologists will work together to help guide women to treatment options that are right for them without regard to monetary gain or other self-interests.

Adenomyosis

Adenomyosis is a noncancerous condition of the uterus that can mimic many of the signs and symptoms of fibroids. This condition results from the lining cells of the uterus growing directly into the muscle wall of the uterus. When the lining cells of the uterus bleed at the time of the menstrual period, these misplaced cells in the muscle bleed as well. And bleeding directly into the muscle causes pain. As the blood accumulates, the surrounding muscle swells and forms fibrous tissue in response to the irritation. This swollen area within the uterine muscle wall, called an adenomyoma, feels very much like a fibroid on examination and is often confused with a fibroid on a sonogram. Adenomyosis is present in about 10 percent of women and, therefore, is less common than fibroids.

What Are the Symptoms of Adenomyosis?

Adenomyosis may be mild and cause no symptoms at all, or, in more severe forms, it may lead to heavy bleeding and severe cramping during menstrual periods. If you have heavy bleeding and severe cramping with your periods, adenomyosis is one of the conditions that your doctor may consider as the cause of your symptoms.

How Is the Diagnosis of Adenomyosis Made?

The diagnosis of adenomyosis is suspected if the uterus feels enlarged and tender to the touch during the pelvic examination. However, the diagnosis of adenomyosis based on these findings is often inaccurate, and other causes—fibroids, endometriosis, or polyps—are often found as the cause for the bleeding or discomfort. Sometimes, the diagnosis may be suggested by the appearance of the uterus on a sonogram, although it is often difficult to tell the difference between adenomyosis and fibroids using sonography. MRI is somewhat better at detecting adenomyosis, but the test is very expensive and rarely used for this purpose. Unfortunately, the only way to establish the diagnosis of adenomyosis with certainty is with surgery. Once removed, the tissue can be examined under the microscope, and the uterine lining cells can be seen within the muscle wall.

What Is the Treatment for Adenomyosis?

The medications Lupron or Synarel (see page 123) can cause cessation of the periods and associated menstrual cramping and even lead to shrinkage of the swelling associated with adenomyosis. However, the effect is temporary—when the medication is discontinued, the symptoms return. At the present time, the only treatment for adenomyosis is surgery. In situations where the adenomyosis is confined to isolated areas in the muscle wall, an attempt may be made to surgically remove these areas and repair the rest of the uterus. In situations where the majority of the uterus is affected, hysterectomy may be the only cure.

Can Uterine Artery Embolization Be Used to Treat Adenomyosis?

Only a small number of women with adenomyosis have been treated with uterine artery embolization (UAE), and the results so far have been disappointing. Symptoms appear to improve for a year or two, but most women then have recurrence of symptoms. Adenomyosis is defined as the presence of uterine lining cells within an otherwise normal uterine muscle wall. The blood supply to that muscle is normal, unlike fibroids, and should be resistant to the effects of embolization. Again, further research will be needed to see if better results can be obtained.

REFERENCES

Bulletti, C., V. Polli, E. Negrini, E. Giacomucci, and C. Flamigni. 1996. "Adhesion formation after laparoscopic myomectomy." *Journal of the American Association of Gynecologic Laparoscopists* 3:533–36.

Dionne, C. 2001. *Sex, Lies and the Truth About Uterine Fibroids.* New York: Avery.

Dubuisson, M., L. Mandelbrot, F. Lecuru, F. Aubriot, H. Foulot, and M. Mouly. 1991. Myomectomy by laparoscopy: A preliminary report of 43 cases. *Fertility and Sterility* 56:827–30.

Friedman, A., and S. Haas. 1993. Should uterine size be an indication for surgical intervention in women with myomas? *American Journal of Obstetrics and Gynecology* 168:751–55.

Parker, W., Y. Fu, and J. Berek. 1994. Uterine sarcomas in patients operated on for presumed leiomyoma and rapidly growing leiomyoma. *Obstetrics and Gynecology* 83:414–18.

Parker, W., and I. Rodi. 1994. Patient selection for laparoscopic myomectomy. *Journal of the American Association of Gynecologic Laparoscopists* 2:23–27.

Pitts, E. 2001. Fibroids and infertility: A systematic review of the evidence. *Obstetrics and Gynecological Survey* 56:483–91.

Rein, M., R. Barbieri, and A. Freidman. 1995. Progesterone: A critical role in the pathogenesis of uterine myomas. *American Journal of Obstetrics and Gynecology* 172:14–18.

Reiter, R., P. Wagner, and J. Gambone. 1992. Routine hysterectomy for large asymptomatic uterine lyomyomata: A reappraisal. *Obstetrics and Gynecology* 79:481–84.

Stewart, E., and R. Nowak. 1998. New concepts in the treatment of uterine leiomyomas. *Obstetrics and Gynecology* 92:624–27.

Stovall, T., F. Ling, L. Henry, and M. Woodruff. 1991. A randomized trial evaluating leuprolide acetata before hysterectomy as treatment for leiomyomas. *American Journal of Obstetrics and Gynecology* 164:1420–25.

5

IF YOU HAVE OVARIAN CYSTS

What Are Ovarian Cysts?

An ovarian cyst is simply a collection of fluid within the normally solid ovary. There are many different types of ovarian cysts, and they are an extremely common gynecologic problem. Because of the fear of ovarian cancer, cysts are a common cause of concern among women. But it is important to know that the vast majority of ovarian cysts are *not* cancer. However, some benign cysts will require treatment in that they do not go away by themselves, and, in quite rare cases, some may be cancerous. A cyst may cause discomfort or may be discovered at the time of a routine examination, when you are feeling absolutely fine. The good news is that almost all ovarian cysts will go away by themselves without any treatment.

What Are the Different Types of Ovarian Cysts?

Ovarian cysts can be divided into two categories: those that go away by themselves versus those that need treatment, and those that are benign versus those that are cancerous. Most cysts are benign and will go away by themselves. The distinction that is most important to your health and well-being is whether the cyst is cancerous or benign. Cancerous cysts should be removed as soon as possible. Benign cysts that will not go away by themselves may also need to be removed to prevent further problems. The following chart lists the different types of cysts, and it may be helpful if you refer back to it as you read this chapter. Further explanations of each type of cyst are included later in this chapter.

Cysts That Usually Go Away by Themselves

Benign	*Cancerous*
follicular	none
corpus luteum	
hemorrhagic	

Cysts That Do Not Go Away by Themselves

Benign	*Cancerous*
endometriomas	epithelial cancers
epithelial—serous,	germ cell cancers
mucinous	
dermoid	

What Causes Most Ovarian Cysts?

The most common types of ovarian cysts are called *functional cysts*, which result from a collection of fluid forming around a developing egg. Every woman who is ovulating will form a small amount of fluid around the developing egg each month. The combination of the egg, the special fluid-producing cells, and the fluid is called a *follicle* and is normally about the size of a pea. For unknown reasons, the cells that surround the egg occasionally form too much fluid, and this straw-colored fluid expands the ovary from within. If the collection of fluid gets to be larger than a normal follicle, about three-quarters of an inch in diameter, a *follicular cyst* is present (see fig. 5.1). If fluid continues to form, the ovary is stretched like a balloon filled with water. The normally white covering of the ovary becomes thin and smooth and appears bluish-gray. Follicular cysts may rarely become as large as three or four inches. The majority of these cysts, even the large ones, go away after a month or two as the extra fluid dissolves back into the bloodstream.

At the time of ovulation, the covering of the ovary tears open to release the egg. Within hours, this covering heals, and the cells in the ovary form a structure called the corpus luteum. The corpus luteum pro-

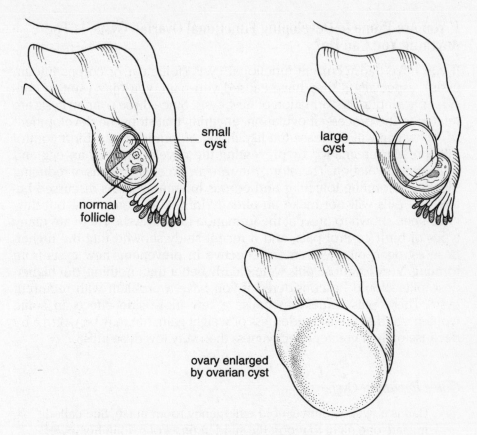

small
cyst

large
cyst

normal
follicle

ovary enlarged
by ovarian cyst

Fig. 5.1. Ovarian cysts

duces progesterone, the hormone that prepares the uterine lining cells
for the arrival of the fertilized egg. Every menstruating woman, every
month, forms a corpus luteum. However, cells can produce fluid within
the corpus luteum and form a cyst. While a *corpus luteum* cyst is usually
no larger than a small marble, sometimes so much fluid is produced
that a cyst of a few inches results. The good news is that, like follicular
cysts, practically all corpus luteum cysts will go away by themselves in a
few weeks. Follicular cysts and corpus luteum cysts are collectively referred to as functional cysts.

A number of other types of ovarian cysts can form as a result of the
abnormal growth of other cells contained in the ovary. These cysts are
less common and are discussed later in this chapter.

If You Are Prone to Developing Functional Ovarian Cysts, Is There Anything You Can Do?

If you have had recurrent functional cysts (follicular or corpus luteum cysts), especially if they have caused you pain, you may want to consider preventing the formation of new cysts. Since these ovarian cysts are related to the process of ovulation, anything that stops the development of a new egg will decrease the likelihood of forming cysts. Birth control pills prevent pregnancy by preventing the development of an egg and preventing ovulation. Therefore, they are an excellent means of reducing the risk of forming follicular and corpus luteum cysts. As discussed below, the pills will not make an already formed cyst go away, but they have been shown to prevent the formation of new cysts. There are many types of birth control pills, and a recent study showed that the higher-dose estrogen pills were more effective in preventing new cysts from forming. Very low-dose pills were clearly better than nothing, but higher-dose pills should be considered if you have a problem with recurrent cysts. These pills sometimes cause a few more side effects in some women, such as breast tenderness or weight gain, but may be worth a try because of their greater effectiveness than very low-dose pills.

Gail's Recurrent Cysts

Gail is a twenty-four-year-old emergency room nurse. She called me late one night to report the sudden onset of pain in her lower abdomen. She had been fine all day but now was having trouble walking because of the pain. I met her at the emergency room. She was visibly uncomfortable, and examining her was difficult because of the pain. We immediately performed a sonogram, which showed a cyst in her ovary and about half a cup of fluid floating around near the ovary. This was pretty good evidence that she had a ruptured ovarian cyst. Reassured that nothing more serious was happening, she decided to go home and back to bed. Within two days, the fluid had dissolved back into her bloodstream, and she was feeling fine and able to return to work. However, one month later she had exactly the same experience. When she had pain again for the third month in a row, we decided to perform a laparoscopy to make sure we weren't missing anything. The laparoscopy showed a benign ovarian cyst that had ruptured, just as we had expected. After the laparoscopy, Gail and I talked about ways to prevent this from happening again. Since she had endured three painful cysts and a laparoscopy, she was already dreading what would happen next month. We discussed the use of birth control pills, which she agreed to start immediately. She has been taking the pills for a few years and has not had another ovarian cyst.

WHAT ARE THE SYMPTOMS OF OVARIAN CYSTS?

Can a Cyst Cause Pain?

Although many cysts cause no symptoms at all, pressure or pain in the pelvic area is a common problem that may cause a woman with an ovarian cyst to see her doctor. As fluid collects in a cyst and makes the ovary expand, the covering of the ovary is stretched. This stretching can cause discomfort or pain. Also, the fluid within the cyst can weigh the ovary down, causing a pulling sensation when a woman moves. In very rare cases, the covering of the ovary tears opens, or ruptures, releasing the cyst fluid into the abdominal cavity. This ruptured ovarian cyst usually results in pain.

Jane's Painful Ovarian Cyst

Jane is a twenty-five-year-old woman who felt some pain on the right side of her lower abdomen one morning when she awoke. The pain was mild at first but then became more bothersome over the next few days. The pain seemed to be worse when she was walking or being active and was better when she was still. Even though her job as a secretary allowed her to sit much of the day, the pain bothered her when she had to get up from her desk and lift or move things. She made an appointment to come to our office. During the pelvic examination, a small cyst about the size of a walnut was felt on her right ovary. The cyst was slightly tender when touched during the examination. We performed a sonogram, which suggested a simple, follicular-type cyst. Jane's discomfort was not too bad overall, and she was reassured that nothing serious was going on. I suggested she limit her activity at work to avoid aggravating the discomfort. She made an appointment for another examination in two weeks, with the instructions to call if the discomfort got worse. Two weeks later she came back to the office feeling fine, and the examination showed that the cyst was already entirely dissolved. Jane was relieved and has not had another cyst.

Can an Ovarian Cyst Cause Severe Pain?

In rare cases, an ovarian cyst can twist the ovary all the way around, a condition called ovarian torsion. The twisting prevents blood from getting to the ovary, and the cells in the ovary begin to deteriorate, releasing chemicals that cause severe pain. Often the pain is so bad that you are not able to stand up straight, and emergency surgery may be needed.

Sometimes the diagnosis is not entirely clear, but surgery is recommended to discover the cause of the pain and to correct it. At the time of surgery, the ovary can be seen twisted around, and it is usually discolored from the lack of blood. The ovary can be untwisted and can be saved. If you have a painful cyst, it is unlikely that it is ovarian torsion, which is a very rare occurrence. See your physician if you experience acute or persistent pelvic or abdominal pain.

Sara's Laparoscopy for Her Ovarian Cyst

Sara is a thirty-five-year-old woman who felt a pain on her right side that was strong enough to awaken her from a sound sleep. She noticed that if she turned toward her right, the pain was better, but if she turned to the left, it became more intense and sharper. She called the office, and we asked her to come right in. The examination was difficult because she was so uncomfortable, but it felt as if her right ovary was enlarged to the size of a lemon. A sonogram showed a large ovarian cyst that was entirely filled with fluid and appeared benign. Unfortunately, Sara was in so much pain that she was crying and couldn't move. She and I agreed that immediate surgery should be performed to relieve her discomfort.

We chose to perform a laparoscopy (see page 165) so that we could examine the ovary first and determine what the problem was without making a large abdominal incision. In the hospital, under general anesthesia, a small telescope was placed through a half-inch incision in Sara's navel to look into her abdominal and pelvic areas. During the laparoscopy, we found a large ovarian cyst that was twisted around itself, causing all her pain. We were able to safely untwist the ovary and then remove the cyst, all with laparoscopic techniques.

Sara felt better immediately after surgery. The sharp pain was gone, and despite being groggy from the anesthesia, she was able to go home that afternoon. Since laparoscopic surgery uses small incisions, the postoperative pain is usually much less than with an abdominal incision. At the time of her two-week postoperative visit, Sara was feeling entirely normal and had already returned to work and exercise.

Can an Ovarian Cyst Destroy the Normal Ovary?

The ovary has a remarkable ability to expand without damage to the small eggs contained within its tissue. As an ovarian cyst develops, the normal ovarian tissue containing the eggs spreads out over the cyst. If the cyst goes away by itself, as most of them do, then the ovary shrinks back down to its normal size over a period of a few weeks without any residual effect. If the cyst needs to be surgically removed, we try to leave as much normal ovarian tissue as possible so that the ovary can heal with healthy eggs remaining. Even with large cysts—those that are more than three inches in diameter—normal ovarian tissue can *almost always* be saved. The ovaries contain hundreds of thousands of eggs, so that the loss of a small number should not make any difference in your fertility or the age at which your menopause will begin.

Can a Cyst Interfere with Your Menstrual Cycle?

The ovaries produce estrogen and progesterone, the hormones that regulate your menstrual cycle. Therefore, when an ovarian cyst disrupts the ovary, it may not produce hormones normally, and the result can be abnormal periods. The bleeding may be heavy or light, long or short, or irregular. Abnormal amounts of hormone can cause water retention, breast swelling or tenderness, and even PMS-type symptoms. Once the cyst resolves, your periods and body should return to normal within a cycle or two. As always, if you have abnormal bleeding, you should contact your physician.

Can a Cyst Cause Infertility?

There are two types of cystic conditions that are associated with infertility: the cysts of endometriosis and polycystic ovarian syndrome (PCOS). If endometriosis cells get inside the ovary, they will cause blood to collect within the ovary itself, forming an ovarian cyst called an *endometrioma*. Endometriosis can interfere with a woman's fertility, although the reasons for this are not entirely clear. The current theories suggest that the endometriosis cells produce chemicals that either interfere with the ovary's ability to release the egg from the ovary or interfere with the sperm's ability to fertilize the egg. In addition, if the endometriosis is severe, it may cause bands of scar tissue to form that block the passage of the egg into and down the fallopian tube. Endometriosis is discussed in chapter 7.

Polycystic ovarian syndrome, also known as Stein Leventhal syndrome, is the result of complicated hormonal changes that are associated with infertility. That is to say, the cysts are not the cause of infertility, but rather result from the same problem that causes the infertility. This condition is discussed on page 70. The most common symptom of polycystic ovarian syndrome is infrequent periods. Notable acne, oily skin, and obesity are also symptoms associated with this problem. As the hormonal abnormalities become established, the ovary forms multiple small cysts (about one-quarter inch) that can make the ovaries two or three times larger than normal. These small cysts can often be detected by sonography.

The drug clomiphene is used to treat infertility associated with polycystic ovarian syndrome. This medication fixes some of the hormonal imbalance long enough for the ovary to produce and release an egg. Clomiphene causes only minimal side effects, and it must be taken for a few days every month until you get pregnant. The success rate is fairly good; about 60 percent of women became pregnant. If pregnancy does not occur in the first three months of using clomiphene, other treatments should be tried. Interestingly, another part of the hormonal imbalance associated with polycystic ovarian syndrome includes an inability of the cells in the body to use insulin properly. New medications designed to help diabetics utilize insulin have also been found to help women with PCOS. These medications may restore normal ovulation and reduce acne and oily skin. Weight loss helps correct some of the problems with insulin and has also been found to be very helpful in restoring ovulation in women with PCOS.

For women who do not respond to medication, treatment with a laser aimed through a laparoscope to puncture the cysts may be effective. This technique has been shown to temporarily bring hormone levels back to normal and often reestablishes ovulation.

How Are Ovarian Cysts Diagnosed?

At the time of a pelvic exam, your doctor will feel next to the sides of the uterus, where the ovaries are located. The ovaries are normally no larger than a small walnut. But if a cyst forms, the ovary can swell to a few inches or more. The doctor is often able to feel a cyst as a soft, movable lump. Regardless of the type of cyst, most feel alike to the physician. Sometimes they are tender, but often they cause no discomfort or pain, and you may be surprised to be told that there is even a cyst present.

If you are not menopausal and the cyst is not bothersome, nothing needs to be done because most of these cysts will go away by themselves. A repeat examination can be scheduled in two or three weeks to make sure that the cyst is dissolving. If the cyst is gone by that time, no further treatment or follow-up is needed. If the cyst is still present at the follow-up visit, I usually order a pelvic sonogram. This test can help to determine the type of cyst present and help plan further treatment.

What Can a Sonogram Show?

The most accurate way to get a picture of the ovary and cyst is with a vaginal sonogram. A small instrument passed comfortably into the vagina bounces harmless sound waves off your uterus, fallopian tubes, and ovaries, forming a picture on a monitor. A sonogram allows the doctor to accurately determine the size of the cyst and to "see" inside it to detect whether it is filled with fluid or solid areas. This can help determine the type of cyst. Depending on which cells in the ovary are overgrowing, certain types of ovarian cysts will make fairly reliable patterns on a sonogram (see fig. 5.2).

On the sonogram, functional cysts usually appear entirely clear in the middle and with smooth walls. The cyst of endometriosis looks like a circle with speckles (blood) floating within. A dermoid cyst (see page 162) may have very white areas, representing the sound waves bouncing off calcium in teeth or bone. A hemorrhagic cyst (see page 162) often has thick areas of blood clot within the cyst that dissolve in a few weeks. Abnormal cysts often have an overgrowth of cells that stick out from the inside of the cyst wall, making the inside of the cyst appear jagged on the sonogram. Many of these irregularly shaped cysts are benign, but cancer can also appear this way. Unfortunately, the sonogram cannot make a definite diagnosis of benign versus malignant cysts. So, if the sonogram shows solid areas within a cyst, surgery will be needed to remove it in order to rule out ovarian cancer.

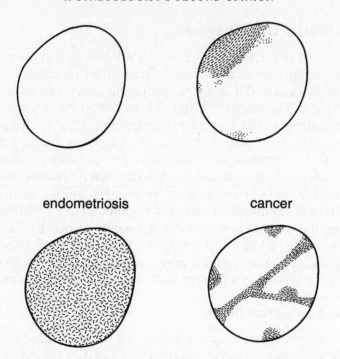

Fig. 5.2.   Sonogram appearance of ovarian cysts

If You Have a Cyst, Should You Have a CT Scan or MRI?

Some doctors may recommend a CT (computer tomography) scan or MRI (magnetic resonance imaging) to get "a better look" at an ovarian cyst. However, neither the CT scan, which is a high-tech X-ray, nor the MRI, which uses magnetic forces to form a picture, can give more helpful information than a sonogram. In addition, each of these tests is five or six times as expensive as a sonogram. The CT or MRI may be helpful in diagnosing a dermoid or hemorrhagic cyst if the sonogram result is uncertain. But no test can flawlessly predict benign or cancerous cysts, and surgery will be required to remove any questionable cyst so that a definite diagnosis can be made.

If You Have a Cyst, Should You Get a CA-125 Test?

The CA-125 blood test was developed in an attempt to detect ovarian cancer at a very early stage. Theoretically, cancer cells should produce chemicals that differ from those produced by normal cells. The hope was that these different chemicals could be detected in the blood, and cancer found before it spread. However, these hopes have not been fulfilled. Unfortunately, the CA-125 test received a lot of inaccurate publicity following the sad death from ovarian cancer of comedienne Gilda Radner. Many press reports suggested that *all* women have the CA-125 blood test as a preliminary test for ovarian cancer to make an early diagnosis. But the CA-125 is a terrible test for determining who has ovarian cancer among premenopausal women.

In addition, studies show that in women under the age of fifty who had an ovarian cyst and an abnormal CA-125 result, no cancer was present 65 percent of the time, meaning the test was inaccurate. Conditions commonly found in younger women, such as endometriosis, fibroids, pelvic infections, benign cysts, and pregnancy all can lead to falsely abnormal results. Perfectly healthy women can have an abnormal CA-125 value as a result of normal variations that occur with the menstrual cycle. Needless to say, getting such a test result would scare you and your doctor. Unfortunately, this fear often leads the patient into unnecessary surgery with all of its attendant risks, expense, and time needed for recovery. Therefore, I feel strongly that the CA-125 test should *not* be done in women younger than fifty years of age who have an ovarian cyst.

The CA-125 test is, however, somewhat more accurate in menopausal women who have an ovarian cyst. For those women, a normal test is reassuring, while an abnormal test still does not mean that ovarian cancer is present. However, the cyst must be removed to be sure there is no cancer. A great deal of research, time, and money are currently being devoted to finding a method of early detection for ovarian cancer, but unfortunately we do not have the answer yet (see chapter 10).

What Is an Epithelial Ovarian Cyst?

The ovary contains many types of cells that are able to form growths within the ovary. At the time of ovulation, the ovary bursts open to release the egg, leaving behind a hollow, raw area inside the ovary. Sometimes, the epithelial cells that make up the outside coating of the ovary get trapped inside the hollow area as it heals. The trapped cells may form fluid that collects within the ovary and produces an epithelial cyst. There are two types of epithelial cells and thus two types of epithelial cysts. One type, called serous cells, produces a clear, straw-colored fluid within the cyst. The other, called mucinous cells, produces a thick mucous fluid. Because the epithelial cells are trapped within the ovary, they must be removed to stop the production of the fluid and prevent further growth of the cyst. Unfortunately, there is no way to treat epithelial cysts other than to remove them surgically.

What Is a Hemorrhagic Cyst of the Ovary?

Sometimes, during the growth of a follicular or corpus luteum cyst, the tissue within the ovary tears as it is stretched and begins to bleed. Like the fluid from the cyst itself, this blood becomes trapped within the ovary. This is called a hemorrhagic cyst. Because the bleeding may occur quickly, it can rapidly stretch the covering of the ovary and result in pain. As the blood collects within the ovary, it begins to form clots, which can be seen on a sonogram. This type of cyst will almost always go away by itself, but it may take a few weeks to do so. Waiting is fine if you feel well, but in rare cases the cyst causes enough discomfort so that surgical removal of the cyst may be desirable.

Sandy's Painful Ovarian Cyst

Sandy is a thirty-seven-year-old woman who was awakened from sleep one night with a sharp pain on her left side. The pain persisted during the night, and she came to the office first thing in the morning. Upon examination, I could feel a swelling in her left ovary. This ovary was also fairly tender when I touched it. Because of her discomfort, we performed a sonogram immediately. The sonogram showed a fluid-filled cyst, but there were some other shadows on the picture that looked like clotted blood. It seemed pretty clear that Sandy had a hemorrhagic cyst, which usually would go away by itself. We discussed whether she would be comfortable enough to stay off her feet for a few days until this cyst settled down. The only other alternative was surgery, and Sandy was naturally not too happy about that. We agreed to do nothing for a while and see how she felt in a few days. She spent the next few days in bed and came back to the office feeling slightly better. We repeated the sonogram, which showed a slightly smaller cyst and some shrinking of the blood clots inside the cyst. Within a few more days, Sandy was feeling better and was able to go back to work. It took about one month for the cyst to go away entirely. The sonogram had helped Sandy avoid surgery.

What Is a Dermoid Cyst?

The idea of a dermoid cyst is somewhat startling. The ovary contains eggs that, when fertilized, have the ability to form a human being. However, for reasons we don't understand, the cells of the ovary can, all by themselves and without the presence of any sperm, start to produce hair, teeth, fluid, and other growing tissues to form a cyst. When removed during surgery, these tissues can be clearly seen within the cyst, which is called a dermoid cyst. Dermoid cysts are fairly common, occurring most often before menopause, and are almost never cancerous (less than 1 in 1,000).

Because of all the unusual types of cells within these cysts, a fairly characteristic appearance on a sonogram can be seen, and often the diagnosis can be made just from this test. Unfortunately, these cysts do not go away by themselves. If dermoid cysts are not removed, they can continue to grow and may crowd out the normal cells to the point where no healthy ovary remains. In rare cases, the cyst can cause the ovary to twist around and stop blood flowing to the ovary, causing severe pain and the need for emergency surgery. Therefore, these cysts should be surgically removed.

Can Endometriosis Cause an Ovarian Cyst?

At the time of the monthly menstrual flow, the lining cells of the uterus are normally shed through the cervix into the vagina. In some women these cells go out the wrong way, through the fallopian tubes, and end up in the abdominal cavity. If these cells survive, they may attach to the outside of the uterus, fallopian tubes, or ovaries, and begin to grow. This is called endometriosis (see chapter 7). During subsequent menstrual cycles, these cells are stimulated to grow and bleed just as the lining cells within the uterus continue to do.

If endometrial cells get trapped within the ovary, the blood has nowhere to go, so it collects within the ovary, forming a cyst called an endometrioma. As the blood ages within the cyst, it becomes dark brown and thick, with a strong resemblance to chocolate syrup. For this reason, endometriosis of the ovary has been referred to as a chocolate cyst. The pattern of this old blood looks distinctive on a sonogram, so the diagnosis can often be made by that test. Sometimes endometriosis within the ovary causes pain, but it may also be painless and only discovered at the time of a routine examination. If endometriosis forms in one ovary, it may also be present near the uterus, fallopian tubes, and other ovary. While this condition is not dangerous, endometriosis can lead to pelvic pain and/or infertility and should be appropriately treated. The treatment for endometriosis of the ovary involves removal of the cyst, often by laparoscopic surgery (see chapter 7).

Do Benign Ovarian Cysts Become Cancerous?

We really don't understand ovarian cancer very well, and we certainly do not know what causes it. Research shows that benign cysts do not turn into cancerous cysts, so if you have an ovarian cyst that seems to be benign upon exam and on a sonogram, waiting for it to go away for two months or so is not risky. Research also shows that women who form benign ovarian cysts are not any more likely to develop ovarian cancer than women who have not had cysts.

What Types of Cysts Are Cancerous?

Ovarian cancer is a rare disease. Only 1 out of every 15,000 women will have the disease at the age of thirty. At forty, only 1 of every 10,000 women have this disease, and at sixty, only 1 of every 1,500 women will have it. Therefore, if a premenopausal woman is found to have a cyst in her ovary, the odds are overwhelming that it is benign. Even in postmenopausal woman, an ovarian cyst has more than a 70 percent chance of being benign. Therefore, if a cyst is found on your ovary, it is most likely a *benign* ovarian cyst. However, cancer can develop in the ovary, and its diagnosis and treatment are discussed fully in chapter 10.

TREATMENT FOR OVARIAN CYSTS ▬▬▬▬▬▬

The appropriate treatment for an ovarian cyst depends on the type of cyst, the symptoms you have, and whether you are pre- or postmenopausal. As noted before, if you are premenopausal, if you are not having bothersome symptoms, and if your cyst appears benign on a sonogram, watchful waiting will often allow the cyst to dissolve by itself within four to ten weeks. However, if your symptoms are very bothersome or the cyst appears suspicious for malignancy, then it should be removed.

As discussed earlier, during the normal menstrual cycle small collections of fluid routinely surround developing eggs, and these functional cysts are common. After menopause, no eggs develop, and, therefore, no functional cysts should form. When a cyst forms after menopause, it usually needs to be removed to determine what type of cyst it is and to make sure cancer is not present.

Should You Take Birth Control Pills to Help Make Your Ovarian Cyst Go Away?

The short answer is no. In 1973, a study was published that included 286 premenopausal women with ovarian cysts who were placed on the pill for six weeks and then reexamined. The pill was used because the doctor who performed the study felt it would help to stop ovulation and quiet the ovary down. After treatment with the pill, 90 percent of the cysts disappeared, and the doctor concluded that the pill was the reason why. Unfortunately, the study did not have a control group, a group of women who had cysts but were not treated with the pill. Twenty years later, in 1993, a study was done that included a group of women not treated with anything. Interestingly, just as many women had their cysts disappear without taking the pill. Clearly, if the cyst is going to disappear, it will do so by itself. Consequently, we no longer use the pill to treat a premenopausal woman who is found to have an ovarian cyst. However, the pill can be used to prevent new ovarian cysts from forming (see page 154).

When Is Surgery Needed for an Ovarian Cyst?

Surgery may be considered necessary if a cyst appears suspicious for cancer on the sonogram, if it causes severe pain, if it continues to grow, or if it does not go away in eight weeks. A number of studies show that cysts that persist longer than eight weeks without decreasing in size have a greater likelihood of being abnormal. This does not mean cancer, but rather an abnormal growth of cells within the ovary that will never go away. If left in place, these cysts may continue to grow and cause discomfort or twist the ovary around and destroy it. Also, in very rare instances (less than 5 percent), these cysts may be cancerous, and early detection and removal are important.

Can Laparoscopic Surgery Be Used to Treat an Ovarian Cyst?

Instruments are now available that enable the gynecologist to remove a cyst, while preserving the normal, healthy ovary, through small incisions in the abdomen. This type of procedure, known as laparoscopic surgery, provides the benefits of outpatient surgery and a quick recovery. Using a telescope placed through the navel and small instruments placed near

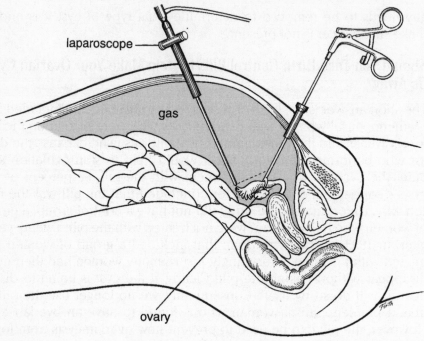

laparoscope

gas

ovary

Fig. 5.3. Laparoscopy

the pubic bone, the gynecologic surgeon can remove either the cyst alone or the entire ovary (see fig. 5.3).

An ovarian cyst, which looks like a small balloon filled with water, grows from within the ovary and stretches the normal ovarian tissue over it (see fig. 5.1). Removal of the cyst, called a cystectomy, is like taking a clam out of the shell. The thinned-out ovarian tissue is cut open, and the cyst is gently peeled away from inside the ovary (see fig. 5.4). The cyst fluid is then removed with a suction device. The cyst now looks like a deflated balloon and can easily be removed through the small laparoscopy incision. Sometimes the normal part of the ovary that remains needs to be sutured closed, and there are special instruments the surgeon can use to do this. Because recent studies show that the ovary may heal better if it is left alone, we usually allow the ovary to heal by itself.

Rarely, if a cyst has destroyed all the normal ovarian tissue, it may be necessary to remove the entire ovary. A number of ways have been developed to allow the removal of the entire ovary with the laparoscope. Using either special sutures or electrosurgical instruments, the surgeon can block the blood vessels going to the ovary, and then cut away and remove the ovary. In most situations, laparoscopic surgery

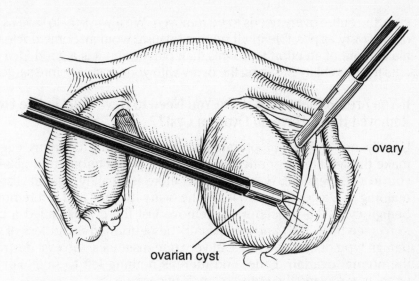

ovary

ovarian cyst

Fig. 5.4.   Laparoscopic removal of ovarian cyst

takes no longer than standard surgery. The benefit of laparoscopic surgery is that you may leave the hospital the same day and return to normal activity within a week or two.

When Is Major Surgery Needed for an Ovarian Cyst?

The goal of all surgery is to take care of the patient in the safest and most expeditious way possible. Based on the examination and sonogram, if the likelihood of a cyst being benign is very high, then laparoscopic surgery has the advantage of a quick and easy recovery. If a cyst is cancerous, then more extensive surgery is needed through an abdominal incision, and laparoscopy is not appropriate. If cancer is suspected, there is no reason to subject a woman to the added time, risk, and expense of a laparoscopy only to find that it is necessary for the doctor to switch, while the patient is anesthetized, to the standard abdominal surgery. Therefore, if there is a possibility that a cyst is cancerous based on the examination and sonogram, abdominal surgery should be performed.

Do Large Ovarian Cysts Need to Be Removed?

Most ovarian cysts don't get any larger than two to three inches in diameter. Infrequently, they can get to be five or six inches or larger. When a cyst gets this large, it almost never goes away by itself, and surgery is needed because it may crowd out and destroy most of the normal ovary. In that case, the entire ovary needs to be removed. We always try to save as much of the ovary as possible in all premenopausal women. Some doctors may make more of an effort to do this than others, and it is a good idea to discuss the possibility of saving the ovary with your doctor before surgery.

If You Are Premenopausal, Do You Need to Have Your Entire Ovary Removed If You Have an Ovarian Cyst?

Usually no. If you are premenopausal, the ovary contains eggs that make the female hormones estrogen and progesterone and also allow you to get pregnant. So, as long as there is healthy ovarian tissue remaining, it is a good idea to leave the ovary in place and just remove the benign cyst. The procedure to remove just the cyst is called a cystectomy (see page 166) and can usually be performed regardless of which benign type of cyst you have. In very rare instances, the cyst destroys all the normal ovarian tissue, and there is nothing left to save. For those women, removing the entire ovary is necessary.

Laurie's Large Ovarian Cyst

Laurie is a twenty-one-year-old college student who was seen by the student health service doctor for lower abdominal aching. The doctor performed a pelvic examination and noted that something felt abnormal near the left ovary. The doctor sent Laurie to have a pelvic ultrasound, which showed a four-inch cyst on the left ovary.

From the look of the cyst on the ultrasound, the radiologist thought this might be a dermoid cyst, which is benign. Nevertheless, because dermoids cannot dissolve on their own, it would need to be removed to prevent further growth and damage to the ovary. Dermoid cysts often have fat within them, and the radiologist suggested a CAT scan, an accurate way to tell if fat was present in this cyst. The CAT scan indeed showed the presence of fat, confirming the diagnosis of a dermoid cyst.

Laurie's student health service doctor recommended she see a gynecologist to have the cyst removed. After an examination, the gynecologist suggested that Laurie have an abdominal incision to remove the cyst. Unfortunately, the recovery for that operation would take six weeks, and she might end up missing a good portion of the semester, forcing her to drop some classes. "This was terrible news to me," Laurie said. "I was trying to graduate on time, but needing a six-week recovery time would make graduating impossible." Laurie was upset about this, but the surgery was clearly necessary. During the next week, Laurie's mother mentioned the upcoming surgery to a friend who was a doctor. The friend asked why the surgery wasn't being performed laparoscopically and suggested they get a second opinion.

Laurie and her mother came into the office two days later. I examined her and reviewed the ultrasound pictures. While the cyst was large, I saw no reason why laparoscopic surgery could not be safely performed. When I mentioned this, Laurie looked very relieved. "Maybe I won't have to miss school after all!" she said with a glowing smile. We planned Laurie's surgery during her spring break. Surgery went extremely well, and we were able to remove the cyst and preserve the entire ovary, which was healthy. The amount of bleeding during surgery was very small, and the procedure was over in about an hour. Laurie went home that afternoon, slept through the night, and was up walking the next morning. Her recovery was quick, and she returned to school one week later, just as classes were starting back up after spring break.

Can an Ovarian Cyst Form After Menopause?

The ovary no longer produces eggs after menopause, and, therefore, it is not possible for a follicular or corpus luteum cyst to form. But other types of benign ovarian cysts do still occur after menopause. In fact, the most likely types of ovarian cysts after menopause are still benign cysts. However, because the incidence of ovarian cancer increases with age, any cyst or growth in the ovary after menopause should be evaluated with a sonogram. Once again, the sonogram can be helpful in predicting whether the cyst is benign, or if it is suspicious for cancer. In addition, if you have a cyst *after* menopause, the blood test CA-125 should be done. As previously noted, the test is inaccurate in premenopausal women, but it is more accurate in postmenopausal women. After menopause, women do not usually have endometriosis, fibroids, or other conditions associated with menstruation that yield a false positive result. If the sonogram shows a benign pattern and the CA-125 test is normal, then the ovarian cyst is probably benign.

A very interesting recent study found benign ovarian cysts to be much more common in postmenopausal women than anyone had realized. Ultrasounds were performed on 7,700 healthy postmenopausal women as part of a study designed to find early ovarian cancers. Small ovarian cysts, two inches or less, were unexpectedly found in 450 of these women.

Because the cysts were benign-appearing on ultrasound, and CA-125 tests were normal, the women had the ultrasound repeated in two months. Surprisingly, half of the cysts had already disappeared by that time.

The other women were given a choice of having surgery to remove the ovary or having another ultrasound performed a few months later. Half of the women chose surgery, and *none* of them had cancer found at the time of surgery. Also, *none* of the women who had repeated ultrasounds and were followed over the next few years were found to have ovarian cancer. It should be understood that benign cysts do not turn into cancer, so you do not need to worry about cancer developing in a benign cyst. This study shows that benign ovarian cysts in postmenopausal women are common. Women and doctors still have varying degrees of comfort about not removing an ovarian cyst. But based on this study and others, a discussion about options should take place. Some women may choose surgery, and others may choose careful follow-up. At this point, both options are reasonable.

If the sonogram looks suspicious or if the CA-125 test is abnormal, then the cyst may still be benign. In some cases, depending on the test results, your circumstances, and the comfort of your doctor, laparoscopic surgery may be performed to examine the ovary. We detach the ovary and place it in a sterile bag inside the abdomen. The bag containing the ovary is brought out of the incision and handed to the pathologist for immediate analysis. If this test, called a frozen section, is benign, no further surgery is needed. If the frozen section shows cancer, an abdominal incision should be made and more extensive surgery should be performed. A larger incision allows the doctor to remove all the cancer, especially if it is present in other organs.

Molly's Ovarian Cyst

Molly is a seventy-five-year-old woman who went to see her internist because of a vague sense of discomfort and pain on the left side of her abdomen. She had no other symptoms, no nausea or vomiting, no fever, no problems urinating or moving her bowels. In fact, at first she chose to ignore the discomfort, but after a while decided to see her family doctor. At the time of her pelvic examination, the doctor felt a swelling near her left ovary and ordered a sonogram, which showed a large ovarian cyst about five inches across. Mollie was pretty nervous by the time she got to my office the next day. When I examined her, I could feel the cyst as a soft, smooth swelling where her left ovary was. It wasn't at all uncomfortable for Molly to have the cyst touched. Because of Molly's age, it was clear that surgery would be necessary to remove the cyst to make sure it wasn't malignant. This was recommended even though this cyst didn't feel the way cancer often feels. Cancer usually grows irregularly, not in the smooth way that this cyst felt. Cancer also often feels hard, and this cyst felt soft. Lastly, cancer sometimes gives off a clear fluid into the patient's abdominal cavity, which causes swelling and bloating. Molly had none of this, and I thought she probably had a benign cyst. I looked at her sonogram, and it did not show any of the features of a cancer. Two days later the CA-125 test came back totally normal. All of the signs now pointed to a benign cyst, but this was a very large cyst and, unfortunately, none of these tests is 100 percent accurate. Surgery would still be needed to remove the cyst and make a diagnosis.

Since we felt the cyst was probably benign, I talked to Molly about the possibility of removing her ovary with laparoscopic surgery rather than through a larger abdominal incision. She was thrilled about the low risk of cancer and eager to try laparoscopic surgery so that she could get out of the hospital quickly and back to her normal routine. At the time of her surgery, we removed her left ovary and sent it immediately to the pathologist, who viewed it under the microscope. Within ten minutes, the pathologist confirmed that the cyst was benign. We removed her right ovary as well, to prevent the future occurrence of either benign or cancerous ovarian cysts. The surgery had taken less than an hour, and that afternoon a relieved and elated Mollie went home.

If You Are Postmenopausal, Should Your Entire Ovary Be Removed If You Have a Cyst?

If you have gone through menopause, two things need to be considered when making a decision about removal of the entire ovary if you have a cyst. First, as you get older, the risk of ovarian cancer, while still not great, increases. If the entire ovary is removed, the pathologist can examine it completely to make sure no cancer is present. And if the ovary is removed, then the possibility of it developing cancer in the future is eliminated. For the same reason, you might also consider having the other (normal) ovary removed during the same surgery. This takes very little additional time and prevents growths, both benign and malignant, from forming in the future.

The other issue relates to hormone therapy. After menopause the main function of the ovary, the production of estrogen, ceases. If you already take hormone replacement therapy, then the removal of your ovaries will not change the way you will feel because your body is already getting estrogen from the medication. If you do not take hormones, no change will be noted either, since your ovaries are not producing estrogen anyway. However, after menopause the ovary does continue to produce some testosterone, a male hormone that increases libido. Some women who have had their ovaries removed notice a decrease in sexual feelings after surgery. If this happens, testosterone pills can be given along with estrogen to enhance sexual feelings. Women always cringe when I mention this, imagining that their voice will deepen, and they will soon grow a beard. However, the amount of testosterone needed to enhance sexual feelings is *very small*, and side effects are extremely rare. In addition, some women note that testosterone has a positive effect on their mood—they feel better and more energetic than if they just take the estrogen alone.

Is a Hysterectomy Needed If You Have an Ovarian Cyst?

In the past, if a woman had completed her family and had a benign cyst that needed to be removed surgically, a hysterectomy was routinely performed at the same time. Doctors felt that performing a hysterectomy made sense because the woman's abdomen was already cut open, and the healing would be the same no matter what additional surgery was performed. Also, if the uterus were removed, then it could not go on to develop a cancer at a later time. This practice has recently been questioned by a scientific study that showed the risks of surgery were greater if, in addition to removing the ovary, a hysterectomy were also performed to remove a normal uterus. This makes sense—more surgery leads to more risk of blood loss, more risk of injury to other organs, and more time under anesthesia. Also, the risk of developing uterine cancer is fairly low. About 3 percent of American women will get this disease in their lifetimes, and it is often diagnosed at an early stage. Hopefully, the idea of limiting surgery to just the problem area will be adopted by more gynecologists. If you have an ovarian cyst and your doctor is recommending hysterectomy, ask why he or she thinks that it is necessary. If you are not satisfied with the answer, you should consider getting a second opinion. The issues concerning hysterectomy are discussed fully in chapter 12.

REFERENCES

Bailey, C., F. Ueland, G. Land, P. DePriest, H. Gallion, R. Kryscio, and J. van Nagel. 1998. The malignant potential of small cystic ovarian tumors in women over 50 years of age. *Gynecologic Oncology* 69:3–7.

Canis, M., G. Mage, J. Pouly, A. Wattiez, H. Manhes, and M. Bruhat. 1994. Laparoscopic diagnosis of adnexal cystic masses: A twelve-year experience with long-term follow-up. *Obstetrics and Gynecology* 83:707–12.

Finkler, N., B. Benacerrat, F. Lavin, C. Wojciechowski, and R. Knapp. 1988. Comparison of serum CA-125, clinical impression, and ultrasound in the preoperative evaluation of ovarian masses. *Obstetrics and Gynecology* 72:659.

Gambone, J., R. Reiter, and J. Lench. 1992. Short-term outcome of incidental hysterectomy at the time of adnexectomy for benign disease. *Journal of Women's Health* 1:197–200.

Jacobs, I., and R. Bast. 1989. The CA-125 tumour associated antigen: A review of the literature. *Human Reproduction* 4:1.

Maiman, M., V. Seltzer, and J. Boyce. 1991. Laparoscopic excision of ovarian neoplasms subsequently found to be malignant. *Obstetrics and Gynecology* 77:563.

Parker, W. 1995. The case for laparoscopic management of the adnexal mass. *Clinical Obstetrics and Gynecology* 38:362–69.

Parker, W., and J. Berek. 1990. Management of selected cystic adnexal masses in postmenopausal women by operative laparoscopy: A pilot study. *American Journal of Obstetrics and Gynecology* 163:1574.

Parker, W., and J. Berek. 1993. Management of the adnexal mass by operative laparoscopy. *Clinical Obstetrics and Gynecology* 36:413–22.

Parker, W., R. Levine, F. Howard, B. Sansone, and J. Berek. 1994. Laparoscopic management of selected cystic adnexal masses in postmenopausal women: A multicentered study. *Journal of the American College of Surgeons* 179:733–37.

6

IF YOU HAVE PELVIC PAIN

What Is Pain?

We all know what pain means. You are hurt or injured, and you feel pain. Yet what seems so simple, something that hurts, is actually quite complex. Pelvic pain, in particular, often bewilders both those who suffer from it and those who attempt to treat it.

It may be helpful to know the general medical thinking on pain to get the full picture. The classic view of pain is defined as the sensation of discomfort that results when a part of your body has been damaged. We also expect that the amount of pain is related to the degree of damage. A major injury, it is thought, should result in severe pain, while minor injuries should be less painful. And yet, this "classic view" may not always be accurate.

The sensation of acute pain begins with the stimulation of a nerve, either from extreme heat or cold, severe pressure, or the inflammation of tissue. These nerves then send pain signals to the brain, and both the number and types of nerves that carry these signals influence what message the brain receives. However, to "feel" pain, your brain must also interpret the signals it receives. Brain chemicals, called neurotransmitters, influence the way your brain interprets the signals. Two main neurotransmitters, endorphins and serotonin, are involved in the perception of pain. Some people are said to have a high or low threshold of pain, and some studies have found that people who feel more pain actually have less endorphins.

These same neurotransmitters are also involved with the regulation of mood. Therefore, your perception of pain and your mood are inter-related. We all know that there are times in which we are able to ignore or withstand more pain. For example, when you are fatigued, you are likely to feel pain more intensely. If you have spent time with a cranky, tired child, you know that the smallest injuries can cause huge howls simply because the child is tired. This process is at work in adults as well. As you can see, the perception of pain involves the interplay of different elements, which can sometimes become quite complicated.

Let me give you two examples of how complicated and intriguing pain can be. The first example is called referred pain. The best-known example is the pain associated with a heart attack. When the heart does not receive enough oxygen, the heart muscle deteriorates and releases biochemicals into the surrounding area that cause pain—the body's warning signal that something is wrong. However, the individual often feels pain in the left arm or abdominal discomfort similar to indigestion. Clearly, nothing is wrong with the left arm or stomach—why do they feel pain there? It turns out that the nerve from the heart and the nerve from the left arm and stomach run into the spinal cord next to each other, and the brain may not be able to tell exactly where the pain is originating. This type of referred pain is very common in the pelvis because the nerves from the bladder, uterus, fallopian tubes, ovaries, intestines, and internal muscles are all wired close together as they enter the spinal cord on their way to the brain (see fig. 6.1). You may think there is something wrong with your uterus, but the pain may actually be coming from an entirely different area.

Another interesting example of referred pain was illustrated in an experiment performed on women having mini-laparoscopy performed while they were only lightly sedated. The doctor used an instrument to touch either the left or right ovary and asked the patient to identify what had been touched. You would think that the brain should be able to tell left from right. However, 30 percent of women identified the wrong area; either the other ovary or the middle of the abdomen.

Another interesting phenomenon is called phantom pain. It is not uncommon for people who have had limbs amputated to have pain in the absent limbs. The brain may be remembering pain present before the amputation, and this memory has become ingrained. Tissue injury in the pelvis—for example, prior infection, which may be long since healed—may still cause chronic, bothersome pain.

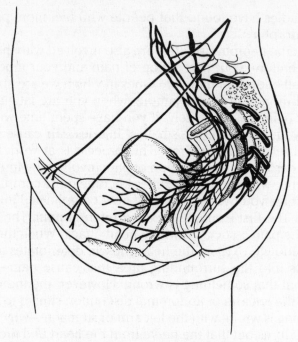

Fig. 6.1.   Pelvic nerves

For all these reasons, as well as the large number of organs present in the pelvis bunched closely together, identifying the exact cause of pain in the pelvis can be a very difficult task.

There are two basic types of pain: acute and chronic. This chapter will discuss acute and chronic pelvic pain, both as the result of gyneco-logic and nongynecologic causes. Medical science is starting to pay much more attention to the causes of pain, the way people perceive pain, and treatment for people who have pain.

What Is Acute Pain?

You feel acute pain after your body has been injured, and an immediate release of chemicals in the skin or deeper muscles excites the nerves in that area. The nerves carry the pain signals directly to the brain. With acute pain, the amount and duration of the pain usually will be related to the severity of damage that has occurred. The greater the injury, the more chemicals released in the skin and muscle, and the more pain you feel. As long as the chemicals are stimulating the nerves, you feel pain. As you start to heal, the amount of these chemicals is reduced, and the sensation of pain decreases. As noted above, your psychological state and mood can alter your perception of pain because your brain is responsible for interpreting these signals. When you are tired or upset, you generally feel acute pain more intensely.

What Can Cause Acute Pelvic Pain?

The relatively sudden onset of pain in the pelvis, the lower part of your abdomen, is called acute pelvic pain. The most common gynecologic causes of acute pelvic pain are twisting or rupture of ovarian cysts; infection of the uterus, fallopian tubes, and ovaries; degeneration of fibroids; and tubal pregnancy. Women often describe acute pain as sharp or stabbing, and it may be so intense that normal activity is impossible. Often, causes of acute pain are associated with other symptoms such as nausea, vomiting, fever, or diarrhea. Many of the causes of acute pelvic pain are fully described elsewhere in this book. Acute pain resulting from ovarian cysts is discussed in chapter 5, pain from ectopic pregnancy is discussed in chapter 3, and pain from fibroids is discussed here and in chapter 4.

Can Fibroids Cause Pelvic Pain?

Most fibroids, in and of themselves, do not cause pain. However, if fibroids grow to be large, they may press on nearby organs, such as the intestines and the bladder, which can result in discomfort. But it would be unusual for this to be severe enough to cause pain. Very rarely, fibroids undergo a process of degeneration, or cell decomposition, which causes the release of chemical substances that produce pain. This type of pain often starts suddenly and may be severe, but usually goes away by itself over a few days or so. Fibroids that form on a stalk (pedunculated fibroids) can twist around on the stalk and cause sudden and severe pain. These very rare cases need to be treated by surgical removal of the fibroid. These problems can cause acute but not chronic pain. Fibroids, including their symptoms and treatments, are fully discussed in chapter 4.

What Can Cause Pain with Intercourse?

There are a number of causes of pain with or following intercourse. A vaginal infection that irritates the lining of the vagina can cause pain, often right at the beginning of intercourse. Signs of infection, such as discharge or odor, are usually present. Infections may be either yeast or bacterial, and the diagnosis can be made by examining the discharge under a microscope to see which organisms are present. Infections are usually easily treated with specific antibiotic or antifungal creams or oral medication.

The tissue of the vagina needs estrogen to stay healthy and elastic. Many months, or even years, after menopause, vaginal lubrication decreases, and this tissue becomes thinner and less elastic. As a result, the vagina is unable to stretch during intercourse, and pain results. If taken when menopause begins, estrogen, either vaginal cream or pill form, is very effective in preventing these changes. If you have already gone through menopause and the tissue is already thin, reversing the process with estrogen can be successfully accomplished, but may take six to twelve months. Alternative remedies such as calendula cream, vitamin E oil, or progesterone cream can also be helpful for women who cannot or do not want to take estrogen. Frequent intercourse or manual stretching of the vaginal tissue also helps to maintain its elasticity.

Vaginal dryness can also lead to pain with intercourse. Normally, if a woman is sexually aroused, a lubricating fluid is produced that coats the vaginal walls and protects the tissue from irritation. Sometimes infection or other irritation can cause the vagina to make less fluid, and discomfort during intercourse results. The hormonal changes that result from breast-feeding, taking birth control pills, or menopause may have the same effect. As a consequence of this discomfort, some women may anticipate pain with intercourse. This feeling of anxious, fearful anticipation of pain is thought to bring on a further reduction in the amount of lubrication and adds to the discomfort.

Liberal use of a nonpetroleum lubricant for every sexual encounter over the course of a few weeks often provides comfort and allows a woman to relax and experience sexual intercourse as pleasurable again. After a while, the lubricant can be discontinued, or used when you think it will help you enjoy your sex life more fully.

Another cause of painful intercourse is an involuntary spasm of the vaginal muscles, called vaginismus. For some women, this may occur to such a degree that intercourse is not possible. Vaginal infection, irritation, or dryness that causes pain with intercourse may lead to vaginal muscle spasms in response to the pain. Another source of vaginal muscle spasms may be prior sexual or physical abuse. Fear of intercourse, regardless of the reason, may also lead to the same problem. For women who have this condition, exercises that contract and relax the vaginal muscles, called Kegel's exercises, can teach improved muscular control and may result in comfort during intercourse. Emotional questions and issues that result from abuse are best resolved under the care of a thera-pist trained to deal with sexual problems.

Scar tissue near the uterus, fallopian tubes, or ovaries from pre-vious infection, surgery, or endometriosis may also cause pain during intercourse. Pain from these causes is usually felt deep in the pelvis rather than in the vagina. Scar tissue is discussed on page 182 and en-dometriosis on page 184.

CHRONIC PELVIC PAIN

What Is Chronic Pain?

Acute pain and chronic pain are very different. Chronic pain, unlike acute pain, persists after your body has had a reasonable time to heal from injury. It appears that chronic pain results from changes in your nervous system that cause the brain to feel pain, even when the original injury is over. Common examples of chronic pain include low back pain, frequent headaches, and chronic pelvic pain. Chronic pain can cause a change in your ability to do physical activity and/or cause a change in your mood. It also can lead to fatigue, sluggishness, insom-nia, and depression. Anyone who is forced to endure long-term pain will be worn down by it and will likely find that their life has been changed by the pain. Fortunately, increased understanding of chronic pain in general has given us a better grasp of chronic pelvic pain.

By the time pain becomes chronic, there are usually both physical and psychological factors contributing to the pain. Let me make it clear that this does *not* mean that people with chronic pain are "crazy," or that the pain is "all in their minds." The pain is real and is conveyed by chemicals made by the brain, called neurotransmitters, which regulate both pain perception and mood.

But having said that pain is not all in the mind, it must also be stated that the way you feel pain depends on psychological factors. For example, if you are afraid that pain is the result of a serious problem or is likely to be long-lasting, that fear about your condition may heighten the way your brain perceives the pain. Therefore, in addition to medical therapy, the best approach to chronic pain may be a multidisciplinary approach that often includes medical and psychological methods, as well as modification of diet and physical activity.

What Is Chronic Pelvic Pain?

Pelvic pain that lasts six or more months, and is not associated with the menstrual period, is called chronic pelvic pain. (Menstrual pain is discussed in chapter 3.) Chronic pelvic pain is a fairly common problem. It is estimated that about 20 percent of the visits to gynecologists are for pelvic pain, and one out of every seven hysterectomies are performed for this reason. A recent telephone survey of over 5,000 women found that 15 percent reported chronic pelvic pain and over 60 percent of the women with pain did not have a diagnosis or know the cause of the pain. Chronic pelvic pain can lead to significant distress, depression, and even disability. In recent years, a great deal of effort and research has been focused on helping women with chronic pelvic pain and people suffering from all types of chronic pain. Because of this, we are often able to help people diminish the effects of pain.

What Can Cause Chronic Pelvic Pain?

Interestingly, when you were developing as a fetus, the same type of cells that went on to form the uterus, fallopian tubes, and ovaries also developed into the bladder. Furthermore, the bladder, the intestines, and the pelvic organs share similar nerves, and your brain may not be able to differentiate pain in one area from that of another area. Lastly, the bladder, the intestines, and the pelvic organs are close together in the abdominal area (see fig. 1.1), and it may be difficult for you to tell exactly where a pain originates. Therefore, gynecologic problems, as well as bladder problems, intestinal problems, and neuromuscular problems can all be felt as "pelvic" pain. In this chapter we will discuss all these causes in detail.

What Can Be Done to Evaluate the Cause of Chronic Pelvic Pain?

Finding the cause of pelvic pain sometimes can be thought of as a puzzle that requires careful and methodical examination until the correct solution comes to light. There are many different causes of pelvic pain, and many of them are nongynecologic.

The best way to start to solve the puzzle and get to the source of your pain is to provide your doctor with a detailed description of the pain. Keeping a daily pain diary that you fill out in the morning, afternoon, and evening can help you track the pain: Where is it? When does it occur? What makes it better or worse? Does eating affect it? Do you have nausea, vomiting, bloating, or diarrhea along with the pain? Do you have any bladder symptoms? The location of the pain, its severity, and any relationship to physical activity or eating will help determine what organs could possibly be involved. The presence of other symptoms may also help focus on particular areas of the body that may need further testing.

A thorough physical examination is the next order of business and should include evaluation of the bladder, intestines, abdominal wall muscles, and the pelvic organs. Often, a "multidisciplinary approach" will be the most helpful way to approach the pain. This method uses a team of medical professionals, combining their experience and problem-solving skills to solve the puzzle, find the source of the pain, and treat it. The team often consists of a gynecologist, a specialized pain-management physician or physical therapist, and a mental health counselor. While "pain clinics" have been developed for this purpose, your primary care physician or gynecologist can assemble this team of professionals to care for you. The gynecologist is responsible for evaluating possible gynecologic causes of pain, and the pain-management physician should be skilled in the diagnosis and treatment of other causes of pain. In addition, consultants such as a urologist (urinary system), gastroenterologist (stomach and intestine), physical therapist or orthopedist (muscles, joints, and bones) may be needed. A mental health specialist is trained to evaluate stress, family, or marital problems, or feelings of helplessness or depression, which all can affect pain. Both the physical therapist and the mental health counselor can also help design an effective plan for stress reduction and pain relief. This may sound like a lot of work, but a pain-free life is a goal worth working toward.

Can Pelvic Infection Cause Chronic Pain?

Infection of the uterus, fallopian tubes, or ovaries is usually associated with fever, nausea, and sometimes vomiting. While infection can certainly cause acute pelvic pain, it is almost never the cause of chronic pain.

However, many women who have chronic or recurrent pelvic pain are often assumed by their doctors to have chronic pelvic infections and are treated with repeated courses of antibiotics. Many of these women are later found to have endometriosis or other causes for their pain. Consequently, they were inappropriately treated, sometimes for years, while their real problem went undetected. Often, viewing the pelvis by means of laparoscopy can make the correct diagnosis for women who are suspected of having chronic pelvic infection. If infection is suspected, a culture of the fallopian tubes for bacteria and chlamydia can be performed at the time of laparoscopy.

Can Pelvic Scar Tissue (Adhesions) Cause Chronic Pelvic Pain?

An injury to the pelvic organs can result from infection, endometriosis, or wounds from surgery. Following an injury, the body forms scar tissue as part of the healing process. Unfortunately, this scar tissue, called *adhesions*, may form between areas of the body that are not normally connected. For example, the fallopian tube may stick to the ovary (see fig. 6.2), or the intestine may stick to the top of the uterus.

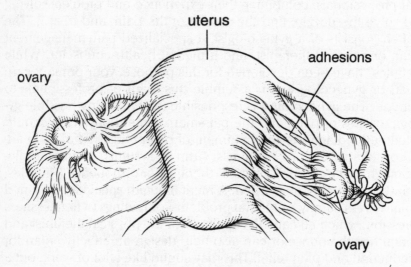

Fig. 6.2.   Severe pelvic adhesions

Although the uterus is anchored inside your body near the cervix, weak, thin ligaments form the only connection for the top of the uterus, fallopian tubes, and ovaries. These ligaments normally allow some movement of the pelvic organs during activity or intercourse. But scar tissue is not elastic like normal tissue; it doesn't stretch easily. If inflexible adhesions form around the pelvic organs, their normal motion may be impaired. Then, the pulling and tugging of scar tissue on normal tissue, which is filled with nerve endings, may lead to pain. Consequently, scar tissue may lead to pain during activity or intercourse.

Adhesions form within a few weeks following an infection or surgery, and once they form, they do not get any better or worse over time. It is common to have adhesions without having any pain, especially if the scar tissue forms in areas that do not normally move during activity. Some areas are just less sensitive. However, if the adhesions are the cause of chronic pelvic pain, removal of the adhesions can be performed surgically. Traditionally, this has been done by abdominal surgery, but now laparoscopic techniques (see page 185) are effective and have the benefit of a shorter recovery period. Nonsurgical techniques such as biofeedback and relaxation techniques should also be considered. These techniques are often helpful for the relief of pain from adhesions.

Dianne's Pelvic Pain

Dianne is a thirty-three-year-old woman who felt lower abdominal and pelvic pain for the past six or seven months. The pain was crampy and came and went from time to time. She seemed to have the most discomfort a few hours after eating, although she did not have any other symptoms of bowel problems such as nausea or diarrhea. She had seen her family physician, who treated her with a medication to help relax any spasm in the intestines, but this had not helped. Because the symptoms seemed to most likely be intestinal, her family physician referred her to a gastroenterologist.

The gastroenterologist agreed that the problem seemed to be intestinal and performed a series of X-ray tests of the small and large intestines. These tests were also normal. I was asked to see Dianne at this point to determine if any gynecologic problem could be found to explain her pain. The only significant part of her gynecologic history was a vague and mild pelvic infection that she had a year ago. The infection had been quickly diagnosed and treated with antibiotics, and she was able to return to work in about two days.

Dianne's pelvic examination was normal, but to be sure that I wasn't missing anything, I ordered a pelvic sonogram. The sonogram was also normal. The only thing left to offer Dianne to try to determine the cause of her pain was a diagnostic laparoscopy. Even though her pain was not severe, Dianne was frustrated and worried, so she decided to have the laparoscopy performed. During surgery, the cause of her pain became immediately apparent. Probably as a result of her prior pelvic infection, numerous thick bands of scar tissue had formed from her uterus and fallopian tubes to her intestines. The intestines were kinked in such a way that as digested food passed through them, the movement of the food caused the scar tissue to pull on the uterus, thus causing the pain. This explained why her pain seemed to be worse following meals. Using laparoscopic scissors, we were able to carefully cut away the scar tissue from the intestines and the uterus and fallopian tubes. The surgery was difficult and required patience. The end result looked good. She appeared to be free from all the scar tissue. In addition, the ends of Dianne's fallopian tubes appeared to be fairly healthy, and we were hopeful that she would be able to get pregnant in the future. Surgical removal of scar tissue relieves pain about two-thirds of the time. In this case, the surgery relieved Dianne's pain, and it has never returned.

Can Endometriosis Cause Pelvic Pain?

As described in chapter 7, endometriosis results from the growth of uterine lining cells outside the uterus. These cells remain under the influence of hormones made by the ovary and, to some degree, go through the changes of the menstrual cycle.

At the end of the menstrual cycle when bleeding occurs with your period, the misplaced cells cause a small amount of bleeding inside your body. The blood and other chemicals released from these cells, which do not belong in this area, irritate the pelvic organs. Over time, this irritation leads to injury of the cells covering the pelvic organs, and scar tissue can result, causing pain.

How Can the Pain from Endometriosis Be Treated?

One form of effective treatment for the relief of pain from endometriosis involves the surgical removal of the areas where the endometriosis has begun to grow. Once the source of the misplaced bleeding is removed, pain often improves. Removal of areas of endometriosis can now be accomplished by laparoscopic surgery using a laser, electrosurgical instruments, or laparoscopic scissors. All of these techniques are equally effective. Thorough removal of the diseased tissue seems to give the best results, but surgery for extensive endometriosis is difficult to perform. Therefore, it is probably best to choose a gynecologist who has experience treating women with this condition.

Should You Have a Laparoscopy Performed?

Laparoscopy is a surgical procedure that involves placement of a thin telescope through an incision in the navel to see inside the abdomen and pelvis. It is often utilized to help establish the cause of pelvic pain and, in many cases, can be used to treat the cause of the pain as well. The procedure is performed in a hospital or outpatient surgery center under general anesthesia. With the laparoscope, the doctor is able to see the uterus, fallopian tubes, ovaries, intestines, appendix, gallbladder, and liver. With a careful inspection, gynecologic problems such as endometriosis, pelvic infection, adhesions, ovarian cysts, and tubal pregnancy can be diagnosed. Inflammation or infection of the appendix, intestines, or gallbladder may also be detected, so that appropriate treatment may be started. In addition, by using specialized instruments during the laparoscopy, many of these problems may be treated at the same time. Adhesions and endometriosis may be cut away, and ovarian cysts or a tubal pregnancy removed.

Although new adhesions can sometimes form as part of the healing process after any surgery, many women found to have significant adhesions at the time of the laparoscopy will feel better after the adhesions are surgically removed. Also, laparoscopic surgery for moderate or severe endometriosis has been shown to provide pain relief about 70 percent of the time. However, the presence of thin adhesions or a small quantity of endometriosis does not often cause pelvic pain, and, therefore, surgery for these problems should be approached cautiously.

In as many as 30 percent of women who have laparoscopy for chronic pelvic pain, a normal uterus, fallopian tubes, and ovaries are found. A normal pelvis may suggest that other tests need to be performed to determine the source of the problem. But if the findings during the laparoscopy are normal, it is extremely unlikely that any serious problem exists with the pelvic organs, and this information can be very reassuring.

While not a major abdominal surgery, laparoscopic surgery does have risks and should be considered only when other nongynecologic causes of the pain have been excluded. Be sure that any surgery is warranted and will provide the relief you are seeking. However, the information acquired at the time of laparoscopy can be valuable. Nothing else—not ultrasound, nor CT scan, nor MRI, nor blood tests—can diagnose problems such as endometriosis or adhesions at an early stage. Therefore, the procedure can be helpful when used appropriately.

Is There a Relationship Between Sexual or Physical Abuse and Pelvic Pain?

Women who have been physically or sexually abused are more likely to suffer from chronic pelvic pain than women who have not been abused. It has been estimated that 30 percent of all women in the

United States have been sexually abused by the time they reach their midteens. At least one study shows a link between sexual abuse before the age of fifteen and a higher frequency of pelvic pain in those women later in life. The understanding of the relationship between sexual or physical abuse and physical symptoms or emotional problems that may be experienced at some point later in a woman's life is a relatively new concept. Abuse is probably evidence of only one of a family's many failures to provide the quality of emotional comfort and support needed for emotional development and growth. Women who have been abused are more likely to have frequent doctor visits, unexplained medical symptoms, and a higher incidence of surgery.

You should consider discussing any history of abuse with your physician or with a therapist. Appropriate counseling can provide the support and guidance that you need to help with your chronic pain, your emotional state, and your recovery. Counseling will allow you to actively participate in the management of your pain and have some control over it, rather than having the pain control you. This support is essential to emotional healing and helps to pave the way toward relief of your pain.

Sandra's Confusing Pelvic Pain

Sandra is a thirty-year-old woman who was first referred to me for evaluation of chronic pelvic pain that had been present for about a year. At first the pain had been infrequent, but now it was occurring almost daily. There was no apparent relationship between the pain and her physical activity, eating, or menstrual cycle. Pain medications had failed to help, and Sandra was understandably frustrated. She had alternated between trying to be philosophical and stoic about the pain, to being depressed and angry that her life had become so entrapped by discomfort. She was hoping that I would find something that her other doctors had missed.

Her pelvic examination and the rest of her physical examination were entirely normal, and a sonogram, performed just to make sure we were not missing anything, was also normal. Since she had a long history of pelvic pain that was increasing in intensity and frequency, Sandra and I discussed performing a laparoscopy to enable me to truly "see" if there was something wrong. She and I both agreed that laparoscopy was a reasonable thing to do at this point. Sandra was becoming increasingly worn down by her pain and frustrated that no cause had been found. Being only thirty years old, she had begun to wonder what the rest of her life was going to be like with this amount of daily discomfort. Her usual optimism was diminishing, and she had been unable to make any plans in terms of her career or her personal life. It was time to try something else.

During the laparoscopy, we looked at her uterus, fallopian tubes, and ovaries as well as her appendix, liver, gallbladder, and intestines. Everything appeared normal and healthy. When I discussed this with Sandra after surgery, she was both relieved and disappointed. It was good to know that all her organs were healthy, yet what could be causing this pain? I reassured Sandra that everything appeared to be perfectly normal and suggested that we allow some time to see if the pain would resolve by itself.

For the next year or so, Sandra's family doctor took care of her health. At times her pain was better and at times worse, but it never went away. Tests of her intestines were performed but were also normal. Then one day she developed the sudden on-set of sharp and severe pelvic pain. She came back to see me. On examination, she was extremely tender. Because of the severity of the pain, we felt that another laparoscopy was indicated to diagnose this problem. We performed the surgery that day and found a twisted and dying appendix, which we were able to re-move with laparoscopic instruments. This seemed to be the cause of this episode of pain but did not explain her more chronic pain. In fact, shortly after the surgery, her chronic pain reappeared. Now we were all depressed. My heart went out to her, but unfortu-nately my medical expertise and experience were not enough to provide her with the pain relief she so badly needed.

Sandra continued to see her family doctor for her regular medical care. But at her next gynecologic visit with me, she ap-peared to be more relaxed and told me that her pain was gone. She then went on to tell me that she had been having a problem in her relationship with her boyfriend and had begun therapy. Dur-ing the therapy, she discussed the fact that as a child she had been sexually abused on multiple occasions by a close relative. Work-ing through this problem with her therapist culminated in a con-frontation with the abusive relative. This had gone a long way toward helping her deal with the pain and fear she felt. Her pelvic pain also began to go away during this time. By the time I saw her, she felt entirely pain free. She and her therapist thought that the pain was a manifestation of the abuse that had occurred years before. I have seen Sandra every year since, about fifteen years in a row, and she has never had the pain again and is now happily married.

I learned a great deal from Sandra's experience. I had been unfamiliar with the association of abuse and pelvic pain before seeing Sandra's recovery. Now I am very aware of the issues of sexual and physical abuse and discuss the subject with women who have chronic pelvic pain. For most women, abuse has not been part of their lives, and the discussion ends there. If, however, someone has experienced abuse and is interested in getting help, I refer them to a therapist who is specially trained to deal with these issues. Many women benefit from this therapy.

OTHER COMMON CAUSES OF PELVIC PAIN

It is not uncommon for women suffering from pelvic pain to have more than one cause of the pain. Interstitial cystitis, irritable bowel syndrome, musculoskeletal spasms and pain are often present in women who have pelvic pain, painful periods, endometriosis, or pain with intercourse. Once again, the intertwined wiring of the nerves in the lower abdomen and pelvis may be responsible for the relationship of these syndromes. Therefore, diagnosis and appropriate treatment of all the components may be necessary for you to get better.

What Types of Bladder Problems Can Cause Pain?

Bladder infections can cause pain that is commonly felt just below the pubic bone. However, the pain usually develops quickly and is associated with other symptoms such as frequency of urination, the feeling of urgency to urinate, pain with urination or, rarely, blood in the urine. These symptoms differentiate a bladder infection from pain that originates in the pelvic organs or intestines. The diagnosis can be made by examining a urine sample under the microscope for the presence of bacteria and white blood cells.

Chronic mild infections of the urethra (the tube that you urinate out of) may also cause pelvic pain. These urethral infections are also often associated with urgency, frequency, and pain with urination. But sometimes irritation of the urethra occurs in the absence of infection. This discomfort, which may be an early form of interstitial cystitis (see below), may result from eating spicy foods or drinking caffeinated or alcoholic beverages that end up in the urine and cause irritation as they pass through the urethra. This diagnosis is often made when, despite treatment with antibiotics, the urethra remains tender, and the feeling of urgency persists. Your doctor will discuss dietary changes with you that restrict irritating foods, like spicy foods, alcohol, or caffeine. Often, these changes will relieve the symptoms without any medication. Some women find help with Kegel exercises (see page 244), which tighten and then release the vaginal muscles. This helps them to relax the muscles around the urethra, reducing spasm and pain.

What Is Interstitial Cystitis, and Can It Cause Pelvic Pain?

Interstitial cystitis is a condition that causes chronic inflammation of the bladder lining, without any evidence of infection. Women with interstitial cystitis have almost constant bladder or pelvic pain or pressure and feel the urge to urinate when there are even small quantities of urine in their bladders. This frequent urination often leads to sleepless nights.

The cause of this condition is unknown. Researchers suspect that the coating layer inside the bladder, which normally protects the bladder from irritation, may be absent or defective in women with this problem. A urologist can diagnose interstitial cystitis by looking inside the bladder with a small telescope, called a cystoscope. The procedure is performed while you are under anesthesia. After examination with the cystoscope, the bladder is filled to capacity with water. If interstitial cystitis is present, small areas of bleeding will appear in the bladder wall. A biopsy of the bladder wall examined under the microscope may confirm the diagnosis. Another test, called the potassium chloride test, may help make the diagnosis. While the patient is awake, a solution of potassium chloride is introduced into the bladder through a catheter. If the bladder lining is healthy, the patient will not feel anything. However, if interstitial cystitis is present, the potassium chloride will irritate the lining cells and cause discomfort.

What Is the Treatment for Interstitial Cystitis?

Treatment for interstitial cystitis is difficult because no available therapy can permanently restore the missing inner protective layer of the bladder. There are a number of treatments presently available to treat interstitial cystitis, each of them helpful to some women and not others.

Dietary changes, hydrodistention, medications, and pain management all have a place in the treatment of this condition.

A relatively new medication called Elmiron does seem to help restore the lining cells and is very effective for many women. Some medications can help with urinary frequency and urgency, while others can provide pain relief. Medications placed directly into the bladder with a small catheter can also be helpful.

Filling the bladder during the cystoscopy with large amounts of water while you are under anesthesia, called hydrodistention, often will relieve discomfort and urgency for months. This treatment can be repeated, if needed. Learning to relax the pelvic floor muscles by performing Kegel exercises may also help relieve symptoms for some women.

Further research into the causes and treatments for interstitial cystitis are under way, and we're optimistic that doctors and patients will soon have more treatment tools at their disposal.

What Types of Intestinal Problems Can Cause Pelvic Pain?

We all know that even simple constipation can cause a fullness or sense of pressure in the pelvis. Intestinal conditions such as irritable bowel syndrome and inflammation or infection of the intestines can also cause lower abdominal and pelvic pain. Oftentimes, we can clearly point to the intestines as the cause of pelvic pain because of the presence of intestinal symptoms such as nausea, vomiting, diarrhea, or constipation. Likewise, a decrease in appetite, a sensation of bloating, or a visible swelling of your abdomen is often the result of intestinal problems. Any blood or mucus in the stool are virtually always the result of intestinal rather than gynecologic disease. Specific intestinal problems are discussed below. If you suspect you have any of these problems, you should be evaluated by a primary care doctor or a gastroenterologist (a specialist in conditions of the stomach, intestines, and liver).

What Is Irritable Bowel Syndrome?

Irritable bowel syndrome is one of the most common causes of lower abdominal and pelvic pain. Some studies have shown that up to 66 percent of women with chronic *pelvic* pain actually have irritable bowel syndrome. The cause of irritable bowel is uncertain. However, as food and gas move through the intestines, people with irritable bowel seem to be overly sensitive to the stretching of the intestines that normally occurs. This leads to crampy pain about an hour or so after eating and seems to be worse at times of stress. The pain may be accompanied by bloating and may last for hours, days, or even weeks. Constipation or, rarely, diarrhea may also be present.

What Is the Treatment for Irritable Bowel Syndrome?

The most effective treatment for irritable bowel syndrome combines medication, dietary changes, and stress reduction. Diets high in fiber (fruits and vegetables), in addition to medications that increase fiber and water in the stool, will help promote normal movement of stool through the colon and lessen the discomfort. Therapy designed to reduce stress, such as relaxation techniques or biofeedback, has also been found to be very effective in decreasing the frequency of attacks. In some women, medications to reduce stress may also be helpful.

Kathy's Pelvic Pain

Kathy is a twenty-eight-year-old women who first saw me for lower abdominal and pelvic pain and bloating that had been getting worse over the past few months. The pain was crampy and came and went without much warning or apparent reason. Kathy assumed the pain was from her ovaries because it seemed to be in that general area. As we talked, it became apparent that the pain was not related to her menstrual periods, her activities, or to intercourse. In fact, the one thing that seemed to make the pain more likely to occur was stress. Kathy had been under an increasing amount of stress on her job, as continuing layoffs of other workers had increased her workload and made her worry that she might be next. She had also mentioned some diarrhea recently but felt this was due to her increased nervousness about her job and her health.

The examination of her uterus, fallopian tubes, ovaries, and abdomen was normal. Kathy was relieved that she didn't have anything wrong with her ovaries because she now admitted that she often worried that she had ovarian cancer. She thought that if she had mentioned that possibility, she would have somehow increased the likelihood of having the disease simply by uttering its name. But despite that enormous relief of knowing her ovaries were healthy, she was still physically uncomfortable, and we discussed having her get further evaluation. Because of the diarrhea, I recommended that she see a gastroenterologist. When this consultation was completed, the gastroenterologist agreed that her examination was totally normal. Based on Kathy's symptoms, he concluded that she probably had irritable bowel syndrome. Before beginning a series of X-ray tests, the doctor recommended that she try a medication to increase fiber and water in her intestines, and to begin some stress reduction exercises. Kathy's symptoms got better over the next few weeks. The diet changes and medication made her move her bowels more regularly, and the crampy pain gradually seemed to disappear. In addition to the relief of knowing that nothing serious was wrong with her, the relaxation exercises really helped to decrease her stress level. What had appeared to be a gynecologic problem, and in Kathy's mind was ovarian cancer until proven otherwise, turned out to be a common and fairly easy to treat intestinal condition. Within a year, even her job seemed to be more secure, which certainly helped to keep her stress to a minimum.

What Is Inflammatory Bowel Disease?

Two uncommon conditions, Crohn's disease and ulcerative colitis, produce inflammation of the inside lining of the intestines and cause abdominal pain. Crohn's disease often begins between the ages of fifteen and thirty but occurs in less than 2 out of 10,000 people. It is usually associated with diarrhea and sometimes rectal bleeding, and fever is common. Episodes of pain and diarrhea may last for days, or even weeks. Ulcerative colitis is also a rare disease, occurring in about 4 out of every 10,000 people, most often near the age of thirty or forty. It is usually associated with acute abdominal pain that is often relieved by a bowel movement. Diarrhea and rectal bleeding are common.

Because both of these conditions cause predominantly intestinal symptoms, we commonly suspect the cause to be intestinal disease rather than pelvic problems. Evaluation by a primary care doctor or gastroenterologist should lead to the diagnosis. Once a diagnosis is made, appropriate treatment can get started.

What Is Diverticulitis?

Diverticulosis is a condition common in both men and women as we get older. Forty percent of people over the age of sixty have this condition, which often causes no symptoms. Diverticulosis develops as a consequence of weakening in the wall of the large intestines. With progressive weakening, small folds and pockets appear in the intestinal wall. These pockets can trap stool, and when stool and the swarm of bacteria contained in it get trapped, an infection may result.

The resulting infection is called *diverticulitis* and leads to abdominal pain and fever. But this infection is rare, and diverticulitis occurs in fewer than 20 percent of people with diverticulosis. Sometimes, a smoldering type of infection may develop and cause a more long-lasting form of pain. The diagnosis of diverticulitis can be made with a specialized X-ray test called a CT scan. Antibiotics are successfully used to treat this illness.

Can Intestinal Cancer Cause Pelvic Pain?

The most common symptoms of colon cancer are a change in bowel habits, either diarrhea, constipation, or a narrowing of the stool. Abdominal pain and rectal bleeding occur in about half of the people with colon cancer. Colon cancer becomes more common with age, and it is uncommon before age forty. A history of a close family member with intestinal polyps or colon cancer can increase your risk of developing this disease. Yearly tests for blood in the stool should be performed after the age of forty. If it is positive, or if you have bowel symptoms that persist, an inspection of the colon and rectum with a small flexible telescope should be performed to make the diagnosis.

Can Muscle Problems Cause Pelvic Pain?

The abdominal muscles are situated over the pelvis and attach to the pubic bone. Sometimes muscle spasms from a previous injury to a muscle or from muscle tension confuse both the patient and the doctor into believing the pain originates from a gynecologic problem.

The nerves that "talk" to the brain are shared in the pelvic area by the uterus, ovaries, muscles, and joints, and you may not be able to tell exactly what part of your body is feeling pain (see fig. 6.1). Therefore, it is not uncommon for muscle or joint pain to be confused with true pelvic pain. For that reason, the right diagnosis is often hard to establish. It might be helpful to keep a pain diary for a few days to see if there are any patterns as to when and where you feel the pain. Pain from muscles or joints is often dull and aching and is usually worse when you are active. What you learn about your body will help your doctor determine the cause of the pain.

What Can Cause Musculoskeletal Pain?

Your parents probably told you to stand up straight, and they were right. Poor standing posture, slumping while you sit, or other poor sitting habits can overstress both muscles and joints and lead to back pain or pelvic pain.

Any previous back or pelvic injuries from work, falling off a horse, playing with the kids, making home repairs, tennis, aerobics, etc., may cause pelvic pain. Arthritis resulting from an old injury or simply the aging process may lead to spasm in the muscles around the joint and cause pain. Sometimes trigger points, very small areas of muscle spasm, are found near previous incisions or areas of prior injury. Women may also have areas of muscle spasm due to poor posture. Your doctor can detect these trigger points by pressing into the abdominal and back muscles. Tenderness in the muscle, rather than in the underlying pelvic organs, will confirm this diagnosis.

What Can Be Done to Treat Musculoskeletal Pain?

Many physical therapists and chiropractors are well trained to treat the musculoskeletal causes of pelvic pain. Treatment usually involves teaching you how to stand and sit properly, as well as the use of heat, cold packs, ultrasound treatments, and massage. Stretching and exercise can also be used to relieve muscle spasm, as can acupuncture and acupressure. For women who have trigger points (small areas of muscle spasm), an injection of local anesthetic into the tender area is very helpful. The anesthesia relaxes the spasm and can often result in long-term relief, even after the anesthetic wears off. Nerve blocks—injection of local anesthesia to larger nerves carrying pain signals—may also be successfully used for pain relief.

Anne's Persistent Abdominal Pain

Anne is a forty-two-year-old woman who had two years of lower abdominal pain that began shortly after she had a hysterectomy performed for persistent, abnormal bleeding. Since she no longer had her uterus, fallopian tubes, and ovaries, there simply were no pelvic organs present that could possibly cause pain. Her gynecologist had performed a pelvic exam and a sonogram, which were completely normal.

Her internist also evaluated her for intestinal or bladder problems that could cause abdominal pain, but none were found. Anne reluctantly began taking pain medications, but now the pain was worse, and the pills were less helpful. Her gynecologist suggested another surgery to determine if scar tissue from the hysterectomy was the cause of the pain. Before agreeing to another surgery, Anne decided to seek a second opinion. When she came into my office, she was emotionally prepared to face a second surgery but wanted to make sure surgery was her best choice.

As we expected, her pelvic examination was entirely normal. However, an area near the side of her previous abdominal incision seemed to be tender. While she was lying down, I gently pushed my finger into all the areas of her abdominal muscles to pinpoint the exact area of discomfort. A spot near the left side of her incision was tender when pushed, and this reproduced the pain she felt on a daily basis.

It became clear that her pain was from the incision, both with regard to the time the pain began and its location. The most likely causes of this type of pain are muscle spasm or irritation of nerves near the incision. Despite the discomfort the exam had caused her, Anne was elated to find out what seemed to be the cause of her pain. Since the pain was only in the incision, surgery did not seem necessary. That was good news.

I referred Anne to an anesthesiologist in our community who has training in pain management. He began injections of local anesthesia to the area. The first two injections, given about two weeks apart, were only briefly and mildly uncomfortable, and provided immediate and enormous relief. Two more injections were given about a month apart, and by the end of this time, Anne was pain free. When I saw Anne a year later for her routine exam, she had been pain free for ten months. The pain has, thankfully, not returned.

What Is the Best Way to Use Pain Medications for Chronic Pelvic Pain?

The most effective medications for managing chronic pain act by preventing the formation of substances called prostaglandins that cause the pain. Called antiprostaglandins, these medications include Advil, Aleve, and generic ibuprofen and are available over-the-counter in low doses.

These medications are most effective for chronic pain relief if they are taken in small to moderate doses every few hours (see individual instructions), rather than waiting for severe pain to occur. This "scheduled" use of pain medication, which should be started under your doctor's direction, has two major benefits. First, taking the medication on a regular basis prevents the pain from ever getting severe. Second, the reassurance of knowing that the pain will not become severe will free you from the constant worry about pain and allow you to focus on your life and work. Worrying about pain truly seems to make it worse, and, not surprisingly, we experience less pain when we are busy and content.

Should Narcotic Medications Be Used for Chronic Pain?

It is not a good idea to use narcotic medications for the relief of chronic pain. Medications such as Percodan, Percocet, codeine, Dilaudid, and Demerol can all be addictive. These medications also need to be taken in increasing amounts to provide continued pain relief. Furthermore, their use may actually cause an increase in pain, as they deplete chemicals in the brain that prevent pain. You will only make your pain worse if you start taking narcotics.

What Other Medications Are Helpful in the Treatment of Chronic Pelvic Pain?

One of the most exciting areas of medicine today is the science of neurobiology, the study of the chemical events that allow the brain to function. For example, a low level of two brain chemicals, serotonin and norepinephrine, has been linked to some forms of depression and also to the perception of pain. And it appears that the inability to produce adequate amounts of brain chemicals may be inherited and not under an individual's control. Certain medications that act to increase serotonin and norepinephrine have been found to be helpful for some forms of depression and also for people who have chronic pain. While the word *antidepressant* may disturb some women, low doses of these medications can increase serotonin and/or norepineprine levels in the brain and can help relieve chronic pain and improve sleep. If necessary, higher doses of medication may be used to help reduce the depression that often accompanies chronic pain. Doctors knowledgeable in the use of these medications for pain management can prescribe them most effectively.

Can Your Attitude About Pain Influence What You Feel?

As noted above, the first order of business if you have pain is to have a thorough medical evaluation. If that evaluation finds that no identifiable or serious problem exists, then, to some degree, you may feel a sense of reassurance. Not finding answers, however, is frustrating. It is very common for people with any chronic pain to feel helpless and depressed. But if a proper evaluation has ruled out a condition that might be dangerous, you have received good news. If a minor, but not entirely treatable, condition is found, there should be some relief in knowing that nothing serious is wrong.

With this reassurance, you should no longer view your pain as a signal of bodily danger, and this shift away from focusing on pain may help relieve it. If a person frequently thinks about pain, the focus will be on the negative aspects of his or her life and circumstances. After being pleasantly busy and distracted, we often find ourselves forgetting about any pain or discomfort we had been feeling. Being productive and doing the activities you like to do can lead to a more positive feeling about your life. This may decrease your pain and also lead to a feeling of control, something people in pain often say they miss.

This explanation is not meant to negate your true feeling of pain. I respect and understand skepticism about this approach, but a positive attitude does seem to make a difference for people with chronic pain. In studies of women with pelvic pain without any obvious cause, those who were taught the positive approach without surgery felt much better than those who were treated with surgery.

Can Relaxation Methods Be Used to Help Treat Pain?

As noted before, your brain determines how you perceive pain, and this perception is heightened by stress and tension. A number of techniques have been successfully used to help reduce the perception of pain of all types, including pelvic pain, headache, and arthritis. Relaxation techniques that use systematic contraction followed by relaxation of all your muscles are very effective. There is nothing fancy in these techniques, although you will probably need practice before they become effective.

Some of you may remember relaxation techniques from your Lamaze birthing classes. Lie down in a quiet place and start by contracting the muscles in your toes and holding that contraction for a few seconds. Then concentrate on totally relaxing the same muscles. After your toes, you can contract and then relax your calf muscles. By starting at your toes and working your way up your entire body, one part at a time, you can induce a state of total relaxation that will reduce stress. Be sure to spend time contracting your cheeks, your forehead, and your neck, since a great deal of muscular tension is often located in the head and neck area. During this time, deep and controlled breathing will also be calming. As you practice this technique, you should gradually be able to achieve total relaxation.

Techniques that divert your attention away from pain are also helpful to reduce pain. Lie down, close your eyes, and imagine you are in a
pleasant and beautiful place. This can be very relaxing. Like Lamaze techniques, the method helps you focus away from pain and decrease the
brain's perception of pain. To make this technique as effective as possible, you will probably have to practice doing it. Transporting yourself
mentally to another place may sound easy, but it takes a great deal of focus and concentration. When I need to relax, I always picture myself sitting on a beach in Hawaii, feeling a warm breeze. A pleasant daydream
can also reduce tension and stress and help to diminish your perception
of pain. Instructional relaxation and visualization tapes are available at
many bookstores. These techniques are most effective if they are used
either on a regular basis or long before the sensation of pain is strong.

Does Acupuncture Work for Pelvic Pain?

Some women find acupuncture effective for pelvic pain relief. The concept of mind-body connection, long a focal point of many Eastern phi-
losophies, is gaining a great deal of attention in Western medicine. The
connection of the mind and body during the perception of pain is the perfect example of how complex our bodies truly are. As with all types of treatment, if you choose to try acupuncture, you should find a well-trained and
respected practitioner. Your doctor may be able to recommend a skilled
acupuncturist in your community. Acupuncture provides quick relief for
some women; for others, the effect is cumulative over a period of time.

Transcutaneous electrical nerve stimulation (TENS) has also been
used successfully to treat chronic pain. Using a weak electrical current
passed through wires attached to the skin, this technique probably
works as acupuncture does by stimulating some nerves to prevent pain
from other areas. Your doctor may be able to refer you to someone with
experience in this simple and safe technique.

Can Biofeedback Treat Chronic Pain?

Biofeedback has also been found to be effective in relieving pain for
some women. During biofeedback, your pulse, blood pressure, and muscle tension are monitored continuously through small wires attached to
your body. When you are relaxed, your blood pressure, pulse, and muscle tension are at low levels. As you practice relaxing, the monitors report information back to you, usually with a sound signal becoming
lower in tone the more relaxed you become. In this way, successful relaxation is "fed back" to you, and you learn how to bring about this re-

laxed state by yourself, at any time, without the monitors. A psychologist trained in biofeedback is the best person to help you learn this skill.

Lila's Difficult Problem

Lila is a twenty-five-year-old woman who came to see me for a *fifth* opinion. For the past two years she had undergone a series of evaluations, tests, procedures, and surgeries, all of which had failed to help her chronic pelvic pain. When the pain had started two years ago, Lila's gynecologist felt she most likely had endometriosis. She had recommended a laparoscopy, which was performed the following month. At that time, very mild endometriosis was found and easily treated with a laser. Lila and her doctor were confident that the treatment would end the pain, but the pain never improved.

Assuming that the pain was the result of a nongynecologic problem, the gynecologist suggested that Lila see an internist for further testing. Blood tests for liver, gallbladder, and kidney problems were done, but revealed nothing abnormal. X-rays of the intestines and a sonogram of the liver, gallbladder, and pancreas were also normal. By this time, Lila had become frustrated and went to see another gynecologist. The second gynecologist reviewed Lila's records and wondered whether the endometriosis had come back and recommended another laparoscopy. This was performed, and, again, very mild endometriosis was discovered and removed with the laser. Once again, the laser treatment did nothing to help her chronic pain. She then went to see a gastroenterologist, who looked into her intestines with a small telescope called an endoscope. This was also normal. So, four other doctors had cared for Lila, and none had been able to cure her pain. Lila came to my office expecting that another laparoscopy would need to be done for her endometriosis. After reviewing all of her records, sonograms, and X-rays, and after performing a pelvic exam that was normal, I felt that another laparoscopy would probably not be helpful.

I reassured Lila that not only was her examination totally normal, but all the combined previous testing had found only a small amount of endometriosis. Treatment through the laparoscope had failed to make her better. We discussed the process of endometriosis (see chapter 7) and the fact that it would be unlikely to reoccur to a significant degree in such a short period of time. At this point, I suggested that Lila consider measures less drastic than surgery to deal with her pain. She agreed to see a pain management physician in our community.

He, too, reviewed all of Lila's records and performed an examination. He agreed that there was no concern about a serious undetected problem and recommended that Lila consider biofeedback and visualization under the direction of a skilled therapist. Exhausted from all the worry and the running around to different doctors, Lila agreed. After a few sessions to learn to use both biofeedback and visualization techniques, Lila is now pain free on most days. She is able to work and do her normal activities without interruption. And when she feels that the pain is coming back, she has the ability to control the pain through the relaxation techniques she has learned. She sees me every six months, or more often if needed, and her pelvic examination has remained entirely normal. While it is clear that most of the testing Lila had was needed to eliminate any serious cause of her pain, continuing down that path was going to get her nowhere. Now she is happily back in control of her life.

Should You Have a Hysterectomy for Pelvic Pain?

The use of hysterectomy for an initial treatment of pelvic pain should be discouraged. Presently, about 10 percent of hysterectomies in the U.S. are performed because of pelvic pain, but many of these women do not have long-term relief of their pain following surgery. One study found that 20 percent of women who had a hysterectomy for pelvic pain had no improvement following surgery, and 5 percent said their pain was actually worse.

One reason for the lack of effectiveness of hysterectomy is that, as described in this chapter, some causes of pelvic pain are not gynecologic in the first place. For that reason, hysterectomy to relieve pelvic pain should be reserved for women who clearly have a gynecologic disease that requires a hysterectomy. In one study of women with chronic pelvic pain who were fully and properly evaluated for gynecologic, nongynecologic, and psychological causes of their pain, only 5 percent needed to have a hysterectomy.

On the other hand, hysterectomy may be appropriate for some women who do have a significant degree of pain that results from gynecologic causes and who have not responded to other forms of treatment (see chapter 12). Clearly, this procedure is only appropriate for women who do not want to have children. Pain resulting from severe endo-metriosis that has not responded to medical therapy and adequate laparoscopic treatment by a gynecologist experienced in treating endometriosis may respond to removal of the uterus, fallopian tubes, and ovaries. Pain that results primarily from severe adhesions due to prior infection or previous surgery can usually be treated by laparoscopic surgery. However, if this has already been tried without success, or if the amount of scar tissue would make laparoscopic surgery impossible, then hysterectomy may be considered.

Among the women operated on for chronic pelvic pain in the Maine Women's Health Study (see page 348), 5 percent noted more than eight days of pain per month prior to surgery, and 80 percent noted that the pain limited their activity. After surgery, only 13 percent of the women had significant pain. But it is important to note that in the Maine Women's Health Study, none of the women had tried a multidisciplinary approach to pelvic pain. Had this been available, some of the women might have been spared from having a hysterectomy.

The decision to have a hysterectomy should not be taken lightly. Almost all medical conditions have more than one option for treatment. And none of the possible side effects of hysterectomy is entirely predictable for each individual.

It is in your best interest to be educated about the health-care decisions you make. Because of the complexity of chronic pain and the continuing developments in treatment, I believe that chronic pelvic pain is one area where a second opinion from someone who specializes in this field is well worth the time and effort.

REFERENCES

Demco, L. 2000. Pain referral patterns in the pelvis. *Journal of the American Association of Gynecologic Laparoscopists* 7:181–83.

Mathias, S., M. Kuppermann, R. Liberman, R. Lipschutz, and J. Steege. 1996. Chronic pelvic pain: Prevalence, health-related quality of life, and economic correlates. *Obstetrics and Gynecology* 87:321–27.

Milburn, A., R. Reiter, and A. Rhomburg. 1993. Multidisciplinary approach to chronic pelvic pain. *Obstetrics and Gynecology Clinics of North America* 20:643–61.

Rapkin, A., L. Kames, L. Darke, F. Stampler, and B. Naliboff. 1990. History of physical and sexual abuse in women with chronic pelvic pain. *Obstetrics and Gynecology* 76:92–96.

Reiter R., and A. Milburn. 1994. Exploring effective treatment for chronic pelvic pain. *Contemporary Obstetrics and Gynecology* March:84–103.

Rogers, R. 1999. Basic neuroanatomy for understanding pelvic pain. *Journal of the American Association of Gynecologic Laparoscopists* 6:17–25.

Rosenthal, R. 1993. Psychology of chronic pelvic pain. *Obstetrics and Gynecology Clinics of North America* 20:627–41.

Steege, J., A. Stout, and S. Somkuti. 1993. Chronic pelvic pain in women: Toward an integrative model. *Obstetrical and Gynecological Survey* 48:95–110.

7

ENDOMETRIOSIS
by Ingrid A. Rodi, M.D.

Endometriosis is one of the most common gynecologic conditions in the United States. We don't know exactly how many American women suffer from this disease, but best estimates set the number at about five million. Women of all ages, races, and backgrounds have been found to have endometriosis.

Recent information suggests that the number of women with the disease may be increasing. Some two million women had hysterectomies for pelvic pain related to endometriosis between 1965 and 1984. Over that time period, the number of hysterectomies performed per year for endometriosis doubled. In addition, the proportion of all hysterectomies performed because of endometriosis rose from approximately 10 percent to 20 percent.

Endometriosis can also affect fertility, and about 30 percent of infertile women are found to have endometriosis. Pelvic pain and infertility related to endometriosis lead to the hospitalization of a substantial number of women every year.

What Is Endometriosis?

The tissue that lines the uterus and is shed during the menstrual period is called the endometrium (see fig. 1.3). In some women, this same tissue can be found growing outside the uterus, where it does not belong. When this occurs, endometriosis is said to be present. The tissue that normally lines the uterus may be found in or on the ovaries, the fallopian tubes, the outer surface of the uterus, or other areas of the membrane that lines the abdominal cavity and surrounds the internal organs, called the peritoneum. Occasionally, endometriosis may be found on the bowel or bladder. And very rarely, it has been found in locations far from the pelvis, such as in an old abdominal scar or even the lungs.

The lining cells of the uterus normally go through cyclic changes in response to the varying levels of the female hormones estrogen and progesterone produced by the ovary throughout the month. During the menstrual cycle, as estrogen levels rise, the lining cells first grow and build up, and then, as the level of both estrogen and progesterone fall at the end of the cycle, the tissue breaks down and is shed as menstrual blood (see page 65). When a woman has endometriosis, even though the lining cells are present in locations where they are not intended to be, they still respond to hormonal changes to some degree as if they were still within the uterus.

So if endometriosis cells are sitting on the outside of the lower intestine, for example, those cells will grow lush and full as if they were in the uterus preparing for a fertilized egg. During the menstrual period, as normal uterine lining cells begin to bleed, the endometrial cells present outside the intestine—endometriosis—also begins to bleed. This blood and other biochemical substances given off by the endometriosis often cause irritation, and even damage, to the surrounding areas. If these cells are present near the uterus, bladder, or the bowel, the irritation may lead to pain in those locations. The body's natural response to irritation and injury may end with the formation of scar tissue, which also increases the likelihood that discomfort will be experienced (see chapter 6). The scar tissue can also interfere with the passage of the egg into the fallopian tube and lead to infertility. Thus, the abnormal location of uterine lining cells leads to the symptoms and problems that we associate with the condition called endometriosis.

What Does Endometriosis Look Like?

The appearance of endometriosis is variable and changes over time. Areas of endometriosis may be small, only a fraction of an inch, or larger than an inch. We think that new endometriosis appears as small, almost clear, raised areas on the surface of the uterus, fallopian tubes, ovaries, or inside lining of the abdomen. Over time, these areas, called implants, continue to collect the pigment contained in the blood they secrete. As this occurs, the areas become pink, then dark red, and finally a dark brown color. The darker areas have often been called "powder burns" because of their color and spindly shape. To evaluate a woman for the presence of endometriosis, a careful inspection of the entire pelvis and abdomen, usually with the laparoscope, must be performed. The doctor should look for all the possible appearances of endometriosis, some of which are fairly subtle (see fig. 7.1).

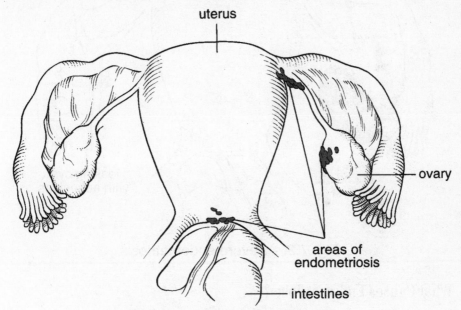

Fig. 7.1.   Mild endometriosis

What Is an Endometrioma?

The cells of endometriosis can get trapped inside the ovary. During the menstrual period, when there is bleeding from this endometriosis, the blood accumulates inside the ovary, forming a cyst. These blood-filled cysts are called endometriomas (see fig. 7.2). As the blood ages and becomes more concentrated, it assumes a dark brown, chocolate color. When these cysts are opened at the time of surgery, they are usually easy to recognize because the dark brown fluid appears quite different than the normal clear fluid of common ovarian cysts. For this reason, the cysts are sometimes called "chocolate cysts." The size of these cysts can range from very small to the size of a grapefruit, and there can be more than one present at a time (see chapter 5). The presence of an en-dometrioma larger than an inch or two may decrease a woman's chances of getting pregnant. Unfortunately, treatment with medication for endometriosis in the ovary is not effective. Surgical removal of an en-dometrioma, usually by laparoscopy, most likely will improve fertility.

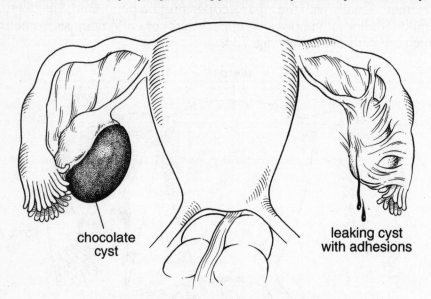

chocolate
cyst

leaking cyst
with adhesions

Fig. 7.2.   Severe endometriosis

What Causes Endometriosis?

A great deal of research and effort has gone into trying to clarify the cause of endometriosis. Several theories have been proposed suggest-ing more than one possible cause, and there is evidence to suggest that any, or all, of these theories may be possible. It may be that endometrio-sis has different causes in different women. At present, the most proba-ble explanations are the passage of menstrual blood out the fallopian tubes and into the abdomen, or the spread of uterine lining cells through the bloodstream or lymph system to other parts of the body. Genetics also appears to play another role—a woman with a mother or sister with endometriosis has a much higher risk of developing the disease. It is likely that an inherited defect of the immune system plays some role in allowing the development of this condition. Some researchers have found links between the development of endometriosis and environ-mental toxins. These concepts are discussed in detail below. The hope is that clarification of the causes of endometriosis will lead to better treatment, or perhaps even prevention, of this common condition.

What Is Retrograde Menstruation?

At the time of the menstrual period, most of the blood and endometrial tissue flows out of the cervix and into the vagina. However, some of the blood and endometrial lining cells can also go out the wrong way, through the ends of the fallopian tubes. This is known as retrograde menstruation and occurs commonly. In fact, if surgery happens to be performed on a woman coincidentally during her menstrual period, menstrual blood and tissue are frequently found at sites outside the uterus, in areas where endometriosis most commonly occurs.

However, even though we know that this "backward" menstruation occurs in most women, the cells usually do not take hold and grow. But when the cells do take hold and grow, endometriosis is the result. Women who have periods closer together, or that last longer, or are heavier, have an increased amount of blood that flows out of the fallopian tubes, and they have a greater chance of developing endometriosis. But still, only in the occasional woman is the tissue able to take hold, grow, and develop into endometriosis. Why the tissue grows outside the uterus in only some women and not in others is not known, although the immune system may be a factor (see page 209).

Can Endometriosis Be Caused by Abnormalities of the Uterus?

Some women have an abnormality of their uterus that may lead to a greater likelihood of developing endometriosis. Very rarely, a girl may be born with a narrowed, or even closed, cervix that prevents the menstrual fluid and lining cells from leaving the uterus during menstruation. A totally closed hymen, also a very rare occurrence, may also block the flow of blood out of the vagina. The only way these cells are able to get out of the uterus is through the fallopian tubes, where they fall into the abdominal cavity. As more menstrual fluid exits through the fallopian tubes, the likelihood probably increases that the cells will take hold, grow, and develop into endometriosis.

In these rare cases, a young woman may experience all the symptoms of a period, including menstrual cramping, without any visible bleeding. These women often see a doctor at a young age because the menstrual fluid and cells start to accumulate after menstrual periods first begin, and pain follows shortly thereafter. The diagnosis of a closed hymen can be made by simple examination of the vagina. Opening the hymen is a simple outpatient surgical procedure.

If no obvious cause of pelvic pain is apparent, a laparoscopy is often performed to determine the cause of the pain, and the diagnosis of endometriosis is made. If the cervix is the issue, surgery can also be performed to open up the cervix and prevent further problems. For reasons that are not clear, it appears that these women have a less aggressive type of endometriosis, with less formation of scar tissue.

Connie's Fibroid Caused Her Endometriosis

Connie came to see me with a history of severe pelvic pain and abnormal bleeding. She was in her mid-twenties and had normal periods until two years prior to her visit, when she noted bleeding in between her periods. She also was experiencing increasingly heavy menstrual bleeding, and she suffered from severe cramping. An evaluation by her prior doctor found nothing abnormal, and she was given some pain medication.

This did not help very much, and she came to see me for a second opinion. When I examined Connie, her uterus was larger than normal, suggesting that a fibroid might be present. On ultrasound examination, a fibroid was seen in the lower part of the uterus, enlarging her uterus and partially blocking her cervix. Most likely, the fibroid was preventing menstrual blood from leaving the uterus through the cervix, and the blood from her period was accumulating in her uterus. When enough blood collected, the uterus would try to squeeze the blood out, and a severe cramp would result.

The pain with her periods was so bad that Connie requested that something be done to end her discomfort. Unfortunately, no medication is available to treat this type of fibroid problem, and surgery was the only answer (see chapter 4). At the time of her surgery, we found a lot of endometriosis around her uterus, fallopian tubes, and ovaries. We suspected that the fibroid had blocked the flow of menstrual blood out of the uterus and forced it out of the fallopian tubes, leading to the development of the endometriosis. We were able to surgically remove all the visible endometriosis. The fibroid was then surgically removed to prevent further obstruction of the cervix.

Connie did very well for a number of years after surgery.

However, a few years later, Connie was found to have a new, even larger fibroid that had grown in the wall of her uterus. This fibroid was pressing on her bladder and causing her a great deal of discomfort, and she again requested surgery. At the time of this second surgery, we noted that this new fibroid was not blocking her cervix, and no new endometriosis had formed. We were able to remove the fibroid, and Connie has done extremely well for the past few years. Stories like Connie's give some credence to the theory that obstructions to the flow of the menstrual blood can lead to endometriosis, and relief of the obstruction can prevent endometriosis from forming.

What Does Your Immune System Have to Do with Endometriosis?

Some researchers feel that a woman's immune system plays a part in the development of endometriosis. Components of the immune system include antibodies, white blood cells that attack foreign invaders, and biochemicals that enhance or reduce the body's response to foreign substances. It is possible that, in most women, when endometrial cells exit out through the fallopian tubes, the body is able to recognize that these cells are in the wrong place, and the antibodies and white blood cells destroy them.

However, recent studies indicate that women with endometriosis often have white blood cells that are not able to recognize and devour out-of-place endometrial cells. These endometrial cells flourish and become endometriosis over time. Some women may also inherit genes that cause the abdominal lining cells to form abnormal amounts of biochemicals that allow the cells to stick to the abdominal lining. Other research found high levels of enzymes in endometriosis cells that caused estrogen to be formed in the nearby area. The estrogen, in turn, feeds the growth of the endometriosis cells. Women with endometriosis also make biochemicals that promote the growth of new blood vessels in the area to feed the endometriosis.

New research in monkeys shows an association between blood levels of dioxin, a chemical found in industrial pollutants, and the frequency and severity of endometriosis. Although the research is still controversial, dioxin has been shown to alter the genes that are responsible for cell growth and tissue inflammation, both important to the development of endometriosis. Further studies are under way to see if this correlation is also present in humans and if there is actually a causal relationship to endometriosis.

Although many research studies have examined the immune system in women who have endometriosis, none have found any clear evidence of cause and effect. Yet these findings reveal the complexity of the possible causes of endometriosis. It is important to understand that women with endometriosis are not more likely to get any other conditions or illnesses, suggesting that the immune system otherwise works normally.

Is Endometriosis an Inheritable Disease?

It is probable that some women are more prone to develop endometriosis because of a genetic predisposition. A woman who has a mother or sister with endometriosis has an approximately 7 percent risk of developing the disease compared to a 1 percent risk in the general population. The reasons for this are not clear but may be related to an inherited tendency to provide abnormal amounts of biochemicals that make the endometrial cells stick to the abdominal lining, and abnormal white blood cells that can't remove endometrial cells that are in the wrong place. It is also possible that genetic factors may interact with environmental factors to increase susceptibility to this disease.

Can Endometriosis Spread Through the Bloodstream or Lymph System?

The body has a vast network of veins and arteries that distribute blood to the body. It also has a separate, but similar, network that carries lymph, a fluid involved in the body's defense system, throughout the body. Some researchers think that endometrial tissue can be carried through either the bloodstream or lymph system to distant locations. This mechanism has been proposed to explain how endometriosis gets to areas remote from the uterus. In fact, endometriosis has been discovered at the time of surgery in areas such as the navel or the lung. However, it is extremely uncommon to find endometriosis in distant locations.

Can Adolescents Have Endometriosis?

Endometriosis is usually thought to be a disease of women in their twenties and thirties, and the diagnosis is often not considered when a physician evaluates an adolescent with pelvic pain. However, a substantial number of young women who experience chronic pelvic pain have endometriosis as the cause. The onset of endometriosis can be as early as the first few years of menstruation, and the severity of the pain may increase over time. Fortunately, the majority of adolescents with endometriosis have a minimal or mild form of the disease. Therefore, in young women suspected of endometriosis, early treatment with oral contraceptives may be considered. Treatment with synthetic progesterone, called progestin, is not advised because the side effects, including weight gain, bloating, acne, and emotional changes, are intolerable to young women. GnRH agonist, a drug frequently used to treat endometriosis, can interfere with bone development in young women and should not be used until puberty is completed (see page 221). If pain does not respond to birth control pills, surgery for diagnosis and removal of endometriosis may be necessary. Following surgery, treatment with birth control pills should be used until the time the young woman wants to conceive a child.

What Are the Symptoms of Endometriosis?

If you have pain before your periods, chronic pelvic pain, pain during or after sex, premenstrual lower back pain, painful bowel movements, the sudden onset of pelvic pain, or a problem with fertility, your doctor will consider endometriosis as one of the possible causes for your problem. On the other hand, many women with endometriosis have no symptoms at all, and the condition may be discovered inadvertently during surgery for another reason.

Katie's Abdominal Pain

Katie is a thirty-nine-year-old woman who had noted pain under her rib cage on her right side for about two months. The pain came and went, but seemed to be present mostly after she ate. Then it became increasingly severe, and she saw her internist for the problem. A series of tests were done, and stones were discovered in her gallbladder. Although the problem was not serious, the gallbladder pain was very bothersome, and Katie decided to have surgery.

Katie's general surgeon removed her gallbladder using laparoscopic techniques. However, after the gallbladder was removed, the surgeon examined the pelvic area and saw multiple areas of adhesions and endometriosis. The surgeon called me at my office and asked if I could come right over to have a look. Within ten minutes I was in the operating room, looking at Katie's uterus, fallopian tubes, and ovaries on the video monitor. Katie had three children and felt well, so the endometriosis did not appear to be a significant problem despite the fact that it was present near her ovaries and behind the uterus. The endometriosis was also not related to her gallbladder problem. However, thinking that if the condition continued unabated it might cause problems with pain in the future, we elected to gently remove the scar tissue and areas of endometriosis. This took only about twenty minutes, following which the general surgeon finished closing the small incisions. After surgery, Katie was surprised to learn about the unexpected findings of scar tissue and endometriosis, but she was glad they had been treated.

Can Endometriosis Cause Pain with Your Periods?

Painful menstrual periods are very common in women who have endometriosis. We often find that women with endometriosis have pain just before their periods begin. When the ovarian hormone estrogen is produced during the menstrual cycle, it acts on both the normal lining of the uterus and the endometriosis to make all these cells grow. Toward the end of the menstrual cycle, the ovary stops the production of estrogen, and both the lining cells of the uterus and the endometriosis start to break down and bleed. As the endometriosis breaks down, it releases substances, such as prostaglandin, which can irritate the surrounding tissues of the uterus, bladder, and bowel and cause pain. However, endometriosis can lead to other patterns of pain as well.

Can Endometriosis Lead to Adhesions (Scar Tissue)?

Endometriosis causes the release of blood and chemical substances onto the tissue inside the abdominal cavity. This tissue is delicate and easily damaged by blood and chemical substances. Normally, the body heals itself from such an injury by increasing the growth of cells in the damaged area to replace those that have been damaged. This is the process that forms scar tissue to mend a wound. Unfortunately, scar tissue inside the body, called adhesions, may form between areas that are not normally connected.

Sometimes adhesions can make the uterus, fallopian tubes, or ovaries stick to each other or to nearby organs such as the intestines (see fig. 6.2). Because scar tissue is not elastic like normal tissue, it doesn't stretch easily, and the pulling and tugging of scar tissue on normal tissue that occurs with activity or sex may lead to pain (see chapter 6).

Teresa Was Missing Work

An unhappy Teresa came to see me one morning in the office. She told me her period had gotten so bad that she was missing work, and she didn't know what to do. She had been placed on birth control pills by her previous physician, in an attempt to decrease her menstrual cramping (see chapter 3). In addition, she had been given a prescription for a strong pain pill, but the pain continued. At one point in our conversation, she started crying, and she confided that she was afraid she would become addicted to the pain pills.

On examination, I didn't find anything unusual, so I recommended a sonogram so that I could "see" the uterus. The only unusual finding was a small cyst in her ovary, about one inch in diameter. Usually, a cyst that size would be of no concern. However, this particular cyst had an unusual pattern on the sonogram, the kind of pattern we often see when endometriosis of the ovary, called an endometrioma, is present. It appeared that the sonogram might have found the cause of Teresa's pain—endometriosis.

I was concerned because endometriosis of the ovary cannot be cured with medication, and surgery would therefore be needed. I suggested that we take a look with the laparoscope to determine if an endometrioma was, in fact, present. If so, we would then be able to remove the endometriosis with the laparoscope and perhaps treat her pain. She was panicked: "How long will I be out of work? I don't have many more sick days left." I was glad to be able to reassure her that we could do her surgery on a Friday, and she would likely be back to work in a week.

During the laparoscopy, I could see that she did, in fact, have a one-inch-wide cyst of endometriosis deep in her left ovary. There was also some scarring from additional endometriosis around the fallopian tube and ovary. I was able to remove both the cyst and the scar tissue with a laser aimed through the laparoscope. By thoroughly burning away the abnormal cells and scar tissue, pain from endometriosis may often be relieved. During her visit following surgery, I recommended a three-month course of GnRH agonist (see page 221) to shrink any remaining endometriosis that had not been visible during the surgery. We also gave her some oral progestin to lessen hot flashes and some vaginal estrogen tablets to prevent vaginal dryness from the medication. Three months after her surgery, the medication was stopped. When she came for her annual checkup, she was smiling when I walked into the room. "I haven't missed a day of work, and my periods are so easy I don't even have to take an aspirin!"

Can Endometriosis Cause Pain with Sex (Dyspareunia)?

When the endometrial cells come out of the fallopian tubes, they often fall down directly into the pelvis. The pelvis is the most common location for endometriosis, and the menstrual fluid and cells often land on the supporting ligaments that attach the uterus to the back of the pelvis, close to the top of the vagina. The endometriosis may lead to scar tissue in this area. The stretching of the scar tissue during intercourse can, therefore, be very painful.

Can Endometriosis Cause Backache?

If endometriosis is present near the muscles in the back of the pelvis, the cells can secrete chemicals that can irritate these muscles and cause them to go into spasm. This leads to low back pain. In addition, the ligaments that support the uterus are attached inside the pelvis near the back. These ligaments are commonly affected by endometriosis, with pain felt near the back as well. Also, a very large endometrioma can lie against the pelvic muscles and nerves and can lead to low back pain.

Can Endometriosis Cause Painful Bowel Movements?

Very rarely, endometriosis can grow into the part of the bowel that surrounds the uterus, fallopian tubes, and ovaries. If this occurs, the scar tissue that results may lead to pain at the time of bowel movements, when stool stretches the intestines as it moves down. If the endometriosis grows all the way through the wall of the bowel, bleeding that occurs from these cells during menstruation can show up in the bowel movement. This is an extremely rare situation.

Can Endometriosis Cause Painful Urination?

It is not uncommon for small areas of endometriosis to grow on the outside surface of the bladder. And, as long as the endometriosis stays outside the bladder, it causes very few symptoms. Very rarely, the endometriosis can grow into the wall of the bladder, irritating the bladder and causing a frequent urge to urinate. More rarely still, the endometriosis can grow through the wall, to the inside of the bladder. If this occurs, at the time of the menstrual period, the blood produced by these cells can be found in the urine.

Can Endometriosis Cause Chronic Pelvic Pain?

Chronic pelvic pain is one of the most common symptoms of endometriosis. The pain often comes on gradually, and may be sharp or dull, constant or intermittent. Interestingly, there is no correlation between the amount of endometriosis seen at the time of surgery and the severity of the pain experienced. This is because in many instances surgeons are seeing just the "tip of the iceberg," as much of the endometriosis can be beneath the surfaces of the pelvic cavity. And there does appear to be a connection between how far under the surface the endometriosis goes and the amount of pain. Therefore, significant pain may result from what appears to be small, as well as large, areas of the disease. Interestingly, women with large areas of endometriosis may have no symptoms at all, adding to our confusion about this medical condition.

It is important for women with chronic pelvic pain to have other possible sources of pain investigated before concluding that endometriosis is the cause. One a diagnosis is established, appropriate treatment can be directed at the source. More about other causes of chronic pelvic pain can be found in chapter 6. Medications may be used to treat pelvic pain from endometriosis over the short term, but often surgical removal of the endometriosis is the most effective way to achieve pain relief. These treatments are explained below.

Can Endometriosis Cause Sudden Pelvic Pain?

Very rarely, sudden, severe pain can result from the rupture or twisting of a large ovarian cyst associated with endometriosis. These cysts, called endometriomas (see fig. 7.2), are filled with endometriosis and the blood that these cells have produced. Very often, surgery is required when endometriomas are suspected, both to make the diagnosis and to treat the condition.

Robin Missed the Show

I remember first meeting Robin in the emergency room. She was all dressed up, and I asked her where she had planned to go that evening. "I was on my way to the Music Center when I experienced this horrible pain in my side. I told my husband to get me to the nearest hospital, and he brought me here."

On examination, her abdomen was very tender, and a sonogram was performed, which showed a cyst in her right ovary. The sonogram showed that the cyst was about the size of a tennis ball but appeared to be partially collapsed and was surrounded by a lot of fluid. These findings suggested that a ruptured ovarian cyst might be present. Robin was having severe pain; she could not even stand up, and it seemed clear that she would need surgery to remove the ruptured cyst and end the pain.

Once I explained the need for surgery to Robin, she understood and agreed immediately. We performed a laparoscopy, and during the operation, I found that her ovary contained an endometrioma, a cyst that contains a collection of blood and endometriosis. This cyst had burst open, causing Robin the sudden onset of severe pain. We examined all of her pelvic organs and other areas inside her abdomen and could not find any other endometriosis. Using laparoscopic surgery, we were able to remove the cyst and all the fluid that had come out of it. We were also able to repair the remaining healthy portion of her ovary, and the results of the surgery appeared excellent.

The next morning when I told Robin what I had found, she was surprised. "I thought women with endometriosis have pain with their periods, and mine are very easy," she said. I explained that many women do have pain with their periods when they have endometriosis, but that, rarely, women have no pain until the endometriosis forms a cyst that goes on to rupture. Robin has done very well since that time and has not had any recurrence of the endometrioma.

Can Endometriosis Cause Irregular Menstrual Periods?

As described in chapter 3, the menstrual cycle is the result of a finely tuned interplay of a number of female hormones. One of the important parts of this system is the production of progesterone following ovulation (the release of the egg from the ovary). Ovulation may be disrupted by the presence of endometriosis, leading to abnormal amounts of progesterone and a disrupted menstrual cycle. For reasons that are not clear, it appears that even if ovulation occurs, it may be not be normal, and irregular cycles may result.

Can Endometriosis Cause Infertility?

Infertility has long been felt to be associated with endometriosis, but all the reasons endometriosis might cause difficulty getting pregnant have not been established. In fact, it may be that the causes of the endometriosis may also independently cause infertility. We know that about 5 percent of women who have had children and request tubal sterilization will be noted to have areas of old endometriosis at the time of their surgery. Therefore, the presence of endometriosis does not, per se, imply that a woman cannot get pregnant.

However, it does appear that the chance of getting pregnant is decreased somewhat if you have endometriosis, and the more endometriosis you have, the less likely you are to get pregnant. Endometriosis appears to start as small areas of abnormally located endometrial lining cells. If the tissue continues to grow and bleed, scar tissue forms around it, increasing the amount of damaged tissue. The scar tissue may even grow around the fallopian tubes and ovaries in a way that blocks the passage of the egg down the fallopian tube.

The probability of a healthy woman in her twenties getting pregnant is about 25 percent per month. For women with mild endometriosis, where the endometriosis is present in small amounts and has not caused any scarring, the pregnancy rate is about 7 percent per month. For women who have severe endometriosis, where extensive scarring, blockage of the fallopian tubes, and large cysts in the ovaries are present, it is not hard to understand why pregnancy rates are extremely low. Surgical removal of endometriosis, as described on page 223, may increase fertility.

Can Endometriosis Cause a Miscarriage?

Some studies in the medical literature have suggested that women with endometriosis have a higher risk of having repeated miscarriages. However, recent and better-designed studies do not confirm these findings. Our best information today suggests that women with endometriosis do not have rates of miscarriage any higher than other women.

Can Endometriosis Lead to Mood Changes or Depression?

Some women may have pain with endometriosis despite medical or surgical treatment. Relaxation techniques, biofeedback, or acupuncture have been found to be helpful for some women with chronic pain from endometriosis (see page 197). However, living with endometriosis can be difficult. If the symptoms come back after treatment or you are having trouble getting pregnant, the frustration and pain might lead you to become depressed. If you are in this predicament, don't suffer in silence. Discuss your feelings with your family and doctor to get the support and the relief you need. Several options are available including counseling, support groups (see resources at the end of this chapter), and medication.

How Can Endometriosis Be Diagnosed?

Endometriosis may be suspected if tender, thickened areas are felt near the uterus on a pelvic examination. If an ovarian cyst is present, sometimes a sonogram may exhibit the patterns suggestive of an endometrioma (see page 158). Unfortunately, we do not have any test presently available that can reliably predict whether or not endometriosis is present. Neither sonography, MRI, CT scan, or blood tests are accurate in this regard.

The diagnosis of endometriosis can only be confirmed by looking at the pelvic organs at the time of surgery. Areas with the characteristic appearance of endometriosis (see page 204) can then be seen. Most commonly, a surgical procedure called laparoscopy is performed under general anesthesia for this purpose. A small lighted instrument is inserted through the navel, and the surgeon looks through the instrument directly or, with the aid of a camera attached to the laparoscope, a view of the pelvis can be projected on a TV screen.

At times, the diagnosis of endometriosis is made during a laparotomy, abdominal surgery that is performed under either general or regional (such as epidural) anesthesia. The incision in the abdomen ranges from approximately two to five inches in length. This abdominal surgery may be needed when a large endometrioma has been identified by the sonogram or if a pelvic mass of uncertain cause is found on examination. In addition, endometriosis may be incidentally found during an abdominal surgery performed for another reason, such as fibroids, an ovarian cyst, or even surgery for appendicitis.

What Is the Endometriosis Classification System?

A classification system has been developed based on the amount and location of endometriosis seen at surgery and the amount and location of any scar tissue associated with the endometriosis. The system was devised in order to assist in evaluating the success of different treatments in helping women achieve pregnancy. In this system, endometriosis is graded as minimal, mild, moderate, or severe according to established criteria. Endometriosis is classified as minimal when it involves just the surfaces of the ovaries, fallopian tubes, or lining cells within the abdomen (the peritoneum). Endometriosis is classified as severe when it invades deeply into the pelvic tissues or causes thick, inelastic formations of scar tissue called adhesions.

Unfortunately, it appears that the present classification system does not show any correlation between the amount of endometriosis seen and the degree of pain present, nor does it predict a woman's chance of getting pregnant. This enigma may be explained by the fact that endometriosis is often present below the surface, and thus is not included in the scoring system. The need for treatment will therefore depend on the degree of symptoms you experience, rather than on the score of endometriosis as determined by your gynecologist.

TREATMENT

Treatment is aimed at reducing the symptoms of endometriosis, usually either pain or infertility. Treatment is divided into three paths: observation, medication, or surgery.

Observation: Is Any Treatment Needed for Endometriosis?

Women who have minimal or mild endometriosis and do not have pain may not require any treatment other than careful follow-up. In practice, however, if the diagnosis of endometriosis is made during laparoscopy, most gynecologists will burn or cut away these cells. However, a few studies have demonstrated that this treatment of mild endometriosis does not enhance fertility. For women with minimal or mild endometriosis, fertility rates are good even if no treatment is performed.

Can Medication Be Used to Treat Endometriosis?

It is known that estrogen causes endometriosis to grow. Endometriosis is extremely rare before a young woman begins to produce estrogen and starts to have periods, and the disease usually disappears after menopause, when estrogen production stops. Therefore, one goal of treatment with medication is to lower, or stop, the production of estrogen. Reducing the levels of estrogen "starves" the endometriosis and causes it to shrink and sometimes even disappear. Two classes of drugs have been developed which lower the amount of estrogen in a woman's body: Danocrine and GnRH agonist (see below). Progestins or birth control pills can also be used to help the symptoms of endometriosis.

Can Progestins Be Used to Treat Endometriosis?

Synthetic progesterone, called progestin, was the first medication used in an attempt to control the pain from endometriosis and is still used today. It can be given by injection or pills. Progestin acts to shrink the cells of endometriosis and thereby decrease the amount of blood and other irritating substances released by the cells. Thus, pain relief can be achieved over a period of time. However, pain often recurs after the medication is stopped. In addition, fertility rates do not seem to be improved following the use of progestins. Side effects of progestins include bloating, water retention, and weight gain, and are frequently tolerable. More bothersome side effects are irregular bleeding and depression. Decreasing the dose of progestin may help alleviate these problems, and adding small doses of estrogen may also be used to alleviate side effects once pain relief has been provided.

Can Birth Control Pills Be Used to Treat Endometriosis?

Oral contraceptive pills have been used for many years as a treatment for endometriosis. The pills contain progestin that acts to shrink endometriosis cells. While taking birth control pills is not quite as effective as Danazol or GnRH agonists (see pages 221), they work fairly well for pain relief, have very few bothersome side effects, and are inexpensive. It also appears that women who have been taking birth control pills for contraception have a lower chance of developing endometriosis in the first place. However, it is still unclear whether a woman who has had endometriosis can prevent the disease from returning by taking oral contraceptives. Although the FDA has not approved oral contraceptives solely for the treatment of endometriosis, they are commonly used for this reason. Some physicians prescribe the active pills every day for three to six months before the placebo pills are taken and bleeding occurs. This schedule avoids any pelvic pain associated with bleeding for much of the year.

What Is Danocrine?

Danocrine (trade name Danazol) is a man-made steroid similar to the male hormone testosterone. It lowers the body's production of estrogen, increases the amount of male hormone in a woman's body, and stops the growth of endometrial tissue. Pain relief is improved in up to 90 percent of women taking the medication, but after the danocrine is discontinued, pain often returns within six months. Pregnancy rates, unfortunately, seem to be unaffected following treatment with danocrine.

One of the advantages of danocrine is that it can be taken orally. However, the medication can cause a number of unpleasant male-hormone–related side effects that include weight gain, decreased breast size, acne, growth of facial hair, or deepening of the voice. One of these symptoms occurs in 80 percent of women who take the drug, but only 10 percent of women have side effects to the degree that leads them to stop the medication. Nevertheless, these unpleasant side effects do limit the use of this medication, and today doctors rarely prescribe it.

What Are GnRH Agonist Medications?

Gonadotropin-releasing hormone (GnRH) agonists stop estrogen production in the ovary. The medications work by preventing the pituitary gland from sending the signals to the ovary that causes the production of estrogen. Three preparations are available in the United States. Leuprolide (trade name Lupron) and goserelin (trade name Zoladex) are usually administered by a monthly injection given in the arm, and nafarelin (trade name Synarel) is given by nasal spray twice a day.

The medications all cause similar side effects, which are a direct result of the reduced levels of estrogen. This effect is sometimes referred to as "medical menopause" because the symptoms are similar to the ones many women experience during natural menopause. However, the symptoms go away after the treatment has been completed and the medication wears off. To some degree, women experience side effects that may include hot flashes, night sweats, insomnia, vaginal dryness, headaches, mood changes such as irritability and sadness, and loss of interest in sex. However, these medications do not produce any male-hormone–related side effects such as weight gain, acne, or hair growth. Because decreased estrogen levels may also lead to osteoporosis, some women may have a small reduction in bone mineral density if the treatment is given for longer than six months.

What Is "Add-Back Therapy"?

The side effects of GnRH agonist therapy often limit the use of these medications. One of the concerning side effects is the loss of bone associated with use of the medication for more than six months. To prevent bone loss, small amounts of progestin can be "added back" by giving an oral progestin to the patient. Progestin helps maintain bone density and may decrease the severity and number of hot flashes.

On occasion, low doses of estrogen may also be added back to decrease side effects of GnRH such as hot flashes or vaginal dryness. The dose of estrogen should be low enough to avoid regrowth of the endometriosis. The estrogen can be given orally or by the skin patch. If vaginal dryness is a problem, vaginal estrogen creams, tablets, or ring are often helpful.

Can Some Women Be Treated with Medication Without First Having a Laparoscopy?

Women who are suspected of having endometriosis based on symptoms and pelvic examination may sometimes be treated without a definite diagnosis based on laparoscopy. Women who have mild or moderate pelvic pain can be treated with birth control pills for three months to see if they improve. If so, the pills can be continued until fertility is desired. If pills are not helpful, treatment with GnRH, as described below, or laparoscopic surgery can be considered.

A recent study examined the possibility of treating women with pelvic pain with GnRH agonist before a firm diagnosis was made by laparoscopy. There were a number of conditions for women participating in the study: Pelvic pain other than menstrual cramps must have been present for at least six months. Women must have also tried oral analgesics and birth control pills for pain relief without any success. And women must have had a thorough evaluation to rule out other causes of pain, through careful gynecologic examination, ultrasound, laboratory tests, and referrals to urologists and/or gastroenterologists where appropriate.

Women were then given either GnRH agonist or a placebo for three months, and the amount of pain was assessed and compared to pain before treatment. Women treated with GnRH had a significant decrease in pain compared to the women treated with a placebo. As part of this study, *all* women then had a laparoscopy performed to determine a diagnosis. Interestingly, almost all the women who met the qualifications to be in the study, as described above, had endometriosis.

Let's consider the implications of this study. First, a thorough evaluation, including consideration of bladder and intestinal causes of pain, can accurately determine women who are likely to have endometriosis. Second, the response to treatment with GnRH is very good and may avoid the need for surgery. Other studies indicate that gynecologists do not always recognize endometriosis, or the full extent of endometriosis, at the time of laparoscopy. Therefore, all of the endometriosis may not be removed, either because it is unrecognized or because the surgeon may not possess the training or skill to remove it, so the patient will have undertaken the risk and expense of surgery without much benefit.

If, on the other hand, women who meet the criteria for having endometriosis are first treated with GnRH, most (80 percent) will prove to have endometriosis and will respond to the medication and can avoid surgery. Women who do not respond after three months can then have a laparoscopy performed to determine the cause of pain, either significant endometriosis or another cause. Women who do respond can have the GnRH continued for another three months. Adding progestin has recently been shown to guard against bone loss. About half of these women will have a return of pain within six months of finishing treatment. Retreatment with another six months of GnRH can be used if the woman's pain returns at a later time. Otherwise, laparoscopic surgery can be performed at that time. This overall approach may make sense and be appropriate and acceptable for some women. As always, discuss your situation with your doctor.

Can Pregnancy Cure Edometriosis?

The role of pregnancy in curing endometriosis is still uncertain. During pregnancy, the placenta produces large amounts of both major female hormones, but more progesterone than estrogen. Progesterone is known to suppress the growth of endometriosis, and, therefore, it makes some sense that pregnancy would relieve the pain associated with endometriosis. This beneficial effect may sometimes last for many months, or even years, after delivery. It should be noted that studies suggest that the longer a woman delays her first pregnancy, the more likely it is that she will develop endometriosis. This is another reason, in addition to the limits of a woman's biological clock, to consider having children before your mid-thirties.

Can Surgery Be Used to Treat Endometriosis?

Since endometriosis was first described almost a century ago, surgery has been the mainstay of both diagnosis and treatment. Until the middle of the twentieth century, the usual treatment for bothersome endometriosis consisted of removing the uterus, fallopian tubes, and both ovaries. This is defined as *radical* surgery. In contrast, removal of just areas of endometriosis without the removal of the ovaries or uterus is called *conservative* surgery.

What Is Conservative Surgery?

Conservative surgical treatment is considered when a woman needs surgery for pain or infertility associated with endometriosis, and she desires to preserve her uterus, fallopian tubes, and ovaries. The goal of this approach is to remove as much endometriosis and scar tissue as possible and restore the uterus, fallopian tubes, and ovaries to their normal positions. Conservative surgery can be performed using laparoscopic surgery or an abdominal incision. Newer modalities involving laparoscopic surgical techniques allow for surgery to be performed through very small incisions with the benefit of a shorter hospital stay and quicker recovery time. The results of laparoscopic surgery for relief of pain or enhancement of fertility have been shown to be as good as or better than the results from abdominal surgery. To perform laparoscopic surgery properly, a surgeon needs special training, expertise, and experience.

Can Endometriosis Come Back After Conservative Treatment?

Unfortunately, endometriosis recurs quite frequently after either medical or surgical treatment. After conservative surgery, 40 percent of women will have some evidence of return of the endometriosis within seven years after initial surgery for mild disease. Seventy-five percent of women with severe disease have return of endometriosis within the same time period.

The best results for pain relief occur following excision (surgical removal) of all areas of endometriosis by an experienced surgeon. Some women may require more than one conservative surgical procedure before they need to have, or are willing to consider, a more extensive operation. A woman may elect to have conservative surgery to allow time to complete her family, and then, at a later time, she may elect to undergo the more radical surgery, hysterectomy. Yet, for some women, repeated conservative operations may provide relief of symptoms.

If a patient undergoes a conservative surgical procedure for infertility, her chance of getting pregnant is related to the amount of endometriosis found at surgery. Women who have mild endometriosis have about an 80 to 90 percent chance of becoming pregnant within five years, whether they have the endometriosis removed surgically or not. Women who had moderate endometriosis treated surgically have about a 60 percent chance, and women with severe disease have about a 35 percent chance of getting pregnant following surgery.

Some women will need radical surgery—hysterectomy and removal of the ovaries—to prevent recurrence of endometriosis. At the time of menopause, decreasing amounts of estrogen cause endometriosis to become inactive, and symptoms usually resolve. Most postmenopausal women can take estrogen replacement without recurrence of the endometriosis because the doses of estrogen given are less than the level needed for the endometriosis to survive.

Can Medication and Surgery Be Used Together for Treatment of Pain?

Some physicians suggest treatment with medication for women following surgery. If areas of endometriosis have been left behind or if pain persists right after surgery, medication may be helpful. Mild symptoms may improve with birth control pills, but GnRH agonist may be needed for more bothersome symptoms. One study found 50 percent of women not given medication following surgery needed treatment with medication after eighteen months, while only 33 percent of women treated with GnRH after surgery needed such treatment.

Jessica's Story

Jessica came to see me for the first time when she was twenty-nine years old. Her main complaint was severe pelvic pain. Two years before, she had had abdominal surgery for a large endometrioma in her right ovary. The endometriosis had destroyed her entire ovary, and it was removed during the surgery. Following the operation, she was treated with Danazol for about six months, but decided to stop the treatment because of the weight gain and mood changes she experienced.

One year later she developed severe left-sided pain and underwent a laparoscopy to diagnose the cause. The endometriosis had come back and was now found on the left ovary, the bowel, and the bladder. Again, we were able to remove the visible endometriosis using laparoscopic surgery. I discussed the options with Jessica and her husband. Her options included getting pregnant as soon as possible now that the endometriosis had been surgically removed, or a trial of birth control pills, or Lupron. She did not want to get pregnant at this time and opted for the Lupron. She was on that medication for six months. Her pain improved, but the hot flashes were a problem, and she had insomnia and depression.

Jessica started attempting pregnancy, but the pain came back and was so severe she opted to have another laparoscopy, which was successfully performed. Not long after that, Jessica became pregnant, and we were all delighted. Unfortunately, she had a miscarriage (unrelated to the endometriosis). Jessica and her husband knew that the pain would be too severe to attempt pregnancy on their own again. They decided to undergo IVF (in vitro fertilization). The procedure was successful, and she was pregnant.

At first she had a lot of pain, but as the progesterone from the placenta started to cause the endometriosis to wither away, the pain disappeared. She delivered a beautiful little boy and had no pain while she was breast-feeding him. However, after her body returned to normal hormone levels, the endometriosis started to grow again, and the pain returned. Again, it became intolerable. We restarted the Lupron for another six months, which controlled her symptoms. Jessica knew that she would have to postpone having a hysterectomy if she wanted to try for another baby.

She underwent another laparoscopy. Luckily, there was no evidence of active endometriosis, and we were able to remove some areas of scar tissue around her fallopian tubes and ovaries. Two months later she was pregnant, and the pregnancy went extremely well, and she was again pain free. This time she had a beautiful little girl. But, a year later the pain was back. Jessica and her husband had already decided that they had completed their family. She realized that this disease had controlled her life for the past several years, and she now requested radical surgery, a hysterectomy. At the age of thirty-nine, ten years after her first abdominal surgery, she underwent a laparoscopic hysterectomy and removal of her remaining ovary and fallopian tube. Shortly after her surgery, she was placed on hormone replacement therapy and has done extremely well. She is not entirely pain free, but she is able to enjoy her life and her family.

What Is Radical Surgery?

Radical surgery is the term used to define the removal of the uterus, fallopian tubes, and ovaries as treatment for severe pain sometimes associated with endometriosis. In addition, all obvious areas of endometriosis are removed in an attempt to provide a cure. If the uterus alone is removed, thereafter 90 percent of women will have relief from chronic pelvic pain and 70 percent of women will have relief of pain during intercourse. However, within five years about 60 percent of women will have some pain return, and 30 percent will need another operation for pain. If the ovaries—the source of estrogen stimulation for the endometriosis—are also removed at the time of surgery, about 10 percent of women will note a return of pelvic pain and only about 5 percent will require another operation.

Low-dose estrogen replacement therapy can usually be safely taken following surgical removal of the ovaries. However, in rare instances, the pain from endometriosis can return with estrogen, and the medication may need to be discontinued for relief.

What Happens to Endometriosis After Menopause?

Following menopause the ovaries stop secreting estrogen, the endometriosis begins to shrink, and the symptoms of endometriosis go away. Menopausal women who have had endometriosis can usually take estrogen replacement therapy, in that the dose of estrogen needed to relieve hot flashes, insomnia, vaginal dryness, and protect the heart and bones is usually less than the dose that would cause the endometriosis to grow back.

Can Holistic Treatments Be Used to Treat Endometriosis?

Some women have found relief from symptoms of endometriosis with alternative approaches. These include acupuncture, traditional Chinese medicine, and homeopathic remedies. No formal studies have been undertaken to compare the effectiveness of these alternatives with standard Western treatments, so we are unable to say how successful these approaches are.

What Kind of Research Is Being Done on Endometriosis?

There are still large gaps in our knowledge of endometriosis. Ongoing studies are attempting to better define the causes of endometriosis down to the level of the gene. Researchers are investigating an alphabet soup of biochemical substances to see which ones play a part in the development of this disease. IL-1, IL-6, TNF-a, VEGF, PGE_2, RANTES, and Beta-integrin are just a few examples of research targets.

Easier, less expensive ways of making the diagnosis are being sought. Special chemicals that are attracted to areas of endometriosis have been attached to molecules that can be detected by imaging techniques. It remains to be seen whether this can result in a nonsurgical diagnosis of endometriosis. In addition, adapting these chemicals to provide treatment as well as diagnosis might eliminate surgery entirely. Other studies are looking at novel approaches to treatment, and still others are investigating which women need not be treated at all.

Are There Any Places Where You Can Get Help If You Have Endometriosis?

If you want more information or help, consider contacting the following resources:

Endometriosis Association
8585 North 76th Place
Milwaukee, WI 53223
phone: (800) 992-3636
website: www.endometriosisassn.org

The Endometriosis Association is a self-help group with chapters around the country. It offers meetings, crisis counseling, medical resources, a newsletter, and other literature on endometriosis.

The American Society for Reproductive Medicine
1209 Montgomery Highway
Birmingham, AL 35216-2809
phone: (205) 978-5000
website: www.asrm.org

Resolve
1310 Broadway
Somerville, MA 02144-1731
phone: (888) 623-0744
website: www.resolve.org

Resolve is a national organization with member chapters across the country. It is dedicated to supporting people who are having difficulty becoming parents. It offers meetings, lectures, publications, referrals to specialists, and counseling services. In addition, Resolve is involved in lobbying on behalf of it members.

REFERENCES

ACOG Practice Bulletin. 1999. Medical management of endometriosis. Number 11.

Balasch, J., M. Creus, F. Fabregues, F. Courmona, and J. Ordi Martinez-Roman. 1996. Visible and nonvisible endometriosis at laparoscopy in fertile and infertile women and in patients with chronic pelvic pain: A prospective study. *Human Reproduction* 11:387–91.

Crosignani, P., P. Vercellini, F. Biffignandi, W. Costantini, I. Cortesi, and E. Imparato. 1996. Laparoscopy versus laparotomy in conservative surgical treatment for severe endometriosis. *Fertility and Sterility* 66:706–11.

Endometriosis: Candidate genes. 2001. *Human Reproduction Update* January–February 7(1):15–20

Hornstein, M., E. Surrey, G. Weisberg, and L. Casino. 1998. Leuprolide acetate depot and hormonal add-back in endometriosis: A 12-month study. *Obstetrics and Gynecology* 91:16–24.

Ling, F. 1999. Randomized controlled trial of depot leuprolide in patients with chronic pelvic pain and clinically suspected endometriosis. *Obstetrics ad Gynecology* 93:51–58.

Marcoux, S., R. Maheux, and S. Berube. 1997. Laparoscopic surgery in infertile women with minimal or mild endometriosis. *New England Journal of Medicine* 337:217–22.

Schenken, R., ed. 1989. Endometriosis: Contemporary Concepts in Clinical Management. Philadelphia: J. B. Lippincott.

8

IF YOU HAVE BLADDER PROBLEMS
by Amy E. Rosenman, M.D.

Jessica's Story

"Mom, something is really, really wrong with me," a frantic Jessica blurted out in a phone call from her dorm room. "I feel like there's shards of glass inside of me when I pee. And I just saw blood in the toilet! What should I do?" Luckily, Jessica's mother, Susan, recognized the symptoms of a urinary tract infection and didn't join the panic her nineteen-year-old daughter was experiencing. But hearing the despair in Jessica's voice alarmed her. "Mom, I'm doubled over in pain, and I have to run to the bathroom every five minutes. But when I get there, it hurts so bad I can hardly stand it, and there's barely anything there." Susan started to feel awful herself and urged her daughter go to the student health center on campus right away. "When I've had a urinary tract infection," Susan told Jessica, "the doctor first has me pee in a cup, and they do a urinalysis. Then the doctor usually gives me antibiotics and a medicine that turns my urine bright orange but stops the pain right away. Go now and call me later."

Normal Bladder and Kidneys

The urinary system is composed of two kidneys, two ureters, and the bladder. The kidneys are about the size of your fist and lie inside your abdominal cavity, toward your back and just below the level of your shoulder blades (see fig. 8.1). The kidneys filter waste and toxins out of the blood. The waste is mixed with some water and forms urine.

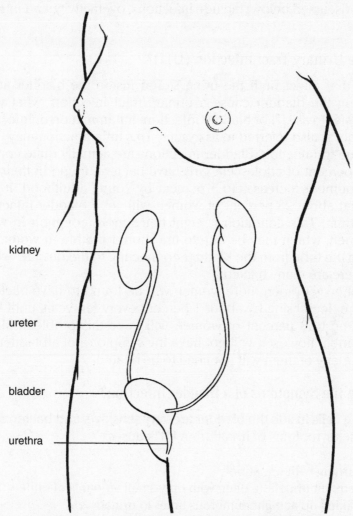

Fig. 8.1. Kidneys, ureters, and bladder

The urine moves down through the ureters—muscular tubes about the diameter of a pencil that run along the spine—and into the bladder. The bladder is a soft, pale pink muscle shaped like a hollow ball that lies in the front of your lower abdomen, right behind the pubic bone. When it is empty, it is about the size of an orange, and when entirely full, it is about the size of a large grapefruit. The front part of the bladder connects to the urethra, the small (about 1½ inches long) muscular tube that carries urine outside of your body. Common problems with the bladder, discussed below, include infections, overactivity, and interstitial cystitis.

What Is a Urinary Tract Infection (UTI)?

Bacteria that infect both the urine stored inside the bladder and the cells lining the bladder cause a urinary tract infection, what we frequently refer to as UTI or bladder infection. Inflammation or infection of the bladder is also referred to as cystitis. This inflammation may or may not be due to infection. Bladder infections are actually quite common. About 1 percent of adolescent girls have bacteria found in their urine, but this number increases to 5 percent by young adulthood. It is estimated that about 25 percent of women will get a bladder infection in their lifetime. This condition is eight times more common in women than in men, which may be due to the shorter urethra in women. The urethra is the tube from the bladder connecting to the outside, which is where there are many bacteria.

As they get older, more women will be found to have bacteria in their urine, increasing by about 1 percent every ten years until by age eighty almost 50 percent of women will have this problem. Many of these women, however, will not have the symptoms of a bladder infection and many of them will not need to be treated.

What Are the Symptoms of a Bladder Infection?

The lining cells inside the bladder are very sensitive, and bacterial infection causes symptoms of irritation. A UTI causes:

- burning with urination
- frequent urination, often with only small amounts of urine
- waking up at night numerous times to urinate
- low pelvic pain, and possibly low back or side pain
- if the infection is more severe, you may see small amounts of blood mixed in with the urine
- a mild fever
- occasionally, the infection may cause such a strong urge to urinate before reaching the toilet that you may not be able to control, and leakage may occur.

Some women have only one of these symptoms; others have a combination of two or more symptoms. Bladder infections generally involve misery and discomfort until you get treated.

Very rarely, a bladder infection can move up the ureters and into the kidneys. Urinary tract infections that involve the kidneys are more serious infections often associated with severe back pain, high fever, nausea, and sometimes vomiting. If these symptoms develop, you should contact your doctor immediately. Untreated kidney infections can cause damage to the kidneys and can lead to spread of infection into the bloodstream and to the entire body.

What Causes Bladder Infections?

The most common cause of bladder infections is sexual intercourse and, as a result, the condition is often called "honeymoon cystitis." About 75 percent of bladder infections start within twenty-four hours following intercourse. All women normally have bacteria on the labia and inside the vagina, and some women have the types of bacteria that are capable of causing a bladder infection. During intercourse these bacteria can be pushed into the urethra and bladder, where they can multiply and cause infection.

Is a Contraceptive Diaphragm a Risk Factor for Bladder Infections?

A number of studies show that diaphragm users are at an increased risk for bladder infections. Although we don't yet fully understand the reasons, it may be that the diaphragm puts pressure on the urethra and causes difficulty emptying the bladder. The longer urine remains in the bladder, the more likely it will become infected with bacteria that also may be present. There may also be some connection between the spermicidal jelly necessary to make the diaphragm a successful contraceptive and the normal, healthy bacteria in the vagina. These healthy and harmless bacteria do not cause bladder infections, but it appears that the spermicide may allow abnormal bacteria to grow in the vagina and gain access to the bladder. The result may be a bladder infection. However, most women who use a diaphragm do not get bladder infections.

Are There More Serious Problems That Can Cause Bladder Infections in Young Women?

Occasionally, a woman may have other medical conditions that increase the likelihood of getting a bladder infection. Diabetes, which causes an increase in sugar in the blood, also increases the sugar filtered into the urine. Since sugar is a nutrient for bacteria and promotes bacterial growth, more bladder infections may occur in a diabetic woman.

Some women are genetically at high risk of forming crystals in their urine that can bind together to form small stones in the kidneys or bladder. If the stones block the flow of urine out of the kidneys, bacteria can grow in the trapped urine and lead to infection. Sometimes, after childbirth, the bladder can bulge or "drop" into the vagina, causing a condition called a cystocele. Urine can remain in the bulging portion of the bladder after you try to empty your bladder. Again, urine that stays in the bladder for a prolonged period of time allows bacteria to grow and can lead to infection. Other uncommon conditions that affect the nervous system and interfere with emptying of the bladder, including multiple sclerosis, paralysis, or spinal cord injuries, may lead to recurring infections.

How Does Our Body Normally Resist Bladder Infections?

Both your anatomy and the nature of urine itself seem designed to help prevent infection. Of course this design is not foolproof, but it has some built-in infection protectors that are always at work. Normally, urine is free of bacteria. It has properties that help to keep it that way. Most bacteria such as the lactobacilli, the bacteria normally found in the vagina, are not able to grow in urine because the acid in the urine kills them. There is also a protein poisonous to bacteria, called urea, which is present in the waste products that are filtered into the urine. These properties of urine all serve to prevent bacterial growth.

Even if a few bacteria get into the bladder, they are flushed out during urination. The design of the bladder wall also has some important defenses that prevent attachment of bacteria to the bladder lining cells. One of these protections is a layer of mucus produced by the lining cells. This mucus keeps the bacteria from sticking to the cells and causing infection.

Why Do Some Women Get Frequent Bladder Infections?

There are genetic differences that affect a person's susceptibility to bladder infections. Scientific studies tell us that women with at least three urinary tract infections per year often have bladder-lining cells that don't make the protective mucus properly. Therefore, bacteria stick more easily to the bladder wall, and infection can be the result.

Other genetic immune factors can increase susceptibility to bladder infections. For reasons that we don't yet understand, women with some subtypes of blood type B or AB have a higher risk of bladder infections than women with other blood types.

How Can a Bladder Infection Be Diagnosed?

We diagnose a bladder infection by examining a sample of urine under the microscope. The urine should be collected properly so that it is not contaminated with bacteria from the skin or vagina. Your doctor should have special wipes in the office bathroom to use to clean around the urethra before giving your urine sample. First you urinate just a little into the toilet to wash out any bacteria near the opening of the urethra. This urine may have bacteria present from the vagina. Then you empty your bladder into a clean container. In rare circumstances, if you are unable to collect a clean specimen, a small tube called a catheter may need to be placed through the urethra into the bladder to collect urine for testing.

Once we obtain a clean specimen of urine, a quick analysis can be performed using a chemical strip known as a "dipstick" that will give information about what's in the urine—red and white blood cells, protein, sugar, pH concentration, and other chemicals. Too much sugar may indicate diabetes, too much protein may indicate a kidney problem. The specimen is then placed in a test tube and spun in a small centrifuge to collect any cells or bacteria at the bottom of the tube. The top portion of the urine is poured out and a drop of the remaining concentrated urine is placed on a slide for viewing under the microscope. If they are present, red and white blood cells as well as bacteria can be seen, and a diagnosis can be made immediately. White blood cells and bacteria are the most common things found in the urine of women with bladder infections. As the body responds to the infection, white blood cells come to the area to devour the bacteria. If the infection irritates the inside lining cells of the bladder, red blood cells may leak out of the irritated areas. About 50 percent of women with a UTI have red blood cells in their urine. When the urinalysis shows bacteria and white blood cells, we begin treatment with an antibiotic immediately.

Another quick test performed in the doctor's office uses a strip of paper containing chemicals sensitive to the by-products of bacteria. If bacteria are present, the paper turns a color. If you have this test combined with a urinalysis, you've had a reasonably accurate series of tests to make a proper diagnosis of a bladder infection. If, however, our view of cells under the microscope is unclear, or the chemical strip test is not clear, or the symptoms differ from the usual, or you have had repeated or difficult-to-cure infections, we will do a urine culture to identify the bacteria and the appropriate antibiotic for treatment.

What Is a Urine Culture and Sensitivity?

The urine culture is a way to take a more precise look at what's causing the infection. The culture involves spreading a small sample of the urine over a gel in a petri dish. This gel is specially formulated to nourish bacteria. Each bacterium in the urine sample multiplies and becomes surrounded by its own offspring. We call this group of bacteria cells a colony. Twenty-four hours later the number of colonies of bacteria that grew in the dish is counted. If there are more than 1,000 colonies, we define that as an infection. The bacteria can be identified by special testing, and they can be tested against different antibiotics to see which will be most effective to destroy them. This is called a sensitivity test. Doing a urine culture and sensitivity involves a bit more time and money. The results are usually back in two days, but sometimes waiting becomes difficult, and the expense is unnecessary. Because of this, most infections are diagnosed with a simple urinalysis.

Do Bacteria in the Bladder Always Cause Symptoms?

No, the vast majority of women who have bacteria in the bladder will not develop symptoms. In fact, more than half of these women will get better by themselves without any treatment. Even if symptoms are present, most women will get better without any treatment. However, since there is no way of knowing which women will not get better, most physicians will treat women who have both symptoms and bacteria found in the urine.

There are some women who have a condition known as asymptomatic bacteriuria. They have no symptoms of UTI, yet on multiple cultures the urine grows a large number of bacteria. These women seldom have significant white blood cells in the urine, indicating no active infection. Sometimes asymptomatic bacteriuria is found on a routine exam. If there are no symptoms, it is not necessary to be treated for this condition.

Is There Any Benefit to Testing Women Who Have No Symptoms?

There are only two circumstances where it is worthwhile to test to see if an infection is present in women who have no symptoms. If a woman is having surgery on the bladder or kidneys, she is at a higher risk of developing an infection after surgery even if there is only a small amount of bacteria found in the urine. Eliminating these bacteria beforehand will reduce the risk of serious infections after surgery. So before any bladder or kidney surgery, we do a urinalysis. Pregnant women should have their urine tested on a regular basis because a simple bladder infection in a pregnant woman is more likely to go up into the kidneys and become a serious infection.

How Is a Bladder Infection Treated?

Although some bladder infections will go away by themselves, most physicians will choose to treat an infection to make sure it does not get any worse or possibly infect the kidneys. Antibiotics, taken by mouth, are the best treatment for a bladder infection. Many types of antibiotics will be effective to cure the most common infections.

Nitrofurantoin (Macrodantin) is an ideal antibiotic for most bladder infections because it becomes very concentrated in the urine while staying at a very low level in the blood. Therefore, it does not reach other areas of the body very well and does not disturb the normal bacteria found in the vagina or intestine. As a result, nitrofurantoin does not lead to vaginal infections or diarrhea. Another advantage of this medication is that even after thirty years of use, very few bacteria have been able to develop resistance to it, so it is still very effective.

Another commonly used medication is the combination of trimethoprim and sulfamethoxazole (TMP-SMX, Bactrim, Septra), a sulfa drug. This combination treats a wide range of bladder infections and can be given conveniently by mouth twice a day. There are very few side effects, and bacteria rarely become immune to these medications. However, these medications have a moderate effect on the normal vaginal and intestinal bacteria, and some women report getting diarrhea or a vaginal infection.

We now have some newer antibiotics that are effective as well. The group of drugs that includes ciprofloxacin (Cipro) and norfloxacin (Noroxin) work well against even more than the usual bacteria. These antibiotics are best saved for those bacteria that do not respond to the routine medications, or for recurring or complicated cases. These newer drugs are very expensive and have no advantage in treating the simple bladder infection over the more standard therapies. Unfortunately, ciprofloxacin is the fourth most commonly prescribed antibiotic in the United States, and its overuse has led to bacterial resistance. Some strains of *E. coli*, the most common cause of bladder infection, are now resistant to ciprofloxacin. Other medications can be used for recurrent or difficult-to-cure infections or for women allergic to the commonly used antibiotics.

Are There Medications That Help with the Burning and Pain of a Bladder Infection?

There are medications designed to collect in the urine and relieve the symptoms of infection while an antibiotic is working to kill the bacteria. Medications such as phenazopyradine hydrochloride (Pyridium) are very effective for relieving bladder pain. These medications are not designed to cure infection; therefore, it is very important to take the antibiotics until they are finished even if you feel well. If you do not finish the antibiotic, you may only kill the weaker bacteria and leave behind stronger, more resistant bacteria. These bacteria will grow back and be much more difficult to treat. Also, drink plenty of water when you are recovering from a UTI. Water will dilute the bacteria and flush them out of your bladder.

How Long Should Antibiotics Be Taken?

There are as many answers to this question as there are petals on a daisy. To treat infrequent bladder infections from common bacteria, the choices vary from one dose of medication to two weeks of treatment. Short courses of antibiotics—three days of medication rather than the usual five to seven days of therapy—have been shown to be very effective in eradicating bladder infections. Even a one-day therapy exists, taken in the form of a powder dissolved in juice. Bactrim or Septra, taken twice a day for three days, is a very effective treatment. Three days of TMP-SMX taken twice a day minimizes side effects and cost. Nitrofurantoin needs to be taken for five to seven days to be as effective, but it is very inexpensive and results in few side effects.

Women with other complicating factors such as diabetes, prior kidney infection, recent bladder infection, or a history of childhood bladder problems should take the longer seven to ten days of treatment to be sure all the bacteria have been killed.

If all the symptoms of a urinary tract infection go away, no follow-up testing is needed. Persistence of symptoms requires further testing, including a urine culture to see if resistant organisms are present in the urine. If bacteria are found that are resistant to the first antibiotic, the sensitivity test will tell us that. It will also tell us what antibiotic is likely to work, and treatment can be changed appropriately. Usually, we then recommend a longer, seven- to ten-day course of the appropriate antibiotic.

Suzanne's Story

Suzanne is a busy stay-at-home mom with three young children. Michael, the youngest, is now five months old and spends his days contentedly nursing, whereas Amy and Eliza attend nursery school and kindergarten. After Michael's birth, Suzanne went to her obstetrician for a six-week postpartum checkup and got the go-ahead to resume sexual relations with her husband. The next morning she needed to urinate every hour and began to feel a burning while urinating.

She immediately went back to see her doctor and was asked to give a urine sample. "That was no problem for me. I felt as if I needed to go every other minute anyway," she told us laughingly. The urinalysis showed the presence of white blood cells, red blood cells, and bacteria. Suzanne was given antibiotics and instructed to take them twice a day for three days. She was also given Pyridium tablets to take three times a day for three days. Pyridium made the urine a bright orange but stopped the burning within a few hours. The urgency and frequency also improved. In twenty-four hours Suzanne was substantially better.

Two weeks later, again after intercourse, the same thing happened. "Tom and I were beginning to think there was a plot against us . . . not getting much sleep because of the baby, and now this—I may never have sex again." This time the doctor did a culture. It showed an *E. coli* infection that should have been cured by the antibiotic that she had taken. We treated her with another antibiotic for ten days. After a few days she felt better, and after a few more days the urinary tract infection was completely gone. After abstaining from sex for two weeks, she once again had intercourse with her husband, and the whole UTI started all over again. "Now I really got worried," Suzanne told us. "I began to wonder if Tom had something and was intentionally infecting me. I started to think he'd been fooling around or something." Suzanne returned to her doctor again. This time the doctor explained that some women are prone to having bowel bacteria grow in the vagina instead of the usual lactobacillus. When the antibiotics are stopped, the *E. coli* are reintroduced into the bladder with sexual activity. Suzanne's doctor prescribed one tablet of an antibiotic to be taken each time Suzanne and her husband had sexual relations. This small dose was enough to kill any bacteria that might be introduced during intercourse. They lived happily ever after.

What If My Infection Comes Back?

Seventy-five percent of women who get a bladder infection will get less than one infection a year. However, 25 percent of women will get two or three a year. For women who are getting repeated infections, a culture of the urine after finishing treatment helps to make sure all the bacteria are killed.

For women who are prone to repeated infections (culture-proven recurrent infections), one of three strategies can be tried. Since infection often follows intercourse, treatment with one antibiotic pill after intercourse often works well to prevent repeated infections. If repeat infections are not related to intercourse, taking one antibiotic pill at bedtime (it stays in the urine overnight and is more effective) for three to six months will often cure repeated infections.

Another choice is called self-start therapy. The patient is given a supply of antibiotics and starts taking them at the first sign of symptoms. The antibiotics are continued for a full course of therapy. The success of these strategies will depend on treating a developing infection right at the beginning with a small dose of medication that will have minimal effect on the normal bacteria of the bowel and vagina. This avoids side effects and the development of resistant strains. Drinking real cranberry juice or extract (not apple juice flavored with cranberry) can also help avoid bladder infections by preventing bacteria from sticking to the bladder lining, allowing them to be flushed out of the bladder before they have a chance to cause trouble.

If the infections might be related to using a diaphragm for birth control, a smaller diaphragm that does not press on the urethra might be tried. Otherwise, another birth control method should be considered. In menopausal women, it is often necessary to treat thinning of the vaginal lining with estrogen to restore normal, healthy bacteria and reduce UTI recurrence. Sometimes women who are breast-feeding and not ovulating also have a low estrogen level, thinning of the vaginal lining, and frequent infections. Vaginal estrogen, available in cream, vaginal tablets, or vaginal ring, works well for them as well.

What Tests Are Required If You Have More Than Three Bladder Infections a Year?

If you have more than three bladder infections in one year, it is a good idea to be evaluated to make sure nothing more serious is going on. We would begin by emptying the bladder with a catheter to ensure that it is not contaminated by bacteria in the vagina. Using the catheter we are also able to measure how much urine is left behind after you try to empty your bladder—called a postvoid residual. Less than three ounces left behind is normal. More than three ounces means you are only partly emptying your bladder, and the urine that sits in the bladder has a greater chance of getting infected. If you are not able to empty your bladder, we may suggest other tests to find out why.

Other tests may also be needed to make sure the kidneys and ureters are not the source of repeated infections. The kidneys and ureters can be evaluated by either ultrasound—a picture of the kidneys made with sound waves—or with an X-ray called an IVP, or a CAT scan of the kidneys. Any of these tests can look for abnormalities of the kidneys and ureters such as stones, abscesses, or tumors, all of which can increase the chance of infection. Cystoscopy, examining the inside of the bladder with a small telescope, will usually be recommended as well. This procedure is performed painlessly in the doctor's office with a local anesthetic gel applied to the urethra. We are looking for a stone, a polyp or, *very rarely*, an early malignancy that might be responsible for repeated infections.

What Is Urethritis?

There are two small lubricating glands, one on either side of the opening of the urethra, called periurethral glands (see fig. 8.1). These glands can become infected and cause symptoms of burning and urgency similar to a bladder infection. However, when the urine is tested, no infection is found. Infection of these glands is called urethritis. The diagnosis can often be made if there is tenderness of the urethra when gently pressed on examination. The cause of these infections is somewhat different than the causes of simple bladder infections. Two bacteria-like organisms called chlamydia and mycoplasma are the most common offenders.

Chlamydia and mycoplasma are difficult to culture, but can be identified with a swab from the urethra that is tested for the DNA of these organisms. This method is accurate and faster than a culture and ideally suited for organisms that are difficult to culture. Once identified, the infection can be treated with appropriate antibiotics such as tetracycline, erythromycin, or azithromycin.

Noninfectious causes of urethral irritation may include allergy or chemical sensitivity to a spermicide or thinning of the tissue due to lack of estrogen. This thinning, as mentioned earlier regarding the bladder, can occur after menopause or after childbirth, when very high estrogen levels decrease rapidly.

What Is an Overactive Bladder?

Most women who drink a normal amount of liquid (four eight-ounce glasses per day) will urinate about eight times in twenty-four hours. Those who urinate more frequently in the absence of other causes have an overactive bladder (OAB). Usually, these women are otherwise healthy but need to urinate about every two hours during the day and get up two times or more every night to urinate. Most cases of overactive bladder have no known or obvious cause. *Very rare* causes of bladder overactivity are nerve damage caused by injury, multiple sclerosis, or stroke.

Allison's Story

Allison strode into the office frustrated and upset. As her story tumbled out, we could hear the fear and anger in her voice. "Two months ago I went away for the weekend—just a simple weekend getaway," she told us. "I needed to stay within three feet of a bathroom the whole time. It was a weekend to forget." Allison phoned her family doctor, who kindly listened to her symptoms and prescribed three days of antibiotics. She felt a little better, but one week later she felt "roped to the bathroom again." She never had any burning, but her family doctor suggested that perhaps she had a bladder infection and prescribed ten days of a different antibiotic. Allison once again felt a little better, but the symptoms never completely went away.

She went to see the doctor. A urinalysis was clear, but since she still had symptoms, the doctor did a urine culture. After two days, the culture was negative—no bacteria, no infection. "Now I was really starting to get scared. If this was not a UTI, what was it? How am I going to get back to normal?" At this point, her family doctor referred Allison to our practice. We asked Allison to keep a voiding diary, which showed that she was urinating frequently and getting up three or four times at night. A complete physical exam with no abnormal signs, coupled with a clear urine culture, added up to a diagnosis of overactive bladder. "Okay," Allison said in both relief and resignation, "now that I have that, what can we do about it?"

Are There Treatments for an Overactive Bladder?

Methods for treating an overactive bladder include dietary changes, pelvic muscle exercises, biofeedback, fluid restriction, timed voiding, and medication. A discussion of each treatment follows.

How Does Diet Affect an Overactive Bladder?

One of the simplest ways to treat an overactive bladder is to see if anything in your diet is causing your bladder to be overactive. Simple dietary changes may bring immediate relief. Some drinks containing alcohol or caffeine act as diuretics. Drinking coffee, tea, and sodas with caffeine will increase the quantity of urine, resulting in more trips to the bathroom.

Some foods irritate the bladder, causing it to want to empty. These are often acidic foods such as citrus or carbonated beverages (they contain carbonic acid). Spicy foods may also irritate the bladder. Eliminating these irritants from the diet may be all that is needed. Experimentation often leads to relief. First, eliminate all the potentially irritating foods for two weeks. If the symptoms go away, the next task is to identify which of the foods is the culprit. Try introducing one of these foods each week to see which one causes a return of the symptoms. Usually, it becomes clear which food or foods irritates you. Then it will be your choice: Eat that particular food and deal with the consequences or forgo it for greater comfort.

What Are Voiding Diary, Timed Voiding, and Fluid Management?

These three elements are essentials of a medication-free approach to the overactive bladder. A voiding diary is a record of trips to the bathroom to urinate. This record can be kept for as little as two days to as long as two weeks. The record may include the time you voided and measurements of urine quantity as well as estimates of how much you drink. It gives your doctor a record and a baseline of bladder activity. This record can be evaluated by a specialized nurse and assessed for the time interval between trips to the bathroom. We then try to systematically lengthen the time between trips. This is done by voiding by the clock or "timed voiding." This method utilizes distraction and Kegel contractions to try to retrain the bladder to be emptied at ever-expanding intervals. Fluid management refers to the regulation of what we drink and when, for what goes in will definitely have to come out at some point. Four glasses of water per day (32 ounces) is plenty of fluids to consume each day. Too much of a good thing will overtax even a healthy bladder. Some magazine articles have led women to believe they need to drink eight glasses of water for the sake of their complexions, their kidneys, and to "wash away toxins." None of this is true, and too much fluid has caused bladder problems and accidents for many women.

How Can Biofeedback and Pelvic Floor Exercises Help with an Overactive Bladder?

If you squeeze your pelvic floor muscles, a natural reflex will cause your bladder to relax and quiet down. This comes in handy when there's no bathroom nearby, and you need a little relief. Strengthening the pelvic floor muscles will also help prevent urinary incontinence as well as add pleasure to your sex life. Dr. Arnold Kegel first described these exercises in the late 1940s. They are simple to do but must be done every day to remain effective.

You can figure out which muscles to contract for the Kegel exercises by sitting on the toilet with your legs slightly apart. Start to urinate normally, but after a few seconds, without moving your legs, try to stop the stream of urine. If you are able to stop the stream of urine, you are probably using the correct muscles. You should contract these muscles ten times in standing, sitting, and reclining positions, at least three times per day—for a total of ninety contractions per day. Once you learn to do Kegels, avoid doing them while urinating, as this may lead to problems emptying your bladder.

Improvement won't be immediate, but in a few weeks to a few months you will probably notice some improvement. The good news is that about 70 percent of women will notice improvement from these exercises within six months.

Biofeedback is a helpful tool that assists with learning pelvic floor exercises. A small sponge with a wire attached is placed in the vagina to sense when the proper muscles are being contracted. When Kegel exercises are performed correctly, the contraction will be displayed on a computer screen. You are using your vision (biologic) to reinforce correct performance of the muscle contraction (feedback).

Sharon Gets in Shape

Sharon was determined to get in shape this year. It was a New Year's resolution for the past three years, but this year she was determined to reach her goal: She would be thin by thirty. Sharon started a sensible diet plan filled with fruits and vegetables and joined a gym. She traveled around town with her water bottle in its handy carrier slung over her shoulder, sipping water constantly throughout the day. Her goal was to finish three one-liter bottles before sunset. All was well. Success was within her reach. She had already lost seventeen pounds and felt she was in the best shape in years when she came in for her annual exam and asked if it was "normal" to urinate every two hours day and night. She was getting up three or four times every night to urinate and was stopping at every public restroom in town.

I explained to her that this was not a normal voiding pattern. Over eight trips to the bathroom in twenty-four hours borders on the excessive, and she was going at least twelve times! We requested she keep a voiding diary for two days. Sharon was drinking almost a gallon of fluids a day, including all her water. The fruits and vegetables were composed of mostly water as well. I explained to Sharon that she was doing too much of a good thing. There was nothing wrong with her bladder, but a little "fluid management" was in order. We asked Sharon to limit her drinking to one liter of water per day instead of three. She was back to urinating every three or four hours and waking up only once to go at night. Problem solved.

What Medications Are Available to Treat OAB?

There are medications that are designed to reduce frequent urination and urgency. These medications interfere with the nerve signals that make the bladder overactive. The most commonly used medications are tolteradine (Detrol), oxybutynin (Ditropan), imipramine (Tofranil), and hyoscyamine (Levsin). Although overactive bladder is a long-term condition, very often medication can be used for about six months, until pelvic floor exercise and behavioral therapy become effective.

All of these medications are part of the solution. They cause mild side effects that include dry mouth, dry skin, slight constipation, and possibly blurry vision. Both tolteradine and oxybutynin are available in convenient once-a-day doses, which have fewer of these annoying side effects. Sometimes, imipramine can be used in combination with the other medications, which may boost their effectiveness. Imipramine was originally developed to combat depression, but it was discovered that lower doses are effective in reducing urination urgency and frequency.

Estrogen may be helpful to the perimenopausal or postpartum woman suffering from OAB. Estrogen can be both taken orally and vaginally. New vaginal delivery systems for estrogen are great improvements over the creams that were the only product available in the past. Estrogen cream was messy to use, and the applicators were difficult to clean. A new vaginal ring (Estring) is made of silastic and contains estrogen. This ring is as effective as the creams are in reducing OAB. The estrogen slowly seeps out of the ring and into the vaginal tissue over a three-month period of time. This ring is comfortable, and you should not be aware of its presence. The only care that is necessary is changing the ring every three months. Another new product, called Vagifem, is a small tablet of estrogen that is placed in the vagina with its own small disposable applicator. The tablet has a bioadhesive on the surface so that it stays put. The tablets are inserted twice a week. The narrow applicator is comfortable to use, and there is not even a trace of the pill noticeable by the user. It is also easy and as effective as estrogen creams.

What Is Interstitial Cystitis (IC)?

Interstitial cystitis (IC) is a bladder condition associated with urgency, frequency, and bladder and pelvic discomfort or pain. For reasons that are not understood, 90 percent of people who get IC are women. This condition has been known by many other names over the years including chronic cystitis, urgency-frequency syndrome, and painful bladder syndrome. Many women with IC are treated over and over again with antibiotics even though urine cultures show no infection.

This condition only became clear to physicians in the 1980s. Prior to that, most of these women were thought to have recurrent or chronic infections that just were not showing up on the cultures. Symptoms of IC may include pain near the pubic bone, the bladder, near the vagina, on the insides of the thighs, or low back pain. The pain is usually worse when the bladder is full. Because the bladder is next to the vagina, pain with intercourse is common.

The cause, or causes, of IC are not clear. Theories include an auto-immune disease, where the immune system may attack the lining of the bladder; an abnormal bladder lining possibly caused by an infection or chemical exposure; or a sensitivity much like a food allergy.

How Is IC Diagnosed?

When we see a woman with the symptoms described above, we suspect IC. To make a definitive diagnosis, it is helpful if a woman keeps a record of how often she urinates during the day and night, called a voiding diary, to help us interpret the frequency issue. Cystoscopy, inspection of the bladder wall under anesthesia, may reveal inflammation or small ulcers sometimes seen with IC. A helpful test is called the potassium chloride challenge test. This is performed by putting a solution of potassium chloride into the bladder with a catheter. Women with IC will have discomfort with the potassium chloride, and women without IC will not. Even though this test is unpleasant, it is helpful to establish the correct diagnosis so that proper treatment can be started.

How Is IC Treated?

Fortunately, there are many treatments now available for IC. The condition is a chronic one, but it can go into remission, and there are a number of medications that can be used in combination to effectively treat it. Elmiron (pentosan polysulfate) is FDA approved for the treatment of IC. This medication may help the bladder lining cells to protect the bladder wall from irritation. It is taken by mouth three times a day and may take three months before results are noticeable. Tolteradine and oxybutynin are medications that reduce the overactivity of the bladder and may also be effective. Hydroxizine (Atarax) is an antihistamine that counteracts increased amounts of this biochemical that can contribute to pain. This medication may also require three months to be effective. Amitriptyline (Elavil) was developed as an antidepressant, but in low doses it has been found to be effective in treating many conditions associated with chronic pain. Neurontin, originally developed to treat seizures, is useful as well with chronic pain. L-arginine, an amino acid, and Cytotec, an ulcer medication, have been helpful to some IC sufferers. Tagamet, an over-the-counter antacid, can give relief by reducing the acidity of the urine.

Some women notice that acidic foods increase the symptoms of IC. Avoiding citrus, apples, grapes, tea, tomatoes, and peppers will often help the symptoms of IC. Also, frequent sips of water will work to dilute irritants and acids in the bladder. However, drinking more than four glasses of water a day may lead to more frequent urination and make the symptoms worse. Calcium citrate, 1,200 to 1,500 mg daily, can also help counteract the acidity in your diet.

There are medications that can be placed directly into the bladder with a catheter. Many women can be taught to do this at home. The medication solution often includes a local anesthetic to immediately reduce the pain. DMSO (dimethyl sulfoxide) is FDA approved for this type of therapy. It appears to reduce bladder inflammation and is effective in about 40 percent of women with IC. Heparin and BCG (a bacterial vaccine) have also proven to be helpful for some women.

Bladder training can also be very helpful for women with IC. Begin by keeping a written record of how often you urinate and how often you feel pain over two days. Next, calculate the average time between urinating. The following day, add fifteen minutes to the average time, and delay voiding until then. If you get a strong urge to void, use Kegel contractions to help delay your next trip to the bathroom. Each week add another fifteen minutes to the time between trips until a comfortable schedule is reached. It may take a few months to reduce urgency and frequency.

Are There Procedures That Can Help with IC?

With a patient under anesthesia during cystoscopy, the bladder can be overfilled with water. This procedure, called hydrodistention, may give relief for up to twelve months. The mechanical stretching of the bladder may interfere with pain signals transmitted by the bladder nerves and result in decreased pain. About 60 percent of women with IC get relief from hydrodistention.

Is This Condition Possibly All in My Head?

Despite years of some doctors suggesting to women that this condition had psychological roots, we are now certain that IC is in the bladder, not in the head. The stress and strain of this chronic painful condition can lead to anxiety and depression, but it starts in the bladder.

Maggie's Story

Maggie was a psychologist with a busy urban practice. She measured her days in fifty-minute "hours" to accommodate the appointments she scheduled for her clients. She had been treated by her internist for multiple bladder infections before coming to see us. She didn't understand why, if her infection was gone, her symptoms still remain. Not only was she still symptomatic with urgency and frequency, but she was developing increasingly annoying pelvic pain as well. In the past three months, even intercourse with her husband caused immediate pelvic pain and was followed by worsening of her bladder pain and irritability. She was distraught and confused. Her workday was a challenge since she could only go to the bathroom in between clients. Maggie struggled to get through each patient session, so she could run to get some relief. "Just to get through a fifty-minute hour is a struggle!" she exclaimed. "I can hardly pay attention to the woes of my clients. I feel like a bladder on two feet! I am always thinking about needing to go." Things were going from bad to worse. "I am at the end of my rope."

After a complete evaluation, a diagnosis of IC was made. At first this alarmed Maggie, but once she started on treatment with Elmiron and some bladder infusions, her symptoms improved. After six months she was in a full remission, able once again to deal with the problems her patients brought her instead of feeling like she was the problem.

RESOURCES

Interstitial Cystitis Association of America (ICA)
51 Monroe St., Suite 1402
Rockville, MD 20850
phone: (301) 610-5300
toll-free: (800) 435-7422
fax: (301) 610-5308
e-mail: ICAmail@ichelp.org
website: www.ichelp.org

National Association for Continence (NAFC)
P.O. Box 8310
Spartanburg, SC 29305-8310
phone: (864) 579-7900
toll-free: (800) BLADDER, (800) 252-3337
fax: (864) 579-7902
e-mail: memberservices@nafc.org
website: www.nacf.org

REFERENCES

Karram, M. 1996. "Lower urinary tract infection." In *Urogynecology and Urodynamics*, edited by Donald R. Ostergard and Alfred E. Bent, pp. 387–408. Baltimore, Md.: Williams and Wilkins.

Lobel, R., and P. Sand. 1996. "Urinary tract dysfunction in adolescents and young women." In *Urogynecology and Urodynamics*, edited by Donald R. Ostergard and Alfred E. Bent, pp. 307–322. Baltimore, Md.: Williams and Wilkins.

9

ABNORMAL PAP SMEARS, HPV, CERVICAL DYSPLASIA, AND CERVICAL CANCER

What Is Cervical Dysplasia and Carcinoma in Situ?

During sexual intercourse, viruses or other as-yet-unidentified cancer-causing agents may get into the cells of the cervix and cause them to grow abnormally. This abnormal tissue growth is called dysplasia. Early on, dysplastic cells stay within the cervical skin. The skin has no blood or lymph vessels that the abnormal cells can invade and, therefore, they have no way to leave the cervix and spread to other areas of the body. Because dysplasia is confined to the skin, it is easy to treat.

In the past, the term *carcinoma in situ* (CIS) was used if the abnormal cells occupied the full thickness of the cervical skin (see fig. 9.1). However, the presence of the word *carcinoma* often implied that the patient had cancer. But carcinoma in situ is not cancer; it is a severe form of dysplasia, and the abnormal cells still remain confined within the skin. CIS cannot spread to other areas of the body. In order to eliminate this confusion, the term *carcinoma in situ* was replaced with the term *high-grade dysplasia* (see page 258). However, if high-grade dysplasia is left untreated over a number of years, the cells may eventually break through the skin layer and invade the layer beneath, where blood and lymph vessels exist. These cells can now spread to other areas of the body and cervical cancer (see page 271) is present.

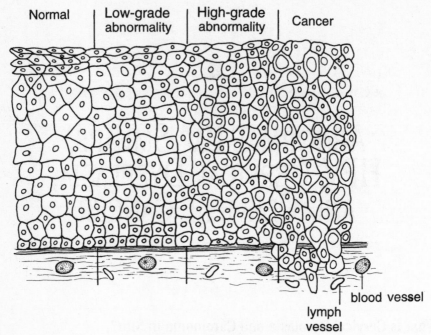

Fig. 9.1. Cervical cells

Where Do These Abnormal Cells Develop?

As previously described in chapter 1, the cervix is the opening into the uterus and can be seen inside the top of the vagina (see fig. 9.2a). The lining cells of the uterus are tall, column-shaped cells, and the cells of the vaginal skin are thin and flat. The area where the lining cells of the uterus meet with the cells of the vagina is called the "transformation zone," i.e., the area where one type of cell changes into another type of cell (see fig. 9.2b). The cells near the transformation zone appear to be particularly vulnerable to carcinogens, substances that can cause cancer. The transformation zone is where cervical dysplasia and cancer develops.

What Causes Cervical Dysplasia and Cancer?

By far the most common cause of abnormal cervical cells known today is a group of viruses called human papillomavirus (HPV). This group of viruses has also been called genital wart virus or condylloma virus. These viruses are very common and have been found in 10 percent of all apparently healthy women. The HPV viruses are actually a group of

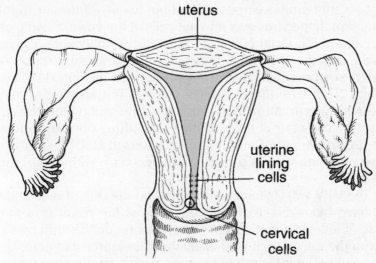

Fig. 9.2a.   The cervix is the opening of the uterus,
found at the top of the vagina.

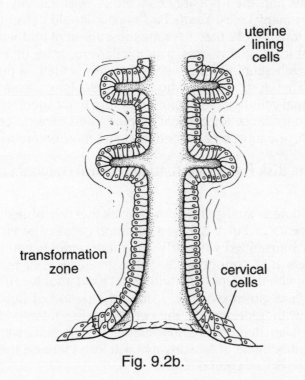

Fig. 9.2b.

about seventy similar viruses, and about twenty of these can infect the genital skin. If the virus gets into the cells of the vulva, vagina, or cervix, it can alter the normal growth of the cells. A noticeable overgrowth of the skin, called condylloma or genital wart, may result. These warts can be felt or seen as small raised, rough bumps on the outside of the vagina or penis. They are almost always painless but sometimes may cause some itching or irritation. If the virus is just present on the cervix, usually no symptoms occur at all, and there is nothing obvious to feel. When there are no symptoms and nothing obvious to feel, the only way to detect whether the virus is present on the cervix is with a Pap smear (see page 257).

The HPV virus is most often found on the skin of men and women who have been infected with the virus as the result of sexual intercourse. While virus particles have been found on the underwear of people with the infection, it is unlikely that this source can actually lead to the spread of the infection to another person. If your sexual partner has the virus on his penis, it may enter the skin cells of the cervix (or vagina or vulva) and cause these cells to grow abnormally, progressing to first precancerous and then possibly cancerous cells. Luckily, this process usually takes many years. Yearly Pap smears should detect the changes in the cells long before they become too abnormal and while they are easily treatable. In other words, with the Pap smear we can see cervical abnormalities beginning long before they are actually a threat to your well-being. Therefore, women who have annual Pap smears are likely to have abnormal cells detected before they turn into cancer. HPV is probably not the only cause for cervical dysplasia and cervical cancer, but it appears to be the most clearly identified and most common cause.

What Are the Risk Factors for Getting Cervical Dysplasia and Cancer?

Having multiple sexual partners increases the risk of getting cervical dysplasia or cancer. Since the most common cause of cervical cancer is the sexually transmitted virus HPV, the more partners you have, or the more partners your partner has had, the greater is your risk of coming into contact with the virus. One additional risk factor for HPV is the age at which you begin intercourse. During the period of hormonal shifts that occurs with adolescence, the cervical cells undergo changes that appear to make them more susceptible to infection with the virus. Therefore, intercourse at an early age will also increase the risk of getting cervical dysplasia and cancer.

While some cancers are more common in certain families, cervical cancer does not appear to be an inheritable disease. So if a family member has had cervical cancer, your risk of getting this disease should be no greater than anyone else's risk.

Can Smoking Increase Your Risk of Cervical Dysplasia and Cancer?

The risk of cervical cancer is definitely higher in women who smoke. Normally, your immune system removes bacteria, viruses, and abnormal cells from your body every day. Smoking appears to have a detrimental effect on the immune system, making it less effective. If not removed by the immune system, the abnormal cells may, over a period of many months or years, develop into cancer cells.

In addition, when you smoke, nicotine is absorbed through your lungs into your bloodstream and then is transported to all the cells in your body. In the body, nicotine breaks down into chemicals known to cause cancer. The cells of the cervix appear to be especially susceptible to these chemicals. For women who have smoked, the risk of developing dysplasia of the cervix is three to four times greater than for women who have never smoked. The risk increases with the amount of smoking, so that the risk of dysplasia is twelve times greater in women who have smoked a pack of cigarettes a day for twelve years. The risk for developing actual cancer of the cervix is two times greater in smokers. Luckily, if you stop smoking, the risk decreases as time goes on.

Smoking has not been shown to increase the risk of breast or ovarian cancer. However, smoking does cause heart disease. The increase in the mortality rate for women from heart attacks has directly followed the increase in the number of women who smoke. As a result, the risk of women dying from a heart attack is now close to being the same as that for men of comparable ages. The health risks of smoking are enormous— there are *many* reasons not to smoke.

How Common Is HPV?

HPV is a very common virus, and can be found in about 10 percent of all women. Some studies have found the virus in as many as 20 percent of women college students. However, the presence of the virus does not necessarily lead to problems, because some types of the virus never cause symptoms or abnormalities shown on a Pap smear. Many women apparently live with the virus without any problems ever developing. In other cases, the virus can be eradicated by the body's own defenses without any treatment at all. In fact, some studies show that about two-thirds of women with the virus will eliminate it over time. Nevertheless, if you have an abnormal Pap smear, you may require some treatment to control the virus.

Fran's Cryotherapy for HPV

Fran is a twenty-five-year-old woman who came to the office for her yearly examination with our nurse-practitioner. On the outside of the vagina, the nurse-practitioner noticed some raised areas that looked like HPV. Fran was unaware of these areas, and they were not tender to touch during the exam. The inside of the vagina was entirely normal, and the cervix appeared clear as well. A Pap smear was taken. In order to determine if the bumps were HPV, the nurse-practitioner injected the area with a very small syringe containing local anesthesia, and a small piece of skin was removed. When the results came back from the lab, they confirmed the presence of HPV. Subsequently, Fran's Pap smear came back entirely normal. Although the abnormal area was small and not causing any problem, we recommended to Fran that the skin be treated. This would prevent any spread of the virus to larger areas of the vagina or to her partner. In addition, we recommended that Fran's partner be evaluated by his doctor for the presence of the virus (see page 261).

Using a small, very cold metal instrument, the skin was frozen for about three minutes. The procedure caused a stinging sensation for a minute or so. After the treatment was finished, we told Fran to soak in a warm tub twice a day if she had any discomfort. Over time, new skin would replace the skin that was frozen and destroyed. When she returned for her next appointment two weeks later, the only evidence of the freezing was a slightly red tint near the area of the treated skin. We checked her again in two months, and there was no evidence of any of the old virus or any new virus. Luckily, Fran's regular, annual gynecologic exam detected the virus early and prevented the problem from becoming too advanced. However, HPV can sometimes be present but undetected. In addition, reinfection with the virus is possible. Therefore, Fran was advised to continue to have routine Pap smears and checkups in the future.

Are Some Types of HPV Worse Than Others?

It appears so. The different types of the HPV virus differ by small changes in their structure. The viral types are numbered 1 to 70, with new types added as they are discovered. The specific type of HPV can be determined only by sophisticated laboratory testing. We currently know that twenty of the seventy types of HPV are capable of causing the cervical cells to become dysplastic or cancerous. The types of HPV have been grouped together according to their risk of causing cervical dysplasia or cancer. HPV types 16, 18, 45, and 56 are aggressive types of the virus and are in the high-risk group for causing dysplasia or cancer. These are the most common types of the virus actually found in cervical cancer cells. On the other hand, viral types 6 and 11 do not appear to cause cervical cancer, even if they are left untreated. Therefore, they are considered low-risk types of HPV.

What Are the Symptoms of Cervical Dysplasia or Cancer?

Unfortunately, cervical dysplasia and early cervical cancer do not cause any warning symptoms. The abnormal cells *do not* cause pain, irritation, bleeding, or discharge early on, at a time that treatment might be easily accomplished. Later, cervical cancer can destroy the cervical cells to the point that bleeding or constant discharge occurs, but at that point treatment is difficult. This is why early detection of abnormal cells by means of the Pap smear is so important.

How Do We Diagnose Cervical Dysplasia and Cancer?—The Pap Smear

In 1948, a Greek immigrant to the United States named George Papanicolaou discovered that the cells shed from the surface of the cervix could be examined under the microscope to see if they appeared normal. Interestingly, he was not a physician, but was working in a pathology laboratory as a technician when he made this discovery. By examining the size and shape of these cells, he was able to detect cancer of the cervix before it was clinically obvious. Later it was discovered that mildly abnormal cells (dysplasia) that could become cancerous were detectable as well. A full description of how the Pap smear is performed can be found in chapter 1.

One of the recent improvements in the Pap smear is the fluid-based Pap smear. For the past fifty years' use of the Pap, cervical cells have been spread on a glass slide in order to be read by the pathologist.

In addition to the cervical cells, the slide also contained cervical mucus, white and red blood cells, and bacteria. These other elements sometimes clouded over the cervical cells and made interpretation difficult. Fluid-based Pap smears eliminate this problem. The Pap smear specimen is placed into a fluid-filled container and sent to the lab. The lab is able to separate the cervical cells from the other elements and just examines the cervical cells. This method is more accurate and is now the preferred way to process the Pap smear.

The wonderful thing about the Pap smear is its ability to see these abnormal cells years before they become cancer, at a time when they can be easily treated. In areas of the world where routine annual Pap smears are extensively used, there has been a dramatic decrease in the rate of death from cervical cancer. This is one of the great success stories of modern medicine.

What Does the Pathologist Look for in the Pap Smear?

All cells have two main parts, the inner part or nucleus containing DNA, and the outer part, called the cytoplasm, producing energy for the cell to function. A normal cell has a small nucleus and a large amount of cytoplasm. When a virus or other carcinogen causes the cell to become abnormal, the DNA in the nucleus starts to grow uncontrollably, enlarging the nucleus so that it crowds out the cytoplasm. This is the abnormality that the pathologist looks for: a large, irregular inner nucleus and a small amount of the outer cytoplasm (see fig. 9.3).

What Do the Pap Smear Results Mean?

The terminology used to describe Pap smear results has changed over the past few years, leading to confusion about what the results of your Pap smear actually mean. Originally, Pap smears were divided into five "classes" based on what the cells looked like to the pathologist. Class I was normal. Class II cells appeared a little irregular to the pathologist, usually representing bacterial infection. Class III and IV Pap smears suggested that dysplastic cells were present and further testing was needed. Class V usually meant cancer. Unfortunately, this class system led to confusion regarding what "number" Pap smear a woman had and what that really meant. Recently, a new system for Pap smear classification called the Bethesda system has been introduced. The term *low-grade* lesion is now used for cells that appear to be infected with HPV or are only mildly abnormal. The term *high grade* is used for more abnormal appearing cells, the type that would have been called class III or IV with

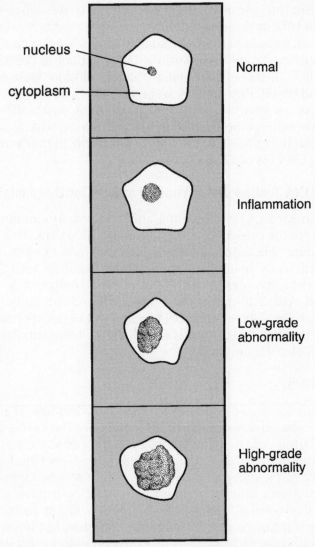

nucleus

cytoplasm

Normal

Inflammation

Low-grade
abnormality

High-grade
abnormality

Fig. 9.3.   Cervical cells as seen on the Pap smear

the old system. A Pap smear that looks like cancer is now labeled "cancer" rather than called class V. A common abnormality reported by the lab is called ASCUS, or atypical squamous (skin) cells of undetermined significance. These cells do not look like true precancer, but do not look entirely normal either. Often the doctor will suggest repeating the Pap smear in a few months to see if the cells appear normal or if they still look abnormal. Another alternative is to have the cells tested for the presence of HPV as discussed below.

A recent update of the Bethesda system includes a category called ASC-H, implying "atypical squamous cells, cannot exclude highly abnormal cells." These cells are often smaller cells that were hard to find before fluid-based Pap smears were available, and colposcopy (see page 263) is necessary to further evaluate their source. The Bethesda system allows the pathologist to actually describe what is seen, rather than just assign a number to the Pap smear result. In that way it is an improvement over the old class system.

Can HPV-DNA Testing Tell If You Are at Risk for Dysplasia?

Most Pap smear labs now have the ability to test abnormal cells on the Pap smear for the presence of DNA from the HPV virus. This testing can also determine whether high-risk or low-risk types of virus are present. That is particularly helpful if the Pap smear result is ASCUS. If the lab finds high-risk virus present with DNA analysis, colposcopy will be recommended. About 40 percent of women with ASCUS on the Pap smear and high-risk virus detected by DNA testing will have dysplasia and need treatment. If only low-risk virus is found, then a follow-up Pap should be repeated in about six months.

What Is AGUS?

AGUS stands for atypical glandular cells of undetermined significance. While the cells on the outside of the cervix are flat cells (called squamous cells), the cells that line the inside of the cervical canal and uterus are thick and fluffy. While squamous cells of undetermined significance are not very suspicious, glandular cells of undetermined significance are worrisome. About half the women with AGUS will have some abnormality of the cervical canal cells or uterine lining cells, and about 10 percent will have cancer. Therefore, complete further evaluation of AGUS is important. Most doctors recommend colposcopy and scraping of the cervical canal to look for cervical abnormalities. A biopsy of the uterine lining cells or full D&C to evaluate any abnormalities of the uterine lining should also be performed. If all of these tests are normal, repeat Pap smears every three months for a year is recommended. If repeat Pap smears show AGUS, cone biopsy (see page 267) may be necessary to find the abnormal cells.

Should Your Sexual Partner Be Evaluated for HPV?

If you have HPV, there is about a 60 percent chance that a male sexual partner may have the virus as well. It is therefore probably a good idea for your partner to see a physician familiar with the evaluation of HPV in men. Some family physicians have the expertise to evaluate men for HPV, and most dermatologists and urologists also have been trained to take care of this problem. Evaluation should include the painless application of vinegar to the penis and examination with a magnifying instrument. The vinegar makes the abnormal cells swell, and the magnification is needed because the changes in the skin cells caused by the virus are sometimes not visible to the naked eye. If skin changes are present, treatment is advised in order to prevent the further growth of lesions both for cosmetic reasons and to prevent any additional spread of the virus. The effect of the virus on men seems to be less dangerous, in that most men with HPV do not go on to develop penile cancer. Treatment usually involves removal of the affected area of skin with a liquid chemical, an electrical instrument, or a freezing instrument. Treatment is usually preceded by a local anesthetic, so discomfort is kept to a minimum.

Condoms play an important part in the prevention of the spread of HPV. If you have been diagnosed with the virus, you should use condoms during intercourse to prevent any spread of the virus to your partner, in case he does not already have the virus. Some women who have been diagnosed with HPV have found that their partner does not want to be examined for the virus. If that is the case, you should continue to use condoms after you are treated in order to prevent any possible reinfection to you in the event that he does have the virus. However, it is best for him to be properly evaluated for his own health, as well as for yours. In order to limit any chance of reinfection, the use of condoms should be continued for at least six months after both of you are free of any detectable virus.

TREATMENT

If You Have an Abnormal Pap Smear, Should It Be Treated?

If the cells on your Pap smear appear to be infected with the HPV virus, and these cells exhibit evidence of high-grade dysplastic changes, then treatment is indicated in order to prevent the cells from becoming cancerous. The time needed for precancer cells to turn into cancer is measured in years, not days. So it is very important to get treatment, but it is almost never an emergency. The treatment options, which are described in the following pages, are aimed at destroying the abnormal cells, so that normal cells can grow back in their place.

If HPV is found, but the Pap smear shows only mildly abnormal cells, then the issue of treatment is controversial. The cervical cells may appear mildly abnormal because they are infected with a low-risk type of virus, which will never turn into dysplasia or cancer. We know that about 60 percent of the time, mildly abnormal cells will be destroyed by the body's immune system without any treatment at all. For those women, follow-up Pap smears over the next few months or year will show a return to normal.

On the other hand, sometimes the cells appear mildly abnormal on the Pap smear because they are only in the *early* stages of an infection with a high-risk virus. These cells, over the course of many months or years, have about a 20 percent chance of becoming high-grade dysplasia or even cancer of the cervix.

We now have the ability to test the cells on the Pap smear to see which type of virus is present, low-risk or high-risk. If no virus or only low risk-virus is present in the cells, then the Pap smear can be repeated in about six months to see if the virus has been eliminated by the body's immune system. If the high-risk virus is present, then evaluation by colposcopy will probably be performed.

Janet's Abnormal Pap Smear

Janet is a twenty-six-year-old woman who has had regular annual Pap smears and pelvic exams, all of which have been normal. At the time of her last examination, her cervix looked healthy, and I expected her Pap smear to come back normal as usual. However, this time the Pap smear results came back ASCUS. When I called to tell Janet about the results, her first reaction was fear that she might have cancer. When I reassured her that this was clearly not cancer and might not even need any treatment, she felt relieved. I suggested we ask the lab to do an HPV-DNA test on the cells to look for high-risk virus, and Janet agreed. About a week later the lab sent us the results—it was a low-risk virus. I called Janet to tell her the good news and suggested she just repeat the Pap smear in about six months. When the Pap smear was repeated six months later, it came back normal. Happily, all the subsequent Pap smears have also been normal. Janet's immune system appears to have eliminated the virus from her body.

What Other Tests Should Be Done If Your Pap Smear Is Abnormal?

The Pap smear is a screening test designed to easily and inexpensively detect cervical dysplasia or cancer in women. Like many quick and inexpensive tests, the Pap smear is not 100 percent accurate. If your Pap smear is found to be abnormal, do not panic! Most Pap smear labs are very cautious, and it is not uncommon for them to "overread" a Pap smear based on any questionable cells they may see. Some abnormal Pap smears turn out to be the result of mild bacterial infections that can be easily treated with antibiotic creams. Other abnormalities are of the type that can just be followed with regular checkups, with very little risk that any treatment will ever be needed. However, if the Pap smear shows dysplasia, or if it shows ASCUS with high-risk HPV, your doctor may want to examine your cervix with a magnifying instrument called a colposcope in order to more accurately determine what kind of problem exists.

What Is Colposcopy?

The colposcope is essentially a set of binoculars attached to the top of a stand. This instrument allows the doctor to see a magnified view of the blood vessels on the skin covering the cervix. As abnormal cells grow, they push the normal blood vessels of the cervix out of their way. These red blood vessels can be seen as they form unusual patterns on the pale pink background of the skin. The patterns typically change as the cells become more abnormal. Your doctor will look for these patterns to determine whether abnormal cells are present, how abnormal they appear to be, and how large or small an area they involve. Colposcopy is an accurate way to check on the results of the Pap smear. If the cells on your Pap smear were slightly abnormal in appearance and a colposcopy shows that the skin looks normal, then nothing may need to be done other than to repeat your Pap smear in three months. However, if abnormal patterns are seen when viewed by the colposcope, then a cervical biopsy will be needed.

What Is a Cervical Biopsy?

A cervical biopsy is the removal of a small area of the cervix. After the tissue is removed, it is sent to a pathologist, who examines the cervical cells under a microscope for an accurate diagnosis. While a Pap smear evaluates the cells that can be scraped off the surface of the cervix, the cervical biopsy removes a thicker area that includes many more cells. Therefore, a cervical biopsy is more accurate than a Pap smear.

Looking through the colposcope, your doctor locates the abnormal area by its appearance. The biopsy instrument is placed against the cervix, and the skin cells are removed. The biopsy instrument is long in order to reach the cervix, but the actual piece of skin removed is extremely small, less than one-eighth of an inch wide. The biopsy takes about a second. Some women may feel a slight pinching, and other women feel nothing. On very rare occasions, a woman may have a very sensitive cervix, and the biopsy may be painful, but any pain lasts only for a split second. If the abnormal cells appear to be growing inside the canal that leads to the uterine lining, a scraping of these cells may also need to be performed. This takes about thirty seconds and can cause menstrual-type cramping, which goes away as soon as the scraping is finished.

In order to allow the cervix to heal, you will probably be instructed not to have intercourse or use tampons for one week after the biopsy. Any irritation to the cervix before it heals may cause bleeding. If that happens, your gynecologist may need to apply a chemical to the cervix to stop the bleeding. However, the site of the biopsy normally requires no care and heals quickly. After three to four weeks, not even a gynecologist could tell that a biopsy had been done. The report from the pathologist takes about a week. Treatment will depend on how abnormal the cells look under the microscope and where they are found on the cervix.

What Are the Treatments for Cervical Dysplasia?

Cryotherapy, LEEP, laser therapy, and cone biopsy have all been used to treat cervical dysplasia with excellent results. The decision about which method should be used will depend on the size of the abnormality, the level of the abnormality, and the comfort and experience of your doctor with the different methods.

What Is Cryotherapy?

The prefix *cryo* means freezing, and cryotherapy uses a very cold instrument applied to the cervix to freeze and thus kill the abnormal cells of the cervix. Some normal cells are destroyed as well, but over the following few weeks, new healthy cells grow to replace all the ones that were destroyed. The procedure takes about seven minutes, and most women feel menstrual-like cramps during this time. As soon as the procedure is over, the cramps go away and there is no further discomfort. For a few weeks following the freezing, the cervix will weep a clear fluid as it heals. This often leads to a clear or yellowish, nonirritating discharge. For the first two weeks after the procedure, intercourse should be avoided so that the cervix can begin to heal. After four to six weeks, the cervix is usually entirely healed.

The good news is that this procedure has a 95 percent cure rate. After cryotherapy, follow-up Pap smears should be taken every three months over the course of the next year to make sure that you are not one of the 5 percent of women who did not get cured. If one of your Pap smears is abnormal again, then the colposcopy is repeated. If needed, you may be retreated with cryotherapy or a different method.

What Is LEEP?

LEEP stands for loop electrosurgical excision procedure. This procedure was developed in Europe years ago and has been frequently performed in the United States since the 1980s. A small wire loop is placed against the cervix, and an electric current is passed through the loop, making it extremely hot. The loop is then able to cut through the cervix in much the same way that a hot knife cuts through butter. The procedure requires special instruments, but it can be performed in the doctor's office and only takes a few minutes to do. Local anesthesia is injected into the cervix, and virtually no discomfort occurs during LEEP. The small portion of the cervix that is removed is then sent to the pathologist for examination. Healing of the cervix occurs over a six-week period of time, but intercourse can be resumed about three weeks after the procedure, when healing is well on its way. LEEP is both diagnostic and therapeutic; the abnormal cells are removed as treatment, and they are also sent to the lab for diagnosis. LEEP removes more tissue than the regular cervical biopsy, and it is also more expensive. Therefore, we use it only when we think that removing more tissue will be necessary.

Susan's Abnormal Pap and LEEP

Susan is a thirty-three-year-old woman who came in for her annual Pap and pelvic examination. Although she had been treated with cryotherapy ten years earlier for precancerous cells of the cervix, all of her Pap smears since then had come back normal. We were both a little shocked when this Pap smear was read as a high-grade abnormality by the pathologist. While none of the cells looked like cancer, we needed to do a colposcopy to evaluate the cells of the cervix and determine which type of treatment would be needed. Susan came back to the office a week later for her colposcopy. Surprisingly, the outside skin of her cervix looked fairly normal through the colposcope. However, the area of cells where dysplasia or cancer usually develops, the transformation zone (see page 252), could not be seen. Sometimes, after cryotherapy, the healing process can cause the uterine lining cells to end up higher in the canal of the cervix where they cannot be seen. This is not dangerous, but it does limit the completeness of the examination.

Because I was not able to see this area of Susan's cervix, I recommended that we remove a portion of the canal of the cervix with the LEEP instrument. Removal would serve two purposes. First, the pathologist could examine the tissue under the microscope and make a final diagnosis of how abnormal the cells appeared. Second, no further treatment would likely be needed since the cells would have been removed. Susan agreed. With an extremely small needle, I injected a small amount of anesthetic, mixed with a chemical to help prevent bleeding, into her cervix. The injection did not bother her at all. Next, the wire loop of the LEEP instrument was used to remove a portion of the canal area from her cervix. Because of the anesthetic, Susan felt nothing. I then scraped the cells high up in the remaining cervical canal for the pathologist to check and make sure that no abnormal cells had been left behind. Then I used an instrument shaped like a metal Q-tip to sear a few blood vessels on the cervix in order to stop them from bleeding. The entire procedure took about three minutes.

The pathology report came back about a week later. It showed that the cells were indeed precancerous and had been growing up inside the cervical canal. Fortunately, all the abnormal cells appeared to have been removed, and the scrapping of cells from the remaining part of the cervical canal was entirely healthy. The follow-up for Susan included Pap smears every three months for a year, then every six months after that. They have all been fine, and no further evaluation or treatment has been necessary.

When Is Laser Surgery Used for Abnormal Cervical Cells?

The medical laser is able to precisely focus high-energy light into a small area, causing intense heat. This heat energy can be used to cut or burn away abnormal cells from the surface of skin. The precision of the laser led to its use in treating the abnormal cells of the cervix. However, this procedure requires a hospital operating room, expensive equipment, and general anesthesia. Recently, LEEP has taken the place of laser procedures because it is performed in the doctor's office, is cheaper and faster, does not require general anesthesia, and is just as effective.

What Is a Cone Biopsy?

A cone biopsy is another procedure available for removal of the portion of the cervix that contains abnormal cells. The cervical cells are both on the outside skin of the cervix and on the inside lining of the cervix that leads into the uterus. The outside cells are usually easy to see with the colposcope, but the cells inside the canal may not be visible. If these cells cannot be seen and properly evaluated, they may need to be removed to make sure all the abnormal cells are eliminated.

A cone biopsy is performed in the hospital, usually with general anesthesia. A scalpel is used to remove a portion of the outside of the cervix as well as the inside canal of the cervix. This portion of the cervix is shaped like a cone, hence the name (see fig. 9.4). Sutures are then placed around the cervix to prevent any bleeding. You may go home the same day. Since there are no abdominal incisions, there is no postoperative discomfort.

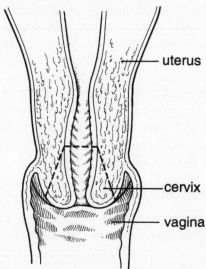

Fig. 9.4. Portion of the cervix removed during cone biopsy

LEEP is performed in much the same way to accomplish the same results as a cone biopsy. Therefore, because of the ease and rapidity of LEEP, most doctors perform the procedure for this situation.

If true cervical cancer is found or suspected on the cervical biopsy, a cone biopsy using a scalpel is the best way to remove the tissue for evaluation. The proper treatment for cervical cancer depends on how deep the cancer goes into the tissue. The extreme heat from the LEEP instrument often distorts the edges of the tissue and makes evaluation of the extent of any cancer difficult for the pathologist. In this situation, using a scalpel preserves the edges of the tissue and allows a better evaluation of the extent of the cancer.

Can the Treatment for Cervical Dysplasia Interfere with Fertility or Childbirth?

The healing that follows cryotherapy, laser, LEEP, or scalpel cone biopsy is usually not detrimental to either subsequent fertility or childbirth. However, about 1 percent of women who have these procedures have scarring in the cervix that interferes with the ability of sperm to enter the uterus. If this problem occurs, a small tube may be inserted through the cervix, and semen may be passed directly into the uterine cavity. This procedure, called intrauterine insemination, is usually successful.

The other problem that may rarely result from treatment for cervical dysplasia is the premature dilation of the cervix during pregnancy. Removal of tissue from the cervix may weaken it, and the weight of the baby may start to stretch the cervix. Since cryotherapy removes no tissue, the risk is very small. LEEP, laser, or scalpel cone biopsies do remove tissue, and care must be taken to remove as little tissue as possible, while still curing the disease. The increased risk of a preterm delivery for a woman who has had one of these procedures is probably about 5 percent. If you have had treatment for cervical dysplasia, you should tell your obstetrician, so that he or she can examine your cervix frequently during pregnancy to check for early dilation.

What Are the Cure Rates for Cervical Dysplasia?

All of the above treatments have virtually the same cure rates, about 95 percent. Therefore, the choice of treatment should depend on the degree of abnormal cells present, the size of the area involved, and the presence or absence of abnormal cells high in the cervical canal. Your doctor will discuss these issues with you and make a recommendation for the best treatment.

Does a Hysterectomy Make Sense for Abnormal Cervical Cells?

If cancer is found on the cervical biopsy, then removal of the entire cervix and uterus—a hysterectomy—is usually indicated. The cervix is actually the lower part of the uterus, and one of the first places cervical cancer spreads is to the rest of the uterus. Therefore, hysterectomy is necessary to remove any other cancerous cells that remain after the biopsy. Cervical cancer virtually never spreads to the ovaries, so the ovaries do not need to be removed, especially in young women, and normal hormonal function can continue.

Hysterectomy may also be presented as an option in a woman with a high-grade dysplasia. But since these conditions can be treated by less drastic means, hysterectomy is not indicated unless there are other compelling gynecologic reasons for the procedure. In some situations, the initial removal of abnormal cells may not be complete. For these women, repeated attempts at removal of the cells short of hysterectomy are often warranted. However, sometimes abnormal cells may persist or recur despite appropriate treatments, and hysterectomy may be considered.

Even hysterectomy does not give a 100 percent guarantee that you will never be affected by abnormal cells again. Since abnormal cells usually result from HPV, some virus-infected cells may be left behind in the vagina after the removal of the cervix and uterus. About 5 percent of women who have a hysterectomy for high-grade dysplasia will have the abnormal cells recur in the vagina. If left untreated over many years, these cells can develop into vaginal cancer. These abnormal cells can also be detected with the Pap smear by scraping the top of the vagina with a small spatula. Therefore, it is important to have an annual Pap smear even after you have had a hysterectomy!

Mindy's Three Cone Biopsies

Mindy, now a forty-two-year-old woman, had had an abnormal Pap smear followed by colposcopy and cryotherapy. In the fifteen years since that initial abnormal Pap smear, her Pap had always been entirely normal. I had been her physician for about five years when her annual Pap smear came back with a high-grade abnormality.

Mindy came in for a colposcopy, but I was not able to see all the cervical cells in order to evaluate them. As sometimes happens after cryotherapy, some of the cervical cells had been pushed high into the cervical canal and were now out of view. In order to remove any abnormal cells that were up inside the cervical canal, I recommended a LEEP cone biopsy (see page 267).

The LEEP cone biopsy was done as an office procedure the following week. After removing the canal of the cervix with the LEEP instrument, I usually take a sample of cells from inside the remaining part of the cervix. These cells are sent to the pathologist in order to make sure that no abnormal cells remain above the part of the cervix that was removed. Unfortunately, when the pathology report came back, it showed that abnormal cells still remained high up in Mindy's cervix. I discussed this with Mindy and recommended that we repeat the LEEP procedure in order to remove a piece of the cervical canal even higher up than what we normally remove. She agreed.

The second LEEP procedure was also uneventful. However, the pathology report again found very abnormal cells in the portion of the cervix that remained. At this point, both Mindy and I were extremely frustrated. The two LEEP cone biopsies had gone well and had removed enough tissue from the cervix, but both had failed to cure the problem. I was not confident that yet another cone would be any more successful, and I discussed this with Mindy. Since Mindy had completed her family, I suggested that she consider a hysterectomy as a way to completely remove the cervix and eliminate any remaining abnormal cells. Mindy felt very strongly that she did not want a hysterectomy. She was afraid that her sexual response and orgasm would be affected if her cervix and uterus were removed. Although this decrease in sexual responsiveness after hysterectomy has not been proven, some women have reported decreased pleasure during orgasm (see page 345). I respected Mindy's desire to avoid the surgery if possible. I discussed the situation with a gynecologic oncologist, who agreed that one more chance of removing the cells would be worth a try. Mindy was delighted with the alternative to hysterectomy but extremely nervous about having yet another procedure.

I recommended that the surgery be performed in the hospital under general anesthesia. This would permit me to take out an extremely large portion of the cervix without having to worry about causing Mindy any pain. I performed the procedure using a laser that enables a surgeon to be very slow and to have precise control over what area to remove. Again I scraped the cells remaining in the cervix. The week of waiting for the pathologist's report was an anxious one. Fortunately, the cells came back from the pathologist all normal. Mindy was extremely relieved, and so was I. I had been reluctant to perform this third attempt at removing the abnormal cells but was now glad that she had asked me to try again. Mindy recuperated nicely from the surgery, and all of her subsequent Pap smears have been normal.

CERVICAL CANCER

Once abnormal cells burrow through the last layer of the skin covering the cervix, cervical cancer is said to exist. Directly below the skin are the blood and lymph vessels that can carry the abnormal cells to other areas of the body. Because these cells may have spread, treatment for cervical cancer requires more extensive treatment than that for high-grade dysplasia. Cervical cancer affects about 15,000 American women each year, and about 5,000 women die of cervical cancer a year. It is most likely to affect women in their late thirties to early sixties, but about 25 percent of women who have cervical cancer are less than thirty years old. In the United States, the number of women who die from this disease has decreased by 70 percent, since the development of the Pap smear. With the routine use of Pap smears, cervical cancer should be a preventable disease.

What Is a Radical Hysterectomy?

If cervical cancer is found on a biopsy and if it has already started to burrow into the cells below, there is a chance that the cancer may have started to spread. Lymph nodes are part of your immune system and cleanse the body of abnormal cells. The lymph nodes are linked to-gether by a chain of lymph vessels that follow along the blood vessels in your body. Removal of the uterus and the lymph nodes and surround-ing tissue near the uterus is advised for women who have cervical can-cer. This procedure is called a radical hysterectomy (see page 337). By surgically removing the lymph nodes and surrounding tissue, the pathologist will be able to tell whether the cancer has already begun to spread. In addition, by removing tissue and lymph nodes that contain cancer, further spread of the cancer may be prevented. If cancer has spread to the lymph nodes, then other therapy in the form of radiation may also be needed after surgery.

Can Radiation Therapy Be Used to Treat Cervical Cancer?

For some women with cervical cancer, radiation therapy may be suggested instead of surgery, or may be needed following surgery. If cervical cancer affects a woman whose advanced age or other medical problems make surgery too risky, radiation may be a safer treatment, and the cure rates are comparable to those of surgery. Radiation uses high levels of X-rays to destroy cancer cells. Two types of radiation are used to treat cervical cancer. Intracavitary radiation uses a device containing radioactive material that is placed through the cervix and into the uterus. This form of radiation is administered in the hospital, but it works quickly so that the device can be removed and you can return home the same day. External beam radiation uses a large machine to aim the radiation at the pelvic area. Administered in an outpatient setting, the radiation is usually given for about twenty minutes a day, five days a week, for six weeks. If cervical cancer is to be treated by radiation alone, both types of radiation must be given. For women who are initially treated with surgery and who are found to have cancer that has spread to the lymph nodes, external beam radiation will be recommended after surgery.

What Are the Side Effects of Radiation?

Radiation is frightening to most people. The machines that administer radiation are large and imposing. Some may fear that the radiation will stay with them and contaminate them; however, this does not happen. Radiation is often an excellent way to treat cancer. It does, nevertheless, have potential side effects. The most common side effect is fatigue. This begins about two weeks after treatment starts and can last for a few months after the treatment has ended. Diarrhea and decreased appetite may also occur, and skin irritation at the site of radiation is not uncommon. The radiation may also affect the skin and lubricating glands of the vagina, and intercourse may become painful. Use of lubricants and gentle self-dilation of the vagina will usually help. Many women with cervical cancer, 75 percent in some studies, will notice decreased sexual feelings after either surgery or radiation. Having a healthy and interested partner and counseling with a therapist skilled in this area will help restore your sexual desire.

What Are the Cure Rates for Cervical Cancer?

As with any cancer, the earlier it is found and treated, the better the cure rate. Due to the extensive use of Pap smear testing, women have been diagnosed with cervical cancer at much earlier stages. At present, the cure rate for early cervical cancer is better than 85 percent. Early detection and treatment have really paid off in the case of cervical cancer. Be sure and get regular Pap smears.

REFERENCES

Berek, J., and N. Hacker. 1994. *Practical Gynecologic Oncology*. Baltimore, Md.: Williams and Wilkins.

Holowaty, P., A. Miller, T. Rohan, and T. To. 1999. Natural history of dysplasia of the uterine cervix. *Journal of the National Cancer Institute* 91:252–58.

Lee, K., R. Ashfaq, G. Birdsong, M. Corkill, K. Mcintosh, and S. Inhorn. 1997. Comparison of conventional Papanicolaou smears and a fluid-based, thin-layer system for cervical cancer screening. *Obstetrics and Gynecology* 90:278–84.

Mitchell, M., G. Tortolero-Luna, E. Cook, L. Whittaker, H. Rhodes-Morris, and E. Silva. 1998. A randomized clinical trial of cryotherapy, laser vaporization, and loop electrosurgical excision for treatment of squamous intraepithelial lesions of the cervix. *Obstetrics and Gynecology* 92:737–44.

Montz, R. 1996. Impact of therapy for cervical intraepithelial neoplasia on fertility. *American Journal of Obstetrics and Gynecology* 1129–36.

Morra, M., and E. Pots. 1994. *Choices: A Sourcebook for Cancer Information*. New York: Avon.

Wright, T., and R. Richart. 1990. Role of human papillomavirus in the pathogenesis of genital tract warts and cancer. *Gynecologic Oncology* 37:151–64.

Wright, T., S. Gagnon, R. Richart, and A. Ferenczy. 1992. Treatment of cervical intraepithelial neoplasia using the loop electrosurgical excision procedure. *Obstetrics and Gynecology* 79:173–78.

Zweizig, S., K. Noller, F. Reale, S. Collis, and L. Resseguie. 1997. Neoplasia associated with atypical glandular cells of undetermined significance on cervical cytology. *Gynecologic Oncology* 65:314–18.

10

OVARIAN CANCER AND THE SEARCH FOR EARLY DETECTION

If *cancer* is one of the most dreaded words in the English language, then for most women, *ovarian* is the worst adjective to place before *cancer*. In all the bad news we sometimes deal with in gynecology, this is the most frightening. Since the death of Gilda Radner, a comedienne who made so many of us laugh, people seem to be much more aware of ovarian cancer. This increase in interest has led to enhanced medical research regarding ovarian cancer. Studies are being done on the cause or causes, the treatment, and a means of early detection. For the 5 percent of ovarian cancer patients for whom the cancer may be hereditary, genetic research is evolving to help determine who is actually at risk. While we still feel as if we are groping in the dark with this disease, when I think back to even a few years ago, I know that we are making strides. This chapter deals with what we now know about the detection, treatment, and prevention of ovarian cancer. If you are anxious and concerned about this disease, I hope that this information allays many of your fears.

How Common Is Ovarian Cancer?

While extremely frightening, ovarian cancer is a rare disease. Only 1 out of every 15,000 women will have the disease at the age of thirty. At forty, about the age that Gilda Radner discovered she had ovarian cancer, only 1 of every 10,000 women has this disease. At the age of sixty, the average

age at which women get ovarian cancer, only 1 of every 1,500 women will have it. In your entire lifetime, if you live to be ninety years old, you have a 1 in 70 chance of developing ovarian cancer. Compare this with the 1 in 3 chance a woman has of dying of a heart attack by the time she is ninety, or the fact that you are more likely to die in an auto accident and twice as likely to die from colon cancer than you are from ovarian cancer. These statistics are not meant to diminish the human toll from this terrible disease. However, all of the interest and media coverage surrounding ovarian cancer have given the impression that the disease is now more common, that there is an epidemic. In fact, the incidence of ovarian cancer is no greater now than it was twenty-five years ago.

Are Most Growths on the Ovary Cancerous?

No. In fact, for a premenopausal woman found to have a growth on her ovary, there is over a 90 percent chance that this growth is benign. In a postmenopausal woman, an ovarian growth has a 70 percent chance of being benign. Therefore, if a growth is found on your ovary, *do not panic*. It will most likely not be a cancer. Chapter 5 is devoted to the most common types of benign ovarian cysts.

What Actually Causes Ovarian Cancer?

Like all cancers, ovarian cancer results from the runaway overgrowth of cells. All the cells in our body have the capacity to multiply—that is how cells grow and how the body repairs damaged tissue on a regular basis. Cells contain numerous genes that control cell division and growth. Some of the genes promote cell growth, while other genes act to suppress runaway overgrowth of the cells. Chance alterations in these genes, called mutations, can cause the genes to malfunction and lead to uncontrolled growth of cells. When the normal controls over cell growth are lost, cancer may result. All the specific genes responsible for causing ovarian cancer to develop are not yet known. However, current research is directed at this problem and may someday allow us to predict which women are at risk for ovarian cancer. In the more distant future, gene therapy may allow alteration of these genes within the body, so that we can actually prevent ovarian cancer from occurring.

Risk Factors for Ovarian Cancer

We know that ovarian cancer is more common in women whose ovaries have continued to produce eggs without interruption over their lifetimes. Every time you ovulate, the surface of the ovary splits open to let the egg out. When the surface cells grow rapidly to heal over the opening, they become more vulnerable to substances (carcinogens) that can cause mutations. To date, the identity of these carcinogens is not certain (see page 284). In order for cancer to develop, it is likely that a number of factors must be present: the presence of a carcinogen, some predisposition to developing abnormal growth of the ovarian cells, and uninterrupted ovulation that increases the chance of the carcinogen getting into the cell.

Events that prevent ovulation, such as pregnancy, breast-feeding, and taking birth control pills, will decrease your risk of developing ovarian cancer. During pregnancy, your ovaries do not produce any eggs for nine months. The hormonal changes associated with breast-feeding keeps the ovaries at rest for a few more months. Birth control pills work by preventing the release of eggs from the ovary. Likewise, the late onset of your periods or early onset of menopause, which result in a decrease in the total number of times you ovulate in your lifetime, will also decrease your risk of getting ovarian cancer. Fewer ovulations lead to fewer vulnerable, healing, rapidly dividing cells and less risk of ovarian cancer.

Genetic factors also appear to play a role in your risk of developing ovarian cancer. Caucasian women have a higher risk than women of African or Asian heritage. And, as discussed on page 277, a strong family history of ovarian cancer may increase your risk.

Can Fertility Drugs Increase Your Risk of Ovarian Cancer?

Some old studies showed an increased risk of ovarian cancer in a small number of women who used fertility drugs over a prolonged period of time. Even in those studies, the risk of developing invasive ovarian cancer for women who had taken at least twelve cycles of fertility drugs was only 1.5 percent, compared to the normal risk of 1 percent. However, a recent analysis of eight studies that investigated whether fertility drugs were causing an increased risk of ovarian cancer found *no such risk*. They did find a small increased risk of ovarian cancer in women who never got pregnant, but this risk had nothing to do with the fertility medications. As noted above, other studies show that never being pregnant increases the risk of ovarian cancer in and of itself, regardless of whether women were trying, or not trying, to get pregnant.

Does Your Diet Influence Your Risk of Ovarian Cancer?

A recent study found that women with a high saturated fat intake had a higher risk of developing ovarian cancer. Most American women consume about 30 grams of saturated fat a day in the form of animal fat, milk products, eggs, and cheese. By decreasing the amount of fat you eat by 10 grams a day, you can decrease your risk of ovarian cancer by 20 percent. If your risk of ovarian cancer is that of the general population, about 1 percent, a decrease in dietary fat can lower your risk to 0.8 percent.

In addition, for every extra 10 grams of vegetable fiber you eat a day, your risk of ovarian cancer decreases by about 40 percent, to 0.6 percent. The reasons for this benefit are not known. In any case, this is another good reason to eat reasonably and to include lots of fruits and vegetables in your diet. Also, decreasing fat and increasing fiber in your diet decreases your risk of heart disease, the major killer of women in this country, and of colon cancer.

Factors That Lower Your Risk for Ovarian Cancer

- Have one or more children
- Take birth control pills (for more than one year)
- No family history of ovarian cancer
- Black or Asian heritage
- Late onset of periods (after age twelve)
- Early onset of menopause (before age forty-five)
- Low-fat, high-fiber diet

What Is Your Risk of Ovarian Cancer If Someone in Your Family Has Had It?

The issue of family ovarian cancer has received a lot of attention from the press and caused a great deal of anxiety for many women. However, less than 10 percent of women found to have ovarian cancer have inherited this disease. Therefore, the vast majority (90 percent) of women who get ovarian cancer have no family history of it. If someone in your family has had ovarian cancer, your risk will depend on how close the relative is to you, how old they were at the time they developed ovarian cancer, and how many of your relatives have had the disease. Knowing the specifics of your family history can either alert you to a possible problem or, more likely, be a source of reassurance.

Women with no family history of ovarian cancer have a 1.4 percent risk of developing ovarian cancer if they live to be ninety years old.

Therefore, about 1 woman out of 100 will develop this disease in her lifetime. To put this in some perspective, about 33 women out of 100 will die of heart disease and 5 women out of 100 will die of lung cancer. If your mother had ovarian cancer, your risk of developing ovarian cancer increases to 7 out of 100 women. If your sister had ovarian cancer, your risk is about 5 out of 100. Having either a grandmother or aunt with ovarian cancer increases your risk to about 3 out of 100. If you have two or more close relatives with ovarian cancer, your risk of developing ovarian cancer increases to 14 out of 100 women.

This information comes from studies of large numbers of women, both Jewish and non-Jewish, who have been diagnosed with ovarian cancer. Through other studies we have learned that the risk of inheriting ovarian cancer is higher in Jewish women of Eastern European (Ashkenazi) descent. In those women, specific ovarian cancer gene mutations have been found to be more common. While only 1 out of 1,000 non-Ashkenazi Jewish women has this mutation, about 20 out of 1,000 Ashkenazi Jewish women have these mutations. A non-Ashkenazi Jewish woman with one close relative with ovarian cancer has a 5 percent chance of having this mutation, while an Ashkenazi Jewish woman with the same family history has a 15 percent chance of having the mutation. For this reason, Ashkenazi Jewish women with a close relative with ovarian cancer might consider getting tested for this gene.

Should You Get Genetic Testing for Ovarian Cancer?

Some women with a strong family history for ovarian cancer have been found to have a mutation in a gene called BRCA, which stands for breast cancer gene. In addition to inheriting a higher risk of getting breast cancer, women with this mutation have a higher risk of developing ovarian cancer. In the general population this mutation occurs in about 1 out of 1,000 women. However, in women of Eastern European Jewish descent the mutated gene occurs in 20 out of 1,000 women. Women who have a BRCA mutation have a 25 to 50 percent chance of developing ovarian cancer in their lifetimes, compared to the 1 percent risk for women who do not have the mutation. Interestingly, women who have this gene mutation and develop ovarian cancer get a less aggressive cancer and survive longer than women who do not have this mutation. As is true for the nongenetic form of ovarian cancer, taking birth control pills substantially reduces the risk of inherited ovarian cancer.

Testing for this gene by taking a simple blood sample is now available for women who suspect they are at high risk because of a family history of ovarian cancer. Deciding whether to be tested is often a diffi-cult decision. There are a number of reasons you might consider having the test done. If it is negative, then neither you nor your daughters need to be concerned about an increased risk of this disease. This often lifts an enormous burden of worry. If the test is positive, then you will have some decisions to consider. With an increased risk of ovarian cancer (and an increased risk of breast cancer), the available options to decrease the risk are drastic: removal of your ovaries and/or breasts (mastectomy). These admittedly limited options lower your risk of cancer but do in-volve a surgical procedure and are emotionally very difficult decisions.

Removal of ovaries can now be performed with laparoscopic surgery as an outpatient, but general anesthesia is necessary. As is true with all surgery, the removal of ovaries includes some risk. In addition, removal of the ovaries will not prevent a very rare form of inherited can-cer that affects the inside lining of your abdomen, the peritoneum. Be-cause this gene mutation also increases your risk of breast cancer, you will need to address the issue of removal of your breasts for preventative reasons. Your age, childbearing issues, your feelings about the possibil-ity of cancer, and your feelings about surgery and removal of integral parts of your body are all important issues. These are extremely difficult decisions and are best made with the counseling and advice of a trained genetic counselor. It is important to see the genetic counselor before you get tested so that these issues can be discussed in advance of the results. Ask your doctor to recommend someone to you, or call a nearby medical center for a referral.

Rebecca's Story

Rebecca is a fifty-eight-year-old woman who was sent to me for a second opinion after her family doctor felt an irregularly shaped mass when he did her annual pelvic examination. I, too, imme-diately felt the mass her doctor discovered and ordered an ultra-sound and a CA-125 blood test. Both test results indicated that cancer might be present, and we scheduled her for surgery a few days later to remove the mass and determine if it was cancerous. As soon as we made our initial incision and looked at her pelvic organs, we knew that Rebecca had ovarian cancer. It had spread to her uterus and fallopian tubes, and the gynecologic oncolo-gist (a gynecologic cancer specialist) and I performed a hysterec-tomy, removal of the fallopian tubes and ovaries, and removal of the nearby lymph nodes. We felt certain we were able to take out all visible tumors. This sense was proven correct when the pathology report came back. It showed that the cancer had not yet spread to her lymph nodes, so chemotherapy might provide a chance of cure.

After recovery from surgery, Rebecca turned her thoughts to her family and her three daughters. Rebecca's grandmother had died of some type of abdominal cancer many years ago, and the family was of Ashkenazi Jewish descent. Rebecca began to wonder if her grandmother's abdominal cancer had actually been ovarian cancer, and she was concerned that her daughters might be at a high risk for the same disease. After we had a long discussion about the risks and issues involved, Rebecca decided to have gene testing performed. She met with a genetic counselor who agreed that this would be a reasonable thing to do for the sake of her daughters' future.

Two weeks later, Rebecca met with the genetic counselor to discuss the findings. Although she thought she had prepared herself for bad news regarding a genetic link, Rebecca was surprised and upset to find that she did indeed have the gene mutation for breast and ovarian cancer. "You know, you just keep hoping for the best, even when the worst happens," she told me. "I'm beginning to come to terms with dying way before I feel ready, but it is devastating to me that my daughters may likely face the same thing. It feels like we've all been handed a death sentence." Her daughters were also shocked to learn the results. Sharon, the oldest, told me, "We've barely come to grips with the idea that our mother is seriously ill, and now we know we're next. The three of us heard the news and panicked." Rebecca set up a meeting with herself, her three daughters, and the genetic counselor to discuss the implications of the test results. In a calm manner, the counselor told them that each one had a 50 percent chance of inheriting the abnormal gene, and the only way to know would be to test them individually. Sharon, the oldest, was thirty-seven, married, and had two young daughters of her own. Natalie was thirty-four, unmarried, unattached, and pursuing a professional career as a singer-actress. The youngest daughter, Leslie, was twenty-nine and engaged to be married in ten months. The discussion with the genetic counselor went on for two hours, and then each went home and continued talking to each other and their friends and family for the next three or four very tension-filled days. By the end of the week, Sharon, Leslie, and Natalie had each come to a decision.

The oldest daughter, Sharon, decided to be tested for the gene. With nine- and six-year-old daughters at home, Sharon did not plan to have any more children. Because she was thirty-seven, Sharon knew she was nearing the time when her risks of breast and ovarian cancer increased. She felt that she could "live with" the recommended surgeries to remove her breasts and her ovaries if that became necessary. Also motivating Sharon to face the results of genetic testing were an urgent need to know if her daughters were at an increased risk and the hope that a negative test would put her mind at ease.

However, neither Leslie nor Natalie felt ready to face further knowledge about their genetic makeup. Both were childless, and both hoped to have children in the future. Removing their ovaries at this point was out of the question. Based on their ages, Leslie and Natalie decided they probably had a few more years to make a decision about their ovaries. When they considered the disfigurement of mastectomy, they just knew they weren't ready to face that either. "We know Sharon's making the right choice for herself, and if we were in her shoes with a solid marriage and two healthy kids to raise, we would do the same thing," Leslie told me. "But neither one of us is there yet."

When the genetic counselor met with Sharon and her husband to disclose the test results, Leslie and Natalie came too. The nervous energy in the room was palpable. With great relief and happiness, the counselor informed Sharon that she did not carry the same gene mutation her mother did. "We all cheered and cried," Sharon said afterward. "My mother was too scared to come with us, and now we wish she had. She missed a joyful celebration. What a moment!"

The negative results also provided a sense of relief for her sisters because they understand what they face but also know that having the gene mutation is not inevitable. "We're just going to make the most of our lives now and deal with this a little later," was how Leslie expressed it to us. "The first order of business is to make sure our mother gets through chemotherapy. We'll take care of our genetics when we have to."

Do Other Types of Cancer in Your Family Affect Your Risk of Ovarian Cancer?

There are a very small number of families who have *multiple* family members with colon, stomach, uterine, or ovarian cancers. These families are said to have hereditary nonpolyposis colorectal cancer (HNPCC). This syndrome was originally called Lynch Family Cancer Syndrome, named after the doctor who first described the genetic basis for these cancers. The genes that cause these cancers appear to be passed on together. They may be passed on through either your mother's or father's side of the family. Women members of these families are at increased risk of developing any of these cancers, while the men are at increased risk for colon cancer. These family cancer syndromes are extremely rare and can only be determined if you know your family history in detail. For example, one study examined the incidence of family cancer syndromes among women who had a mother or sister with ovarian cancer. Of the 391 women who had enough information about their family to participate in the study, only 19 families (5 percent) appeared to have inheritable ovarian cancer, and another 82 families (20 percent) had inheritable multiple cancers. Most of these families showed the prevalence for cancer over two to four generations. The other 75 percent of the women had no basis for inheritable cancer. Women who come from families with HNPCC have a 10 percent chance of developing ovarian cancer in their lifetimes, and the average age for developing the cancer is forty-five, or twenty years earlier than most women develop the disease.

What Should You Do If You Have a Strong Family History of Ovarian, Stomach, Uterine, and Colon Cancer?

If you are a member of one of the rare families where a number of relatives have had these types of cancer, then you should consider seeing a genetic counselor. These counselors are trained to take a detailed family history and then are able to calculate your risk of developing any of these cancers. Your doctor should be able to help you get in touch with the appropriate genetic counselor.

If your family has an increased risk of these cancers, special tests can be performed to evaluate you on a regular basis. In this rare situation, and this situation only, screening tests for ovarian cancer (sonograms and CA-125 blood tests) may make some sense, although their value has not been proven. In fact, a number of screening programs for high-risk women have stopped accepting new patients because the testing has not been helpful. Some women have developed ovarian cancer despite recent normal tests, and others have had abnormal test results, but no cancer was present. If you are felt to be at very high risk, you should discuss screening tests with a genetic counselor and also discuss having your ovaries removed after you have completed your family (see page 291).

Other cancers found in HNPCC syndrome are easier to test for. An annual scraping of the uterine lining cells is a relatively simple office procedure that can detect uterine lining cells in the precancerous stage. Breast exams and annual mammograms should be performed to screen for breast cancer. Screening for colon cancer can be performed by colonoscopy, which enables your doctor to see and remove precancerous polyps before cancer develops.

Discuss all these tests with your doctor or genetic counselor. Early detection saves lives. Have the appropriate screening performed if your family history suggests a higher risk. Genetic testing is now available for families thought to be at high risk for HNPCC. Specific guidelines for screening HNPCC known-positive families for the specific inherited cancers are available and recommended.

Are There Any Medications That Can Decrease Your Risk of Ovarian Cancer?

Yes, believe it or not, birth control pills have been shown to decrease your risk of ovarian cancer. Continuous ovulation during your lifetime increases the risk of ovarian cancer. Birth control pills work by preventing ovulation, and thus decrease your risk. Even taking the pill for just one year will decrease your risk of ovarian cancer by about 10 percent. Taking the pill for five years or more decreases your risk by *50 to 70 percent*. The same decreased risk associated with the use of birth control pills also appears to be true for women considered at high risk of developing ovarian cancer because of a strong family history.

Many people have had a fear or a distrust of taking birth control pills. Early studies, performed twenty years ago when the doses of the pill were extremely high, found a slightly increased risk of heart attack for women on the pill. But for women on the low doses of hormone found in the pill today, the risk of a heart attack is less than 1 in 20,000. For comparison, the high levels of estrogen present during pregnancy increase the risk of heart attack to 1 in 10,000 women.

Some women have worried about taking the pill for long periods of time. There are many who feel that they should give their bodies a "break" by getting off the pill after a few years. The research shows us that this fear is unfounded; the risks of using the pill actually decrease over time. In addition, taking the pill for long stretches may actually have some health benefits for you. Besides decreasing your risk of ovarian cancer, taking birth control pills decreases your risks for developing benign ovarian cysts, heavy menstrual bleeding and anemia, uterine cancer (by 60 percent), and benign breast cysts.

Unfortunately, the medical community has not relayed these positive facts adequately to the public. A recent study of women faculty, students, and employees at Yale University found that 80 percent of these women did not know that the pill could decrease the risk of ovarian cancer. Obviously, we need to provide better education in this area. While the pill is clearly not indicated for, or desired by, everyone, it does have a place in women's medical care. If using the pill interests you, ask your doctor about the positive health benefits of oral contraceptives.

Can Some Types of Surgery Decrease Your Risk of Ovarian Cancer?

Surprisingly, both tubal ligation (getting your "tubes tied") and hysterectomy (without removal of the ovaries) have been shown to decrease the risk of subsequently developing ovarian cancer by almost 50 percent. Although the reasons for this decrease are not entirely clear, here is the current thinking: Blocking off the fallopian tubes (tubal ligation) and removing the uterus (hysterectomy) both prevent any substances in the vagina from moving up inside the uterus and out the fallopian tubes, where they can land on the ovaries. Although these substances have not been identified, the theory suggests that once these substances are present on the ovary, they may induce the development of cancer.

One substance that is a possible candidate for inducing ovarian cancer is talc. Talc has sometimes been found in the ovaries of women with ovarian cancer. Presumably this comes from talcum powder used in hygiene products, which may get into the vagina and then end up on the ovary.

While the association between talc and ovarian cancer is still theoretical, if you are using a powder that is labeled as "talcum powder" or "containing talc," it is advisable to switch to another powder. Professionals in the medical field are still at the supposition and educated-guess stage regarding talc and other substances that may be factors in the development of this disease.

DIAGNOSING OVARIAN CANCER

Why Is Ovarian Cancer So Hard to Detect at an Early Stage?

Your ovaries are very small. Before you reach menopause, the ovaries are about the size of a pecan. After menopause, when they have stopped producing eggs, the ovaries shrink to the size of an almond. The ovaries lie deep within your pelvic area and are covered over by your intestines, your abdominal muscles, and the body layer that contains fat and skin. Considering the small size of the ovaries, positioned under all of this covering, it is understandable that they are sometimes hard to feel.

As the ovaries become affected by cancer, they begin to enlarge. Unfortunately, because of their normal small size and position, growth is hard to detect until it is fairly significant. In addition, the early symptoms of ovarian cancer are vague. Bloating, abdominal discomfort, and pelvic cramps are all early symptoms of ovarian cancer. But, these are also common complaints experienced by countless numbers of people. Bloating, abdominal discomfort, and pelvic cramps may be attributed to intestinal problems and are sometimes ignored by the patient or her physician. Usually these symptoms simply go away without any real illness developing. However, you should report to your doctor any abdominal complaints that persist for more than a week or two, and you should probably be examined.

What Does "Screening Test" Mean?

Medical tests are usually performed when a person has symptoms of a disease and a specific diagnosis is suspected. In contrast, a screening test is performed to detect a disease in people who feel entirely *well*. In order for a screening test to be effective, it must be able to detect the disease in its earliest stages when cure is possible. A screening test must also be relatively easy and inexpensive to perform and be fairly specific for the disease you are attempting to detect. For example, a test that is even 99.6 percent specific for a particular disease will only detect 1 affected woman for every 10 women who test positive.

A Pap smear is a very effective screening test for cervical cancer. The test is easy and inexpensive to perform and can detect abnormal cervical cells in a precancerous form. These abnormal cells can be easily treated, thus preventing the development of cervical cancer. The goal has been to find a screening test just as effective for ovarian cancer.

Is Sonography a Good Screening Test for Ovarian Cancer?

Unfortunately, the answer is no. Sonography is a medical test that uses sound waves bounced off the ovaries to form a picture on a screen, much like the technology used for a ship's sonar. This technique was felt to be a promising method to detect growth in the ovaries that might be the beginning of a cancer. The hope was that this test would detect ovarian cancer before it had a chance to spread. Unfortunately, the test has a hard time distinguishing between ovarian cancer and benign ovarian cysts. These benign cysts are much more common than ovarian cancer, and most of them do not need to be treated at all (see chapter 5).

A study that illustrates this problem was conducted in England. An ad for free ovarian cancer screening was placed in the paper. Within a short period of time, 5,700 women agreed to get this free testing. Of the 5,700 women who had a sonogram of their ovaries, 361 of them had abnormal-appearing ovaries. The 361 women then underwent major abdominal surgery. Three of these women were found to have widely spread ovarian cancer that would have been easily detected by a pelvic exam. And only three women with early ovarian cancer were found and cured. This is wonderful for the three women whose lives were saved by the sonogram. However, 355 women had a major surgery that they did not need. They were subjected to the risks of anesthesia, bleeding, need for transfusion, infection, and injury, in addition to the discomfort of surgery and the time needed for recovery. At this point, for the general population the risk that an abnormal screening sonogram may lead to unnecessary surgery seems to outweigh the benefit.

In addition, it has been calculated that if all 43 million American women over the age of fifty had a pelvic sonogram every year, we might expect to find an abnormality in 2.5 million women. Thirty-seven thousand of these women would be found to have ovarian cancer that otherwise would not have been detected so early. But 2,463,000 women would have had unnecessary surgery. Of those women, 2,500 might be expected to die from the procedure, and 112,500 would have a serious complication. In addition, the cost of the sonograms would be $11.8 *billion* per year. The cost of the unnecessary surgeries would be about $37.5 *billion* per year. So, for all these reasons, a sonogram is not recommended as a routine screening test for ovarian cancer.

Susan's Abnormal Sonogram

Susan is a fifty-eight-year-old woman who saw her family physician after a few weeks of mild abdominal pain and bloating. She felt no nausea or vomiting and hadn't had diarrhea, constipation, or any fever. The examination of her abdomen was normal, as was a pelvic and rectal exam. Blood tests for infection, liver, and gallbladder problems were also normal. Susan and her doctor were both reassured by all this, and she was given a medication to reduce any spasm in the intestines. When the pain and bloating persisted despite the medication, her doctor ordered some X-rays of her intestines and a sonogram of her gallbladder and pelvis. All of these tests were also normal, with the exception of a two-inch fluid-filled cyst seen in her left ovary.

Susan came to our office worried that this test indicated ovarian cancer. On examination, I couldn't feel anything abnormal. In addition, there was no tenderness on examination of her uterus, fallopian tubes, or ovaries, and it seemed unlikely that her original complaints of pain and bloating were related to a gynecologic problem at all. But when I reviewed the sonogram, it was clear that a cystic mass was in fact present. Since Susan was postmenopausal, it was unlikely that this represented a simple ovarian cyst, the kind that would disappear by itself. We performed a CA-125 test (see page 288), which was thankfully normal. At this point, the suspicion of ovarian cancer was extremely low, but because a mass was present, I recommended surgery to remove it. We performed a laparoscopy (see page 165) the next week. During surgery, it was immediately clear that the mass was not her ovary but rather her fallopian tube, which was filled with fluid. This probably resulted from a previous infection that had occurred many years before and had never caused any symptoms or problems. In fact, had the sonogram not been performed, no one would have ever known about the "cyst," and she never would have had surgery.

We removed the fallopian tube through the laparoscope to prevent similar confusion in the future. The pathologist confirmed that this was an old infection that had been cured by the body's defenses long ago. Interestingly, following all the commotion of testing, surgery, and recovery, Susan's pain gradually went away by itself. I do feel that all the right things were done for Susan's problem and that surgery was indicated under the circumstances. However, I think her case illustrates that medical tests are not foolproof and sometimes can lead to other unnecessary tests or procedures. As noted above, the performance of routine yearly sonograms on all women would certainly lead to more situations like Susan's.

What About Doppler Sonography?

Doppler sonography is a special form of sonography that uses sound waves to measure the speed of blood flowing through blood vessels. Blood vessels that form along with cancerous growths have thinner walls than normal blood vessels, allowing blood to flow faster. If the speed of the blood flow can be measured, then the likelihood of cancer can be determined. The theory makes some sense, but unfortunately the results of this technique have not been very promising so far. Some benign ovarian cysts have the rapid flow that we expect from a cancer, and some cancerous cysts have slow blood flow and appear benign. Perhaps with better technology and more experience, the test may become useful, but, at present, it is still considered experimental.

Is CA-125 a Good Screening Test for Ovarian Cancer?

Cancer cells are different than normal cells, and they produce different chemicals. One of these chemicals has been detected in the bloodstream of women with ovarian cancer to a much greater degree than in normal women. The blood test to detect this chemical is called CA-125, because it was the 125th substance that was tested to look for a marker for ovarian cancer.

Like sonography, the CA-125 test can appear abnormal in normal women who do not have ovarian cancer. For women who are postmenopausal, ovarian cancer will only be found in about 5 percent of women with an elevated CA-125 level. The test is even less accurate in women who have not yet reached menopause. Conditions common in young women—endometriosis, fibroids, ovarian cysts, pelvic infections, pregnancy, normal menstrual periods—can all make the level of CA-125 go up in the absence of cancer. In addition, the test can be elevated in entirely healthy women of any age for no apparent reason.

Therefore, it is not a good idea to perform this test on all women in an effort to detect ovarian cancer. If abnormal, the result usually scares the patient. The doctor, also worried about the possibility of ovarian cancer, will more often than not recommend surgery that is likely to be unnecessary.

Also, CA-125 levels are normal in 50 percent of women who *do* have early ovarian cancer, precisely the women we would like to find in order to treat them when the disease is curable. Therefore, we do not recommend CA-125 as a screening test for ovarian cancer.

Olivia's Abnormal CA-125 Test

Olivia is a forty-seven-year-old woman with three children. Recently, her aunt (her mother's sister) was diagnosed with ovarian cancer. Olivia's health was excellent, and she felt fine, but she was concerned and afraid and went to see her doctor. When Olivia told her doctor why she was worried about ovarian cancer, the doctor performed a pelvic examination, which was normal, and then ordered a CA-125 test. The test came back abnormal. At the time I saw Olivia, she was very anxious and had been unable to sleep or relax. I explained to her that the CA-125 test was most likely falsely elevated because of its lack of accuracy in premenopausal women. Unfortunately, this did little to reassure her. I performed another pelvic exam that was completely normal; her ovaries felt fine.

We talked about what to do at this point and decided to try to get more information about her ovaries. Olivia wanted concrete proof that she did not have ovarian cancer. I repeated the CA-125 test and ordered a pelvic sonogram. Normally, I would not have recommended either test, but Olivia was so concerned that I felt if the additional information was reassuring, we might not have to do any surgery. The sonogram came back perfectly normal, but the CA-125 test was still high. Despite long conversations and reassurances based on the medical facts, Olivia wanted an absolute guarantee that she did not have ovarian cancer. Unfortunately, the only guarantee would be the removal of her ovaries and examination of them under the microscope.

Olivia insisted on surgery despite the risks and needed time for recovery. In addition, this was going to be expensive because her insurance company told her they would not pay for the surgery since she did not have a disease to justify an operation. Olivia wanted the surgery anyway. We performed a laparoscopic removal of her ovaries as an outpatient. During the operation her ovaries appeared normal, and immediate examination by the pathologist confirmed that no cancer was present. Despite having to go through surgery and a significant expense, Olivia was so relieved by the pathology report that in the recovery room she said that the ordeal had been worth it. However, I couldn't help but wish that the initial CA-125 test had never been done.

Do Screening Tests Make Sense If You Are at Very High Risk for Developing Ovarian Cancer?

Possibly. If you have a very strong family history of ovarian cancer, the goal must be early detection. For those few women who have a ten to fifty times greater risk of developing ovarian cancer (see page 277), it is probably worth the risk of having a falsely abnormal test result, even if it leads to unnecessary surgery. A number of medical programs have been established to test high-risk women with sonograms and CA-125 levels in an attempt to detect ovarian cancer at an early and curable stage and collect information about the effectiveness of these tests. If you are at high risk, you might ask your doctor if a program exists nearby. To date, these programs have found only a few early, curable ovarian cancers. In addition, a number of women have had normal screening tests but go on to develop ovarian cancer within the next six months, before they are due to be tested again. We hope as information continues to be gathered, some methods will be developed that can lead to early ovarian cancer detection. As noted below, women who are at very high risk might consider the removal of their ovaries.

Are There Any New Screening Tests on the Horizon?

There is an enormous amount of money being spent on ovarian cancer research, and much of it is aimed at tests for early detection. The most recent and interesting of these developments is called proteomics. Researchers took blood samples from women with ovarian cancer and compared all the proteins present in their blood to the blood samples from women without ovarian cancer. Using complicated computer analysis, they were able to detect a group of proteins in the women with cancer that were not present in the cancer-free women. Despite not knowing what proteins they had found or what their function was, they were able to determine a pattern of proteins that was consistently found in women with cancer. This pattern of proteins was then checked against stored blood samples from another group of women. Half of these women had surgery for ovarian cancer, and the other half were cancer free. The researchers were not made aware of which blood samples came from which women. All women (100 percent) with cancer were accurately detected by the test. Importantly, all (100 percent) women with early, *curable* ovarian cancer had an abnormal test result. And 95 percent of women without ovarian cancer had a normal test. While this technology is still in its infancy, this kind of analysis appears promising for the early detection of ovarian cancer. If the test continues to be successful, it will probably be available to the public in the next few years.

Other tests for individual proteins in the blood that might signal early ovarian cancer are being investigated. LAPA (the abbreviation for the biochemical it measures) and osteopontin are but two. These are blood tests along the lines of CA-125, and only time will tell if they show any promise.

A new and novel idea for detecting ovarian precancer is comparable to a Pap smear of the ovary. After the patient takes mild sedation, a tiny telescope (the size of pencil lead) is placed through the navel and into the abdominal cavity, and two similarly sized instruments are placed above the pubic bone. This microlaparoscopy allows the doctor to scrape cells off the surface of the ovary for genetic analysis. The hope is that precancerous mutations can be detectable well before cancer actually develops, much as a Pap smear detects precancerous cells of the cervix. Because the procedure involves surgery and some risk of complications, it is presently performed only on women with a strong family history of ovarian cancer.

Should You Have Your Ovaries Removed *Before* They Develop Cancer?

The answer to this question depends on your risk of ovarian cancer and on the level of anxiety you feel based upon this risk. Remember that very few women, less than 5 percent who get ovarian cancer, have inherited this disease. If you have two first-degree relatives (mother or sisters) with ovarian cancer and, therefore, may have as high as a 50 percent risk of developing ovarian cancer, or if you have the BRCA gene, removing your ovaries as soon as you finish having children is recommended. You should also consider having your children at an early age so that your ovaries can be removed before the age when your family members developed the disease. After surgery, you may consider taking hormone replacement therapy to treat bothersome menopausal symptoms or to prevent the development of osteoporosis.

Women who have one first-degree relative with ovarian cancer and one first-degree relative with either breast, uterine, or colon cancer are considered to have about a 12 percent risk of developing ovarian cancer. They should also consider having their ovaries removed after completing their families. Removal of the ovaries may now be accomplished using laparoscopic techniques. This surgery, using tiny incisions and the guidance of a small telescope, has the benefits of outpatient surgery and quick recovery.

All women with a family history of ovarian cancer should strongly consider taking birth control pills as a preventative measure (see page 283).

Janet and Jessica's Family History of Ovarian Cancer

Janet and Jessica are sisters whose mother recently discovered she had ovarian cancer. They believed their grandmother had died of ovarian cancer. Janet is thirty-three and wants one more child, in addition to the two she already has. Jessica is twenty-seven and not yet married, but looks forward to having a family. We discussed the fact that they were probably at a higher risk of developing ovarian cancer, probably around 25 percent. Since they both wished to get pregnant in the future, I recommended that they take birth control pills until they were ready to get pregnant. Since the pill stops the ovary from ovulating, it decreases the risk of ovarian cancer. So Janet and Jessica have started taking birth control pills to decrease their chance of getting the disease. With the knowledge we currently have, it would be reasonable to surgically remove Janet's and Jessica's ovaries after they have completed their families. Perhaps by that time, there will a genetic marker available to tell us exactly who is susceptible to the illness.

What Is the Best Way to Check on Your Ovaries?

For women who do not have a strong family history of ovarian cancer, the best way to check for ovarian cancer is still with an annual pelvic exam by your doctor. Sonograms or blood tests are not very good at finding early, curable ovarian cancer, and if you get a "false positive" result, you may end up with other tests and, at times, surgery (see page 286). In addition to being misleading, the high-tech testing is very expensive. In the near future, a better test probably will be available. But for now, see your doctor for a pelvic exam once a year, or at any other time you have symptoms or problems.

What Should Be Done If the Doctor Feels an Abnormal Ovary on Your Examination?

If your ovary feels enlarged at the time of your pelvic examination, further evaluation will depend on your age and the way the ovary feels to your doctor. As noted in chapter 5, most ovarian cysts are benign and need no treatment at all. This is usually true for women who are premenopausal. For postmenopausal women, the majority of cysts are also benign. However, the risk of ovarian cancer increases as a woman ages. Therefore, cysts found in postmenopausal woman are a little more cause for concern.

Benign cysts often feel smooth and movable to your doctor when your ovaries are examined. Cancer often feels hard, immobile, and irregular. Although the pelvic examination is helpful to determine if a cyst is present, a sonogram is usually required to determine what type of cyst it might be. The patterns that the cells form within the cyst can be seen on the sonogram and may suggest benign or malignant characteristics.

For a postmenopausal woman found to have an ovarian cyst, the CA-125 blood test result can provide additional helpful information. If the CA-125 result is elevated, it should be viewed with concern, and abdominal surgery should be performed. Since neither the sonogram nor the CA-125 test can make a *certain* diagnosis, surgery is needed to remove the ovary so that it may be examined under the microscope.

As noted before, the CA-125 test should *not* be performed in premenopausal women because it is often inaccurate in that age group. Premenopausal women should have a pelvic examination and a sonogram to determine whether surgery is necessary.

Evaluation of an Ovarian Cyst

Premenopausal	*Postmenopausal*
Pelvic examination	Pelvic examination
Sonogram	Sonogram
	CA-125

Is Surgery Necessary If Your Ovary Feels Abnormal?

As described in chapter 5, most ovarian cysts in young women go away by themselves, and no treatment is needed. These cysts tend to appear entirely clear and fluid filled on the sonogram. If the sonogram shows scattered areas of blood within the cyst (endometriosis) or areas of calcium (dermoid cyst), surgery is usually needed because these cysts will not go away by themselves. If the sonogram shows solid areas of tissue mixed with fluid, either a benign ovarian tumor or ovarian cancer may be present. Surgery is necessary. And because of the somewhat higher risk of ovarian cancer, surgery should always be considered when an abnormal ovary is found in a postmenopausal woman.

Are All Cysts Found in Postmenopausal Women Cancer?

When I was in residency training, we were taught that all cysts, in fact all enlarged ovaries, found in postmenopausal women were likely to be ovarian cancer. The thinking was that since these women were no longer ovulating, the simple types of cysts commonly found in premenopausal women should not ever form. Therefore, the risk of a cyst being cancer would be high. It was not uncommon for a cyst to be found upon examination, and surgery performed within a few days to remove not only the ovaries, but also the uterus. However, almost all of these cysts were benign.

As previously noted (see page 169), a recent study of 7,700 healthy postmenopausal women found small, benign-appearing ovarian cysts (two inches or less) in 450 (6 percent) of these women. Each woman had an ultrasound repeated two months later, and, surprisingly, half of the cysts had disappeared.

The women who still had a cyst after two months were given a choice of having surgery to remove the ovary or having another ultrasound performed a few months later. Half of the women chose surgery. *None* of these women had cancer. The other women chose to have repeated ultrasounds, and *none* of them developed ovarian cancer. It should be understood that benign cysts do not turn into cancer, so you do not need to worry about cancer developing in a benign cyst.

This study showed that benign-appearing cysts in postmenopausal women are not uncommon and are almost always benign. Therefore, the option of careful follow-up should be discussed. Some women or doctors may be uncomfortable with not removing an ovarian cyst. Some women may choose surgery, and others may choose careful follow-up. At this point, both options are reasonable.

What Kind of Surgery Can Be Done If You Have an Abnormal Ovary?

As noted in chapter 5, some ovarian cysts are benign but may need to be removed to prevent twisting, rupture, or continued growth. If the evaluation of a cyst with pelvic examination and sonogram (and CA-125 in postmenopausal women) suggests that the cyst is benign but needs to be removed, laparoscopic surgery is an excellent technique (see page 165). This method has the benefit of a very short hospital stay (usually less than twelve hours) and full recovery within a week or so.

However, if there is any concern based on the examination or sonogram (or CA-125 test in a postmenopausal woman) that cancer might be present, then the best choice is abdominal surgery. If cancer is found, standard surgery will give your doctor a better opportunity to remove all of the abnormal tissue. Although some gynecologic cancer specialists have been working on laparoscopic techniques to perform cancer surgery through the laparoscope, these techniques are not fully tested and therefore are not yet accepted as common practice. Abdominal surgery for ovarian cancer is still the accepted standard.

Jacqueline's Enlarged Ovary

Jacqueline is a seventy-three-year-old woman who saw her family doctor for a regular checkup. During the pelvic examination, her doctor felt an enlarged ovary on the right side and referred her for further evaluation. I spoke to Jacqueline about making an appointment and found that she was calm and confident about her health. To save time, I suggested that she get a pelvic sonogram and CA-125 test before coming to see me at the office. When she came for her appointment, she had the sonogram pictures and blood test results in hand for me to review.

When I examined Jacqueline, I could feel the enlarged ovary. The good news was that it wasn't very big, about two inches in diameter, and it did not feel stuck to her uterus or intestines, which may indicate cancer. After the examination, I reviewed the sonogram and was again relieved to see that the cyst on her ovary was totally filled with fluid, just like benign cysts. And her CA-125 blood test was normal. All of these tests pointed to a benign cyst, but it would be impossible to exclude cancer until the ovary was removed and examined under the microscope. However, because the risk for ovarian cancer was felt to be extremely small, I recommended laparoscopic surgery to shorten her hospital stay and encourage a quick recovery.

Jacqueline was admitted for surgery the next week. Using laparoscopic surgery, we were able to first drain the fluid out of her enlarged ovary and then remove the ovary through a small incision. The ovary was sent immediately to the pathologist, who examined it under the microscope and determined it was benign. We then removed her other ovary to prevent the development of any cysts, or even cancer, in the future. Jacqueline was able to go home the same day and was back to normal activity within ten days.

TREATMENT FOR OVARIAN CANCER

What If Cancer Is Suspected?

If ovarian cancer is suspected based on a pelvic examination, a sonogram, or an elevated CA-125 level in a postmenopausal woman, then abdominal surgery should be performed. The objectives of surgery are, first, to make a definite diagnosis and, second, to remove the cancer if it is found.

Gail's Abnormal Ovarian Cyst

Gail is a forty-six-year-old mother of two teenagers who came to the office for her regular annual examination. I felt that her left ovary was enlarged to about the size of a baseball. This was surprising to her because she had felt absolutely no pain or discomfort, although it is not uncommon to have a cyst without being aware of any pain or pressure.

The fact that I felt something abnormal frightened Gail, and her first thought was that this was cancer. I tried to reassure her that most ovarian cysts are *not* cancer, and a sonogram would be helpful to get a better idea as to what we were dealing with. Unfortunately, the sonogram was abnormal, showing what appeared to be solid areas of growth within the ovary—the picture that we sometimes see with ovarian cancer. I became concerned. The good news was that there was no evidence of anything else abnormal on Gail's sonogram or pelvic examination. My thinking was that this growth might not be cancer, but the only way to know was to perform surgery and remove the ovary.

Gail was understandably anxious and wanted the surgery performed as soon as possible. Because of the possibility of cancer, we made a regular abdominal incision. Laparoscopic surgery has not been fully adopted for patients with cancer. At the time of surgery, the first good news was that we did not see any evidence of obvious cancer. Cancer often looks like granular and irregular growths on top of, or embedded in, normal tissue. Gail's ovary was enlarged, but it and the rest of her pelvic organs looked smooth and healthy. Irregular cancer growths sometimes start to weep a clear fluid that collects inside the abdomen (called ascites), and we saw none of this fluid. I immediately started to feel better about Gail's problem.

We removed the ovary and had the pathologist perform a "frozen section" right away. The pathologist examined the ovary and took a small piece of tissue from an area she thought might be abnormal. She then placed the tissue in a special freezer for a few minutes. Once it was frozen, she cut it into extremely thin slices and placed the slices on a slide. The slide was then dipped into a dish of red- and then blue-colored solution that was soaked up by the cells so that they could be more easily seen under the microscope. When she examined the cells, the pathologist confirmed what we had hoped. The ovarian cyst was benign. The frozen section had taken fifteen minutes. After the surgery, Gail and her family were extremely relieved. I shared their relief and happiness, but at the same time I felt frustrated that we do not yet have a simpler way to make the diagnosis of a *benign* growth that would have avoided the anxiety, fear, and surgery that Gail had endured.

What Kind of Surgery Is Performed If Ovarian Cancer Is Found?

Ovarian cancer tends to spread to the organs right next to the ovary. Therefore, the uterus, the other ovary, and both fallopian tubes should be removed to eliminate any cancer cells that may have already spread. In addition, the fat pad surrounding the intestines, called the omentum, should be removed because it hangs directly over the pelvic organs, and cancer cells can easily attach to it. Removing your omentum may irritate your intestines for a few days and delay your ability to eat after surgery (see page 376). Otherwise, there are no side effects or long-term consequences. Biopsies of the inner lining of the abdominal cavity will also be taken to determine if the cancer has spread to these areas. Knowing whether the cancer has spread outside the ovary is important. If the cancer has not spread, then usually no further treatment is needed, and the prognosis is excellent. If the cancer has spread, chemotherapy is usually needed.

Can a Woman Who Has Had Ovarian Cancer Have Children?

If ovarian cancer is found in a woman who wishes to have children, and it appears *entirely* confined to one ovary, your doctor may consider just removing that one ovary to preserve your fertility. There is some risk in this choice in that you really do not know for sure if the cancer is confined to just that ovary until the entire ovary and other biopsies from the pelvis are examined by the pathologist. The complete pathology report takes about two days. If cancer is unexpectedly found in areas other than just the one ovary, then more surgery will be needed to perform a complete hysterectomy and remove any remaining cancer cells (see page 297). However, if all the other biopsies are normal, you do not need any further surgery and can get pregnant. Follow-up with pelvic exams, CA-125 tests, and sonograms may be suggested until you do get pregnant. Pregnancy has no effect, good or bad, on ovarian cancer. However, most gynecologic oncologists would recommend that you have a complete hysterectomy after completing your family to eliminate any future chance of cancer recurrence.

What Is Chemotherapy Like?

If the cancer cells have spread outside the ovary, chemotherapy is virtually always recommended. The goal of chemotherapy is to bathe any remaining cancer cells in the body with chemicals that are designed to destroy them. The drugs are usually given through an IV directly into the bloodstream over the course of a few hours. This treatment is given once every three to four weeks for a total of six treatments. Chemotherapy interferes with the ways that cells divide, and rapidly growing cells are more vulnerable to this effect. Cancer cells, which grow rapidly, are thus usually killed.

However, blood cells, hair, nails, and the lining cells of the intestinal tract are also all rapidly growing and renewing tissues. As a result, these cells often suffer the effects of the chemotherapy as well. The most common side effect of chemotherapy is nausea and sometimes vomiting. Often, the nausea is mild, but if it is a problem, relaxation techniques, changes in diet, or taking specific medications can be used to lessen this side effect. Psychologists who have experience working with cancer patients can help you choose remedies for your side effects.

Hair loss is often an anguishing side effect for anyone receiving chemotherapy. There is no physical discomfort, but it is a constant reminder of loss and illness. Some of the new drugs like Taxol will usually cause hair loss, but it is *temporary*, and the hair will grow back entirely once the treatments are finished.

The white blood cell count of most women decreases during chemotherapy, which makes them somewhat more susceptible to infection during the treatments. Care should be taken to avoid contact with people with colds or other infections. This susceptibility is temporary, and the white blood cells return to normal after about three weeks. The most common and bothersome complaint of women on chemotherapy is fatigue. A decrease in the number of red blood cells, which carry oxygen, lowers the ability of cells in your body to produce energy, and the result is fatigue. Women often describe waves of exhaustion that complicate even the smallest task. The exhaustion may last for a few hours or even a day or two. A good diet, regular exercise, and an ample amount of rest will usually help lessen the fatigue. Medications are now available that increase the white blood cell or red blood cell count, and these may be used if needed.

In general, as time goes on during the course of chemotherapy, you may start to feel worn down, both physically and emotionally. However, within a month of finishing chemotherapy, strength and energy start to return. After a few months, most women feel back to normal, have a more positive outlook on life, and are ready to move forward. Excellent books are available for women with ovarian cancer.

Anne's Ovarian Cancer

Anne is a seventy-two-year-old woman who went to see her internist because of abdominal pain and bloating. She had noted these problems for a few months, but they had been getting worse over the past few weeks. Her clothes were getting tighter around her waist despite the fact that her appetite was not very good, and she was eating less. Her internist felt an abnormal area near her ovaries and referred her for evaluation. On examination, it was clear that there was a mass of extra tissue around both of Anne's ovaries, and her abdomen appeared swollen. Ovarian cancer was my first thought, and this had already occurred to Anne. I asked her to have a sonogram and a CA-125 test, both of which came back abnormal. The diagnosis was almost certainly ovarian cancer, and Anne was very upset and frightened.

I asked Anne to see a gynecologic cancer specialist for a

consultation because I expected the upcoming surgery to be very difficult. The cancer felt as if it was wrapped around Anne's intestines, and I was concerned we might need to remove a piece of the intestine in order to remove all of the cancer. I expected that the oncologist's expertise would be needed. He agreed with the planned surgery, and we decided to perform it together. Gynecologic oncologists are first trained as obstetrician-gynecologists and then spend an extra two years training to take care of women with cancer of the uterus, fallopian tubes, or ovaries. Much of that extra time is spent learning to perform the difficult surgical procedures sometimes involved in removing cancer. We scheduled her surgery for the next week so that she would be able to make arrangements for someone to care for her ill husband.

At the time of surgery, it was immediately apparent that cancer was present. The ovaries were both covered with abnormal growths that extended up to the intestines and entwined them. It was no wonder that Anne's abdomen was swollen and her appetite decreased. During four hours of painstaking surgery, we removed the uterus, fallopian tubes, and ovaries, and a small portion of the intestine that had been encased in tumor. We also removed the fat pad around the intestine, which also had tumor on it. We could see that some cells were still stuck to areas of the intestines and the inside lining of the abdomen, but they could not be safely removed. Because of the extensive nature of the cancer, Anne was going to need chemotherapy. The goal of surgery was to remove as much cancer as safely possible, and we were able to remove about 99 percent of the cancer cells.

Anne was depressed after surgery, both because of the hard reality of having cancer and because of her slow recovery following a long and difficult surgery. Her family was very supportive and helped her through the next few days. Her husband was able to come to the hospital with one of their children, and this cheered her up a bit. The final pathology report came back two days after surgery. It confirmed what was certain, that cancer was present. But, it also showed that the cancer cells did not appear to be very irregular or wildly growing. Because of this, Anne's prognosis was better. This was some good news to soften the bad.

After Anne recovered from surgery, she began treatment with chemotherapy. Other than some fatigue, she tolerated the chemotherapy well. We measured her CA-125 levels regularly, which fell back to normal and, thankfully, stayed there.

If ovarian cancer recurs, it usually does so within the first year or two. For the first few years, Anne had a pelvic examination and CA-125 test every three months. As each year passed (we are now celebrating number ten for Anne), we all became increasingly confident that Anne was one of the fortunate women who have beaten this disease. I still see her every six months for her pelvic examination, and she remains totally healthy and cancer free.

What Are the Cure Rates of Ovarian Cancer?

The most common type of ovarian cancer comes from the cells that cover the ovaries, the epithelial cells. Epithelial cancer is responsible for about 90 percent of all ovarian cancers. If it is found early, before it has spread beyond the ovary (stage I), it is 90 percent curable. The only treatment necessary is removal of the ovary. However, once the cancer spreads outside the pelvic organs, the cure rate drops to around 30 percent despite major surgery and chemotherapy. That is the current predicament with this terrible disease. How can we make an early diagnosis and treat the disease when it is curable? There is an enormous amount of research being undertaken to find ways to prevent ovarian cancer from forming, to detect it early if it does occur, and to treat it more effectively. There is reason to believe that many of these goals will be attained in the near future.

Are There Different Kinds of Ovarian Cancer?

The ovary has a number of different kinds of cells within it, which can turn into cancer. The cells that are destined to become eggs can form a number of different cancers depending on which type of cell grows abnormally. This group of cancers is called the germ cell cancers. These cancers are very rare, accounting for only 5 percent of all ovarian cancers. It is impossible to tell the different types of ovarian cancer before surgery, but a pathologist can determine the type when he or she looks under the microscope. Germ cell cancers tend to occur in younger women, most often before age thirty. Many of these cancers cause early symptoms such as pelvic pain or pressure; therefore, germ cell cancers are often diagnosed before they spread. On a sonogram, germ cell cancers have a different appearance from functional ovarian cysts, which are extremely common in young women, and the diagnosis may be suspected from that test. The good news is that germ cell cancer is extremely curable.

What Are the Cure Rates for Germ Cell Cancer?

One of the major advances in cancer therapy has come in the treatment of germ cell tumors. Previously difficult to treat, almost all of these tumors can be now be *cured* with removal of just the affected ovary, followed by appropriate chemotherapy. Many women who have had germ cell cancers get pregnant and live totally normal and healthy lives.

What Is Borderline Ovarian Cancer?

Borderline ovarian cancer is also an overgrowth of abnormal ovarian cells. Borderline cancer doesn't behave like either a cancer or an entirely benign tumor. These tumors usually grow very slowly and do not spread as aggressively as ovarian cancer does. The entire ovary is usually removed, and the prognosis is very good, approaching a 95 percent cure rate following surgery. We make the diagnosis by looking at the cells under a microscope, and once it is made, no further treatment is needed. Careful follow-up is still important because sometimes tumor cells may have been left behind and can slowly grow back. Another surgery may then be necessary.

Can You Take Estrogen Replacement Therapy If You Have Had Ovarian Cancer?

Estrogen replacement therapy is used after menopause to provide estrogen to your body after the ovary has stopped making it. There is good evidence that estrogen *does not* make ovarian cancer any worse. Because your ovaries must be removed if ovarian cancer is found, you will have lost the main source of estrogen in your body. The loss of estrogen may cause bothersome symptoms such as hot flashes, insomnia, and vaginal dryness, especially if you were premenopausal before surgery. In addition, estrogen reduces the risk of osteoporosis by 70 percent, so estrogen therapy may be a good idea for some women.

If You Have Ovarian Cancer, What About Your Emotional Health?

I have learned a great deal from the women I know who have had cancer. Most importantly, I have learned what helped them get through it.

Many talk about the essential need of emotional support from loved ones. For many women, having someone to complain to, to cry to, or to talk about fears with seems to be a key part of enduring the treatment process. For some, crying is the only thing to do. Other women feel the need to push forward. They may cry at a later time, or not at all. You know yourself best—there is no "right" way to handle dealing with cancer.

This may seem like an inauspicious time to initiate relationships, but there are likely to be others in your community who are also undergoing treatment for ovarian cancer or other forms of cancer. Support groups are sponsored in hospitals, synagogues, and churches. These groups can be enormously helpful in providing support and education. Individual or family therapy may also be useful in helping you and your family get through these difficult times. There are now trained mental health professionals who specialize in working with cancer patients. They can provide methods to help control symptoms of the disease or side effects of medications, as well as help with overall coping.

It is often the case that family and friends rally around someone undergoing cancer treatment. You may want to allow people to help you. Many women who are accustomed to running a business or a career, a home, and a family find it difficult to be on the "needy" end. Some have told me that initially they turned down offers of homemade dinners or help with transportation, shopping, or baby-sitting. Cancer makes us all feel helpless. Some women felt that, by accepting some help, they eased not only their own burden but also helped their loved ones cope by allowing *them* to do something.

Women with cancer often mention the need for a sense of humor. Norman Cousins taught us years ago that laughter is often good medicine. Sometimes the trials and tribulations of the entire process lend itself to a sense of humor. The world of doctors, hospitals, and cancer treatment has a lot of raw material to work with. Look for those moments.

REFERENCES

Biesecker, B., M. Boehnke, K. Calzone, et al. 1993. Genetic counseling for families with inherited susceptibility to breast and ovarian cancer. *Journal of the American Medical Association* 269:1970–74.

Cousins, N. 1991. *Anatomy of an Illness.* New York: Bantam Doubleday.

Droegemueller, W. 1994. Screening for ovarian cancer: Hopeful and wishful thinking. *American Journal of Obstetrics and Gynecology* 170:1095–98.

Hankinson, S., G. Colditz, D. Hunter, B. Rosner, and M. Stampfer. 1992. A quantitative assessment of oral contraceptive use and risk of ovarian cancer. *Obstetrics and Gynecology* 80:708–14.

Kerlikowske, K., J. Brown, and D. Grady. 1992. Should women with a familial ovarian cancer undergo prophylactic oophorectomy? *Obstetrics and Gynecology* 80:700–7.

Ness, R., 2002. Infertility, fertility drugs, and ovarian cancer: A pooled analysis of case-controlled studies. *American Journal of Epidemiology* 155:217–24.

Parazzini, F., S. Franceschi, C. Vecchia, and M. Fasoli. 1991. The epidemiology of ovarian cancer. *Gynecology and Oncology* 43:9–23.

Petricoin, E., A. Ardekani, B. Hitt, P. Levine, V. Fusaro, S. Steinberg, G. Mills, C. Simone, D. Fishman, E. Kohn, and L. Liotta. 2002. Use of proteomic patterns in serum to identify ovarian cancer. *Lancet* 359:572–77.

Rossing, M., J. Daling, N. Weiss, D. Moore, and S. Self. 1994. Ovarian tumors in a cohort of infertile women. *New England Journal of Medicine* 331:771–76.

Stratton, J., P. Pharoah, D. Easton, and P. Ponder. 1998. A systematic review and meta-analysis of family history and risk of ovarian cancer. *British Journal of Obstetrics and Gynecology* 105:493–99.

Struewing, J., P. Hartge, S. Wacholder, S. Baker, M. Berlin, M. McAdams, M. Timmerman, L. Brody, and M. Tucker. 1997. The risk of cancer associated with specific mutations of BRCA1 and BRCA2 among Ashkenazi Jews. *New England Journal of Medicine* 336:1401–8.

11

UTERINE BLEEDING, PRECANCER, AND UTERINE CANCER

What Is Uterine Cancer?

The uterus, the organ that prepares each month to provide a home to a developing pregnancy, has two distinct layers. The main body of the uterus is made of muscle, and the inner lining is composed of the cells that are shed monthly as the menstrual period (see fig. 11.1). Uterine cancer develops within the lining cells, called the endometrial cells, of the uterus and not the uterine muscle itself. For that reason, uterine cancer is often called endometrial cancer. The terms *uterine cancer* and *endometrial cancer* are often used interchangeably.

As in most cases of cancer, we do not fully understand the reason why the uterine lining cells begin to grow in an abnormal and an uncontrolled manner. When the cells become abnormal, they first go through a precancerous stage. The good news is that both the precancer and early cancer usually cause abnormal bleeding and are, therefore, often diagnosed at a time when they are quite easy to cure.

What Is Atypical Hyperplasia?

As the endometrial cells overgrow and become abnormal, they go through a precancerous phase called atypical endometrial hyperplasia. Hyperplasia means overgrowth, and simple hyperplasia is a benign condition. However, if the overgrowth is also associated with changes in the

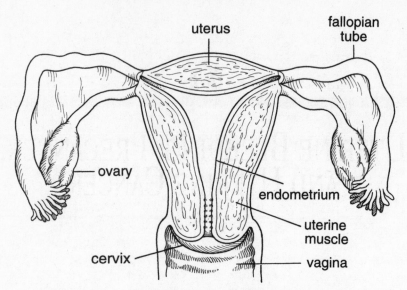

Fig. 11.1. Endometrium (uterine lining cells)

cells that allow it to grow uncontrollably, then a precancerous condition is said to exist. We detect this precancerous condition, called atypical hyperplasia, by observing irregular and dividing lining cells under the microscope. Further uncontrolled growth leads to endometrial (uterine) cancer, characterized by cells that divide wildly.

Is Uterine Cancer Common?

Although uterine cancer is the most common cancer of the female pelvic organs, it is still rare, occurring in only 2 out of every 1,000 women older than fifty. The average age of a woman who has uterine cancer is sixty. It is seen much less frequently in younger women. Only 5 percent of women who develop uterine cancer are under forty years of age, and it is almost unheard of in women under thirty.

What Causes Uterine Cancer?

The actual cause of uterine cancer is not known, but certain things may make a woman more likely to develop it. Imbalances between the two main hormones, estrogen and progesterone, are important factors in this disease.

Estrogen, produced by the ovaries, stimulates the growth of uterine lining cells. In general terms, an uncontrolled overgrowth of cells is defined as cancer. Therefore, if the cells are exposed to too much estrogen over a long period of time, the precancerous condition called atypical hyperplasia may develop. Further exposure to high levels of estrogen can lead to cancer.

Progesterone, the other main female hormone, which is only produced for the two weeks after ovulation, causes the endometrial cells to stop growing. A lack of progesterone like that found in some women who do not ovulate regularly may allow the cells to grow without this restraint and can also lead to overgrowth and abnormal cells. Even though we don't truly know the cause of uterine cancer at this time, it appears that long-standing hormonal imbalances are an important element.

Does Being Overweight Increase Your Risk of Uterine Cancer?

We have come to realize that uterine cancer appears more commonly in persistently overweight or obese women. Normally, the cells that compose fat have the ability to convert adrenal hormones, produced in the small adrenal gland above each kidney, into estrogen. The more fat cells you have, the more adrenal hormone is converted into estrogen, thus raising the total amount of estrogen in the bloodstream. Since estrogen stimulates the growth of the endometrial cells, too much estrogen can lead to overgrowth, precancer, or even cancer. Losing weight will decrease this production of extra estrogen and decrease your risk of developing uterine cancer.

Does Frequently Missing Your Period Increase Your Risk of Uterine Cancer?

Women with a history of many missed periods during their reproductive years are also at an increased risk of developing uterine cancer. Even when you are missing periods, your ovaries continue to make estrogen. However, progesterone is produced in the body only after the release of an egg.

One of the most common causes of irregular periods is a hormonal imbalance that leads to a failure of ovulation (see page 73). Without ovulation, the ovary does not produce progesterone. Without the progesterone around to put a brake on cell growth, the lining cells continue to grow unabated. Over many months or years, these cells may overgrow to the point of forming precancer or cancer.

If you are premenopausal and do not have more than a few periods a year, you should discuss your situation with your doctor. Treatment with progesterone tablets is often indicated and is an easy and safe way to stop this overgrowth.

Do Other Medical Conditions Increae Your Risk of Uterine Cancer?

Women who have diabetes or high blood pressure seem to develop uterine cancer more often than women who do not have these medical problems. We do not understand the reasons for this, although diabetes and high blood pressure are more common in overweight people. And being overweight increases your risk of developing uterine cancer.

Does Taking Estrogen Alone for Menopause Increase Your Risk of Uterine Cancer?

Many years ago, estrogen *alone* was given to postmenopausal women to relieve their hot flashes and other menopausal symptoms. However, in 1975, it was discovered that these women had a higher incidence of uterine cancer. Since we now know that estrogen causes overgrowth of endometrial cells, taking estrogen alone resulted in that increase in uterine cancer.

If you do not take any hormones after menopause, your risk of developing uterine cancer is 2 per 1,000 women. However, if you take estrogen alone after menopause, your risk of developing endometrial cancer increases to about 10 per 1,000 women. If you take progesterone along with the estrogen, your risk decreases to less than 1 per 1,000 women. This decreased risk results from the protective effect that progesterone has on endometrial cells. Therefore, it is recommended that progesterone be taken along with estrogen for postmenopausal hormone replacement.

Janet Has Abnormal Bleeding

Janet is a sixty-nine-year-old woman who was referred to me by her family physician because she had begun having vaginal bleeding. When she had entered menopause twenty years ago, she had initially resisted taking estrogen replacement therapy. At the time, this was not unusual since many women and doctors were skeptical and afraid of hormone replacement. However, severe hot flashes and lack of sleep finally wore her down, and within a year she asked to start estrogen. As was common at that time, estrogen was started alone, without any progesterone. And for the next twenty years, estrogen alone is what her doctor continued to prescribe, and that is what she took.

The bleeding had started recently, but otherwise she felt fine. Her pelvic examination was entirely normal. Since she had not been taking any progesterone, I knew she was at risk for uterine cancer. Therefore, I recommended that she have a D&C and hysteroscopy to evaluate the cause of the bleeding. As usual, we performed the hysteroscopy first. The hysteroscope is a very small telescope that allows us to see inside the uterus to determine what may be the cause of abnormal bleeding. Instead of the normal pale pink, smooth lining of the uterus, a cauliflower-shaped, grayish bleeding area was seen at the top of the uterus. It looked like cancer. (see fig. 11.2).

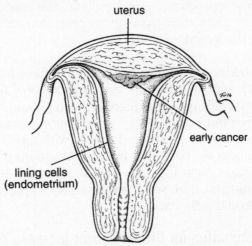

Fig. 11.2. Uterine cancer

The D&C removed a considerable amount of tissue for the pathologist to examine under the microscope. I told Janet what I suspected, and she was shocked because she felt entirely well. It is sometimes especially difficult to come to grips with having a major illness when you feel completely fine. I explained that this was often the case with uterine cancer. It does not cause pain until it is very far advanced. And since this was Janet's first episode of bleeding and she had no symptoms and a normal pelvic examination, I was hopeful that the disease was in its early stages and therefore curable.

A week after the D&C, the pathology report confirmed that uterine cancer was present. But the cells appeared to be slow growing, which suggested an excellent prognosis. For reasons that are not clear, the uterine cancer that results from taking estrogen after menopause without any progesterone is usually a slow-growing disease and often is less aggressive than uterine cancer unrelated to estrogen therapy. We scheduled Janet for surgery the next week. To remove all the cancerous cells, removal of her uterus—a hysterectomy—would be necessary. In all likelihood, this surgery would provide an almost certain cure.

At the time of surgery there was no evidence of any spread of the cancer, and on the morning of her discharge from the hospital, the pathology report from the hysterectomy confirmed that the cancer was the slow-growing type and had not begun to spread. Janet's prognosis was excellent. She was angry about having been given estrogen without progesterone, but was relieved that she would be well.

If you are taking estrogen alone (and you have not previously had a hysterectomy), you should have an ultrasound of the uterine lining cells. If the lining cells appear overgrown, you should have some of the lining cells of the uterus removed by your doctor and examined under a microscope. This can be performed simply with a procedure called an endometrial biopsy (see page 87). If the cells appear normal, then a decision can be made regarding how you should take your hormones. If the cells are abnormal, then you have probably caught the precancer or cancer early, when it is treatable.

Does Taking Tamoxifen for Breast Cancer Increase Your Risk of Uterine Cancer?

Tamoxifen is a medication that is frequently prescribed for postmenopausal women who have had breast cancer. Tamoxifen helps to prevent the recurrence of breast cancer, although the reason for this prevention is not known. However, a possible side effect of the medication is an overgrowth of the endometrial cells of the uterus. In a small number of women taking tamoxifen, precancer or cancer of the uterus may develop.

As is true with uterine cancer in general, abnormal bleeding or spotting will occur in most women who develop precancer or cancer while taking tamoxifen. At one time, annual testing with either biopsy or ultrasound measurements was recommended to help evaluate the uterine lining cells. Unfortunately, these screening tests for uterine precancer or cancer have not proved helpful. Therefore, it is important for women taking tamoxifen to alert their physician if any vaginal bleeding or spotting occurs. An ultrasound of the uterine lining will often show thickening as a result of the tamoxifen, so often a hysteroscopy and D&C are necessary to make sure no cancer is present.

Lillian Takes Tamoxifen

Lillian is a sixty-one-year-old woman who found a small lump in her breast while doing her monthly self-exam during her morning shower. It was now two years since the lump had been removed and diagnosed as cancer. Luckily, this malignancy was discovered fairly early. There was no spread to her lymph nodes, and she had been told her prognosis was excellent. Her oncologist had placed her on tamoxifen to help decrease her risk of recurrence. For two years, she had been doing well and feeling fine. However, she recently noticed a small amount of vaginal bleeding and was sent to me for further evaluation.

As was expected, her examination was normal. In light of the fact that she was bleeding, and especially because she was taking tamoxifen, I recommended a hysteroscopy and D&C (see page 316). This was performed in the office the following week. The hysteroscopy revealed that an endometrial polyp was present. Polyps are also more common in women taking tamoxifen. I was able to remove it easily, and the pathology report showed that it was benign. With that reassuring news, Lillian was able to continue the tamoxifen as recommended.

Is Uterine Cancer an Inheritable Disease?

Most uterine cancers do not appear to run in families. However, some of the risk factors for uterine cancer, such as diabetes, hypertension, and obesity, do run in families and thus may indirectly increase your risk for uterine cancer.

There are also a very small number of families that have a very high incidence of breast, colon, ovarian, and uterine cancers over many generations. This rare syndrome of inheritable cancers is called the Lynch Family Cancer Syndrome, named after Dr. Henry Lynch, who discovered this genetic link. If you are aware of a number of people in your family who have had these cancers, you should consider seeing a genetic counselor who is specially trained to determine your risk of getting a specific disease based on a detailed study of your family history (see page 282). If it is determined that you are at high risk for any of these cancers, appropriate screening tests can be performed for early detection of precancer or cancer. For uterine cancer, an effective screening test is an annual endometrial biopsy.

Does Having Children Decrease Your Risk of Uterine Cancer?

Women who have had a number of full-term pregnancies are at decreased risk of developing uterine cancer. During pregnancy, the placenta normally produces a large amount of progesterone that relaxes the uterine muscle cells and prevents early labor. When the uterine lining cells are exposed to this progesterone, any growth, or overgrowth, of these cells is restrained. This small degree of protection from the development of uterine cancer appears to be lifelong.

What Can You Do to Decrease Your Risk of Uterine Cancer?

Interestingly, women who have taken birth control pills for five years or longer have a 60 percent lower risk of getting uterine cancer. All birth control pills contain more progesterone than estrogen. We know that progesterone decreases uterine lining cell growth. This is apparent to women who have taken the pill because they often notice less menstrual bleeding as a result of this thinner lining. Less cell growth also means a lower risk of overgrowth that might develop to the point of cancer. Another benefit of taking birth control pills is described in chapter 10; the pill decreases the risk of ovarian cancer by 50 percent as well.

What Are the Symptoms of Uterine Cancer?

Abnormal bleeding is an early sign of uterine cancer, but most women who have abnormal bleeding *do not* have uterine cancer. As discussed in chapter 3, there are lots of other, more likely, and nonworrisome causes of abnormal bleeding. But in the rare woman who has developed uterine cancer, the cancer cells often become fragile and are more prone to bleeding.

The bleeding tends to occur irregularly and unpredictably, whenever the cells become fragile enough to break off. Luckily, the blood from these cancer cells can be easily seen as it passes through the cervix and into the vagina. As a result, abnormal cells are often detected at a very early stage, when they are treatable, and long before cancer has a chance to spread.

Uterine cancer in its early stages does not cause pain, nausea, vomiting, or other obvious symptoms. Since they feel entirely well, many women are shocked to find that they have uterine cancer. Also, irregular bleeding may last for only a few days and then, as some of the abnormal tissue temporarily heals, may stop for days, weeks, or even months. Therefore, if you have abnormal bleeding, you should see your doctor, even if you otherwise feel fine, and even if the bleeding stops. This is true for women of any age but is especially true for postmenopausal women, where the incidence of uterine precancer and cancer is higher.

Mary's Uterine Cancer

Mary was a forty-six-year-old woman who had had fibroids for a number of years. When she began to have heavy bleeding, she telephoned her doctor, who reassured her that this was the result of her fibroids and nothing to worry about. About six months later, she began to have bleeding in between her periods, and her doctor asked her to come in for an examination. The pelvic examination showed that her uterus was slightly enlarged from the fibroids but had not changed size in over a year. Again, the doctor told Mary not to worry.

For the next few months, Mary's periods were regular and reasonably normal in flow, and she felt very relieved that the problem had just gone away. However, the following two periods were heavy, and she again began to have bleeding in between periods. At this point, Mary sought a second opinion and came to me for an examination and consultation. Her pelvic examination showed that her uterus was slightly enlarged from the fibroids, but the history of abnormal bleeding suggested that other tests should be performed to determine whether a cause other than the fibroids might be responsible for the bleeding.

We scheduled a hysteroscopy and D&C in the office (see page 316). During the hysteroscopy, a large amount of extra endometrial tissue was seen, which was an indication of some type of abnormality.

A D&C was then performed to scrape out the uterine lining cells for analysis under the microscope. The pathology report from the D&C showed uterine cancer, and, unfortunately, it appeared to be a fast-growing type. Mary was naturally upset and felt distraught that this problem had likely been with her for a while, but she had been told not to worry about it.

We scheduled a hysterectomy for the end of that week. In addition, we planned to remove some lymph nodes near the uterus to make sure the cancer had not begun to spread. Unfortunately, during the surgery, we were dismayed to find many enlarged lymph nodes, which was evidence that the cancer had already spread. We removed the lymph nodes and performed a hysterectomy and sent all the tissue for analysis under the microscope. As we feared, the lymph nodes were full of cancer. And the uterus contained cancer cells, which appeared to be a very fast-growing type.

After the surgery, I joined Mary and her husband to discuss all the implications of these findings. The prognosis was not good since the cancer had already spread to the lymph nodes. Some form of additional treatment would be needed, and I recommended that she see a gynecologic oncologist, a cancer specialist, for further evaluation and treatment. About two weeks later, when she began to feel stronger, Mary went to see the gynecologic oncologist. As soon as she recovered from the surgery, he began to give her high doses of chemotherapy.

Unfortunately, a few months later, a CT scan (a very sensitive X-ray test) showed that the cancer was regrowing—the chemotherapy was not working. The last chance was to place Mary on high doses of progesterone. While this is not expected to cure the cancer, it keeps the cancer controlled for months or even years in some women. A few months later, I saw Mary as she was leaving the hospital following one of her frequent follow-up tests. For the first time, she appeared completely discouraged and worn down. The cancer appeared to be winning. A month later, her husband called to tell me that she had passed away.

Cancer is sometimes unpredictable, and Mary's had been fast growing. I cannot help but wonder, though, whether an earlier D&C and earlier detection of the cancer would have saved her life. Both she and her husband had agonized over that same question. For me, as a gynecologist, the thought of Mary has reemphasized the lesson of never ignoring abnormal bleeding. If your body is signaling you with a symptom, take it seriously and don't ignore it. Make sure your physician does the same.

Does a Pap Smear Detect Uterine Cancer?

Usually not, since this test was designed to detect cervical cancer and was not intended to diagnose uterine cancer. The Pap smear is a scraping of just the cells from the cervix, the lower part of the uterus that connects to the top of the vagina. The uterine lining cells, called endometrial cells, are way up inside the uterus and are not reached during the Pap smear. Therefore, a normal Pap smear does *not* exclude the possibility of uterine cancer.

On rare occasions, the cells from the uterine lining may fall down into the cervix and can be seen on the Pap smear. Although the occurrence of these cells in the cervix can be normal, the cells may be falling down because they are overgrowing. Full evaluation of the lining cells with a D&C should be done to make sure that no precancer or cancer is present, especially if the cells are found after menopause.

Can a Sonogram Detect Uterine Cancer?

A sonogram, a picture made as a result of bouncing sound waves off parts of the body, can be used to examine the uterus. As uterine lining cells overgrow, they form a thicker lining that can be visibly detected by sonogram. Unfortunately, the thickened lining of hyperplasia, which is benign, looks exactly the same as atypical hyperplasia (which is precancer) and the same as uterine cancer. Thus, the sonogram cannot make the diagnosis of uterine cancer. If a sonogram detects a thick uterine lining, then a D&C should be performed to determine whether abnormal cells are present.

Who Should Be Evaluated for Uterine Cancer?

Any postmenopausal woman having abnormal bleeding needs a doctor's evaluation. If you have not had a period for a year or more and then begin to bleed, this is abnormal. If you are taking hormone replacement therapy and bleed at the wrong time, this is abnormal.

How Is the Diagnosis of Uterine Cancer Made?

To diagnose uterine cancer, the lining cells of the uterus must be collected so that they can be examined under a microscope. A simple procedure called an endometrial biopsy is one way to collect these cells. It is performed in the doctor's office, takes about one minute, and is essentially painless. A very thin plastic instrument is inserted through your cervix and into the uterine cavity. As the instrument is removed, it uses a gentle suction to scrape off and collect the endometrial cells. These cells are then placed into a bottle and sent to the lab for examination under a microscope.

As an alternative, an office D&C may be suggested to determine the cause of uterine bleeding. The doctor's recommendation for an office D&C rather than an endometrial biopsy will depend on your age, the amount of bleeding you are having, the findings at the time of your examination, the appearance of the lining cells on ultrasound, and your general medical condition. An office D&C is somewhat more accurate than an endometrial biopsy because it removes more cells for analysis. I think an office D&C is indicated for all women bleeding after menopause, and who have a thickened uterine lining seen on ultrasound, women with very heavy bleeding, or women who have had an endometrial biopsy but have persistent or recurrent bleeding. Women who have an enlarged uterus should have a D&C because adequate sampling of the lining cells may be difficult with an endometrial biopsy.

An office D&C is somewhat more involved than an endometrial biopsy, and a mild sedative medication may be necessary. Usually, a very small telescope called a hysteroscope is first placed through the cervix to examine the uterine lining cells. This helps your doctor see what abnormalities exist and can help identify the area that should be removed for review by the pathologist. Together, the D&C and hysteroscopy take about five minutes. Discomfort, in the form of menstrual-type cramping, is very mild and is sometimes not experienced at all. If you prefer to have general anesthesia so that you feel nothing, a D&C may also be performed in the hospital. A full description of office D&C and hysteroscopy is found on page 86.

What Does Endometrial Cancer Look Like Under the Microscope?

As normal endometrial cells overgrow, the cells become more abundant and crowded together. This is called hyperplasia and is not a worrisome condition. In some women, however, in addition to the overgrowth, the individual cells become irregularly shaped, and the nucleus, the part of the cell that contains the genetic material, starts to divide more rapidly than normal. This is called atypical hyperplasia and is considered a precancerous condition. When these cells are even more overgrown and wildly dividing, endometrial cancer is said to be present (see fig. 11.3).

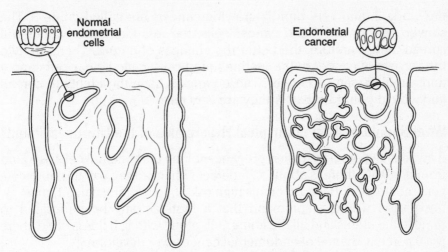

Fig. 11.3. Uterine lining cells

Should You Consider a Second Opinion for the Pathology Results of an Endometrial Biopsy or D&C?

The interpretation of abnormal cells under the microscope is not an exact science, and differences of opinion among pathologists can exist. Pathologists often have areas of expertise, and it is reasonable, especially if there is any question about the findings from a D&C, to have a second opinion from a pathologist experienced in gynecologic pathology. In fact, one study found that 60 percent of biopsies originally thought to represent hyperplasia were normal when reviewed by an expert pathologist. Only 3 percent of these biopsies were found to represent cancer. This is something you might discuss with your doctor. To get a second opinion, the original glass slides prepared by your doctor's lab can be sent to the second lab, and no new tests or biopsies need to be done. If a diagnosis is not clear, I may rely on a specialty pathologist nearby or, sometimes, will even send slides to pathologists in other areas of the country for a second opinion.

Is All Uterine Cancer the Same?

The cells that line the uterus are called endometrial cells, and the cancer that results is technically called endometrial cancer. For reasons that are not clear, some of these cells become fast-growing cancers, and some grow much more slowly. The slow-growing cancers are called grade 1 endometrial cancer. Those that grow somewhat more rapidly are grade 2, and very rapidly growing cancers are called grade 3. The slower the growth of the cancer cells, the less likely the cancer will spread and, therefore, the better the chances of a cure. There are two other types of cancer of the uterine lining cells, called clear cell cancer and papillary serous cancer. These cancers have the ability to spread very quickly, but fortunately they are very rare.

What Should Be Done If Atypical Hyperplasia of the Uterus Is Found?

If atypical hyperplasia, called precancer of the endometrial cells, is found from the D&C, there is about a 25 percent chance they will turn into cancer if not treated. Because of this high risk of developing cancer, most gynecologists would recommend that a hysterectomy be performed to remove the uterus and all the lining cells along with it. If this is done, there is a 0 percent chance of endometrial cancer ever developing.

However, atypical hyperplasia can sometimes be treated by high doses of progestin taken in pill form. Progesterone causes uterine lining cells to stop growing, and in high doses it can even eliminate overgrown abnormal cells. However, the progesterone doesn't always work; in fact, it is only successful about 25 percent of the time. After three months of progesterone treatment, a repeat D&C should be performed to determine if the abnormal cells have gone away. If the pathology report shows that abnormal cells remain, then they have a very high chance of turning into cancer, and a hysterectomy should be performed. For many women, particularly those who are not interested in getting pregnant, the uncertainty of progesterone treatment is so uncomfortable that they choose to have a hysterectomy to eliminate any possibility of cancer.

Terry Gets a Second Opinion

Terry is a seventy-five-year-old woman who had recently noticed some vaginal bleeding, which she reported to her doctor. A D&C was performed, and the pathologist reported that an early cancer was present. Terry was told to have a hysterectomy, but she was unhappy about this recommendation because she wanted to avoid surgery if possible. She sought a second opinion.

When I saw Terry, her pelvic examination was normal. When I read the pathology report, the pathologist had used the words "suggestive of cancer" rather than "cancer." Pathology is not always an exact science, and I felt that the diagnosis might not be certain. Therefore, I suggested that we have the slides reviewed by another pathologist to determine whether a second pathologist thought a cancer was truly present. Our pathologist reviewed the same slides but felt that the cells looked like precancer, not cancer.

Terry's general health was not good, and she wished to avoid surgery if possible. Terry and I discussed the possibility of her taking doses of progestin for three months. Then we could repeat the D&C to determine if the cells had changed back to normal. While this treatment only had a 25 percent chance of getting rid of the precancerous cells, she was adamant about not having a hysterectomy unless it was absolutely necessary. She was aware that if abnormal cells were still present at the end of three months, a hysterectomy should be performed at that time.

She agreed and began to take the progestin. In three months she returned for a repeat D&C. This was performed in the office, and the results were back in five days. The pathology report showed that no abnormal cells remained—the progesterone had worked. Just to be safe, I recommended that we repeat the D&C again in six months. And again, the report showed that all the cells were normal. Terry was fortunate and has continued to do well for the past five years.

TREATMENT FOR UTERINE CANCER

What Happens If Uterine Cancer Is Found?

Uterine cancer is one of the most curable cancers of the body because it is usually found early. If the cancer cells appear to be slow growing based on their appearance under the microscope, and if there is no evidence that the cells have spread at the time of surgery, then the treatment is removal of the uterus. Hysterectomy cures 95 percent of women when the cancer is found early. Women with early, slow-growing uterine cancer may be able to have laparoscopic hysterectomy (see pages 334) with the benefit of shorter hospital stays and faster recoveries.

In some situations, radiation may also be recommended following hysterectomy. If the cancer appears to be the fast-growing kind based on the appearance of the cells under a microscope, or if there is any evidence of the cells spreading into the muscle wall of the uterus, then radiation is usually needed. The purpose of the radiation is to kill any cells that have already escaped from the uterus and were left behind after the uterus was removed.

Barbara's Cancer Is Detected Early

Barbara is a sixty-seven-year-old woman who went through menopause at age fifty-one. She had decided not to take estrogen and progesterone hormone replacement therapy and had not had any vaginal bleeding since that time. However, one day she noticed a brown discharge and called her primary care doctor. Following her examination, her doctor recommended that a D&C be performed to find out the cause of the bleeding. I performed a D&C and hysteroscopy in the office that week. The results of the D&C showed uterine cancer of the slow-growing kind, grade 1.

The cancer had appeared very small at the time of the hysteroscopy and was felt to be very early. Barbara wished to have a quick recovery and requested a laparoscopic hysterectomy (see page 334), and her surgery was scheduled for the following week.

At the time of surgery, the pelvis was inspected with the laparoscope and looked entirely normal. There was no evidence that the cancer had spread. We performed the hysterectomy, and both ovaries were removed as well. Barbara made a quick recovery from the surgery and was able to leave the hospital the next morning. The final pathology report showed that the cancer had not spread and was, in fact, a grade 1 cancer, the type that grew slowly. Barbara was reassured that she was cured and would not need any radiation. Barbara's case met our goal—the early detection of uterine cancer.

Can Your Ovaries Be Left If You Need a Hysterectomy for Uterine Cancer?

If you have slow-growing cancer that has not spread into the muscle wall of the uterus, or outside the uterus, then your ovaries do not have to be removed. Uterine cancer can spread, however, either by traveling through blood and lymph vessels or by traveling down and out the fallopian tube. Therefore, if the cancer cells appear to be fast growing or the cancer appears to have spread into the uterine muscle or elsewhere, the ovaries should be removed. This will allow the pathologist to confirm that the ovaries do not contain uterine cancer cells. Removal of the ovaries can also prevent the future development of ovarian cancer, and women who have had uterine cancer are at twice the risk of developing ovarian cancer as the general population. Therefore, if you have been found to have uterine cancer of any sort and you have gone through menopause, you should consider having your ovaries removed.

Is Radiation Used to Treat Uterine Cancer?

Radiation may be used in addition to hysterectomy if any factors are discovered that increase the risk that the cancer has spread. Fast-growing cancer cells or cancers that spread into the uterine muscle increase the chance that the cancer has already spread. Sometimes this information can be detected at the time of surgery, but usually the risk of spread can only be known after the pathologist has examined all of the removed tissue. If spread of the cancer is seen, or if the risk of undetected spread is present, then radiation should be considered once healing from the surgery is complete.

The goal of radiation is to kill any remaining cancer cells and prevent regrowth of the cancer. The radiation therapy is administered with a large machine that aims the radiation at the pelvis. It is usually given for about twenty minutes a day, five days a week, for about six weeks. It is not uncomfortable but often leads to fatigue that may last for a few months after the treatments are completed. Diarrhea can occur during the treatments but usually resolves shortly thereafter. While no one looks forward to either surgery, or, if necessary, radiation, the cure rate with uterine cancer is good. Therefore, timely and appropriate treatment should be sought.

If You Have Had Uterine Cancer, Can You Take Estrogen Replacement Therapy?

Medical thinking on this question has recently changed, with many doctors believing that the use of estrogen replacement is acceptable after treatment for uterine cancer. We know that if the uterine lining cells are exposed to prolonged periods of estrogen without the helpful effects of progesterone, the lining cells may be stimulated to overgrow and form precancer and cancer. However, once those cells are removed with a hysterectomy, taking estrogen does not appear to have any detrimental effect on the risk of recurrence of the cancer.

A recent study divided women with endometrial cancer into two groups; one group took estrogen and the other group did not. Both groups were equal in terms of the extent of cancer found and the type of treatment given. After seven years, the group on estrogen did just as well as the group not taking estrogen.

While some women will choose not to take estrogen, others have very bothersome symptoms of menopause or are at risk for osteoporosis and may wish to obtain some benefits from estrogen replacement therapy. Progesterone may be taken concurrently with the idea that it may prevent any regrowth of endometrial cancer cells. This is theoretical and has not been scientifically shown to be effective. For now, women who have had uterine cancer should fully discuss this issue with their doctors.

Why Should You Seek Early Medical Evaluation?

For most women who have abnormal bleeding, the cause will *not* be uterine cancer, but if cancer is present and they seek care early, it can often be cured. The moral of the uterine cancer story is that the symptom of abnormal bleeding should be checked out quickly. Sometimes we hope that things that scare us will "just go away." The good news is that if we take care of them early, sometimes even bad problems such as uterine cancer will actually "go away" with prompt treatment. Hiding from the possibility of cancer delays treatment and sometimes makes curing the disease impossible. We all have to fight off the desire to put our heads in the sand. Be aggressive in the maintenance of your good health. If you notice something "new" or "not quite right," let a doctor examine you. Saying to yourself, "Oh, I'm sure it's nothing" is no substitute for the relief you'll feel if there is nothing to worry about or you have caught a problem in time. Early detection and early intervention save lives. Be sure yours is among them.

REFERENCES

ACOG Committee Opinion. *Tamoxifen and Endometrial Cancer.* April 2000, No. 232.

Berek, J., and N. Hacker. 1994. *Practical Gynecologic Oncology.* Baltimore, Md.: Williams and Wilkins.

Fu, Y. 1997. Editorial: Pathologic diagnosis of endometrial hyperplasia. *Journal of Gynecologic Techniques* 3:117–18.

Kurman, R., P. Kaminsky, and H. Norris. 1985. The behavior of endometrial hyperplasia: A long-term study of "untreated" hyperplasia in 170 patients. *Cancer* 56:403.

Lee, R., T. Burke, and R. Park. 1990. Estrogen replacement therapy following treatment for stage I endometrial carcinoma. *Gynecologic Oncology* 36:189–91.

Malfetano, J. 1990. Tamoxifen-associated endometrial carcinoma in postmeno-pausal breast cancer patients. *Gynecologic Oncology* 39:82–84.

Morra, M., and E. Potts. 1994. *Choices: A Sourcebook for Cancer Information.* New York: Avon.

Suriano, K., M. McHale, C. McLaren, K. Li, A. Re, and P. Disaia. 2001. Estrogen replacement therapy in endometrial cancer patients: A matched control study. *Obstetrics and Gynecology* 97:555–60.

12

IF YOU ABSOLUTELY NEED A HYSTERECTOMY

Hysterectomy, the surgical removal of the uterus, is a procedure surrounded by controversy—and for good reason. Hysterectomy is the second most common major operation performed in the United States today, second only to cesarean section. Approximately 600,000 American women have a hysterectomy every year, at a cost of almost $5 billion. By the age of sixty, one out of every three women in the United States has had a hysterectomy. The controversy about hysterectomy arises from the feeling that many of these procedures are unnecessary. And a recent study found that despite efforts to educate gynecologists about alternatives to hysterectomy, the rate of hysterectomy has not decreased in the past decade. I, for one, believe there are now many alternatives to hysterectomy.

The percentage of American women who have a hysterectomy is much higher than that of European women. For example, American women are twice as likely to have a hysterectomy as women in England and four times as likely as Swedish women. French doctors almost never perform a hysterectomy for fibroids, which is the most common reason for hysterectomy in the United States. Many factors contribute to these differences, including cultural attitudes, physician training, the availability of elective surgery in a particular country, and the ability to pay for care. However, overall, it appears that the rate of hysterectomy in the United States is high.

There are differences in the rates of hysterectomy between various parts of the United States. Women in the South are 78 percent more likely to have a hysterectomy than women who live in the Northeast, where the rate is the lowest. The rate is also 40 percent higher in the Midwest and 20 percent higher in the West than it is in the Northeast. And while the rate of hysterectomy is lowest in the Northeast, the proportion of hysterectomies performed with an abdominal incision is highest in that region. Vaginal hysterectomy, which is associated with less discomfort and a faster recovery, is most common in the South, where the rate of hysterectomy is highest. The regional differences in the rate of hysterectomy (the number of procedures per 100,000 women in the population) and the type of hysterectomies performed suggest that factors other than good medical care are involved in the decision to have surgery.

The approach to hysterectomy by some physicians has been cavalier. As recently as 1969, an American physician wrote in the medical literature that, after completion of childbearing, the uterus was a useless organ that should be removed to prevent bleeding and the development of cancer. While this opinion clearly has no place in our thinking today, many physicians consider the current rate of hysterectomy to be too high, and doctors continue to disagree among themselves about the appropriateness of the procedure in given situations. The recent medical literature supports the perception of many women that the rate of hysterectomies currently performed is too high. A number of studies have examined the medical appropriateness of hysterectomies. A review of patient records by a panel of expert gynecologists formed by RAND found that 70 percent of the procedures were believed to be inappropriate due to failure to perform proper diagnostic tests or try alternative therapy prior to recommending hysterectomy.

With a justifiable inquiry, women's magazines and books on women's health by both nonmedical authors and physicians have picked up the diatribe against doctors in the name of women's rights. Some describe individual accounts of bad experiences when having a hysterectomy, the insensitive attitude of doctors, or an aftermath of sexual problems and personal struggle. While no doubt some horror stories exist, some of these authors do a disservice to the cause of health education and to those physicians who do provide excellent medical care to women.

To compound the disservice done by presenting inaccurate science and medicine, some authors attempt to dogmatically coerce their readers, in much the same way that they have accused practicing physicians of doing. To these authors, hysterectomy has become a political issue. Some authors state that only 10 percent of hysterectomies are necessary, meaning only those that are performed for cancer. However, if the other 90 percent of hysterectomies are absolutely unnecessary, that leaves little room for women who are truly suffering from gynecologic problems and who are looking to gain useful and vital information about an often valid way to help themselves.

Symptoms that result from uterine problems, such as severe pain or bleeding, will often respond to medications or other nonsurgical treatment, but sometimes they do not get better. Women with these intractable symptoms that affect their lives may benefit from hysterectomy. As noted later in this chapter, a recent American study done by a female doctor at Harvard found that most women who had a hysterectomy performed for moderate or severe non-life-threatening symptoms were "very satisfied" with the results of surgery. It appears that if you are suffering from symptoms such as severe pain or bleeding, hysterectomy can sometimes offer an improvement in the quality of your life. In England, where hysterectomy rates are low, few hysterectomies are performed for these quality-of-life problems. One question then, often discussed among British physicians, is whether it is a good or bad thing that a means that can improve lives is not utilized to do so.

American women who have had hysterectomies for symptoms they felt were interfering with their lives have been made to feel guilty that they "gave in." One woman, writing in a column in *The New York Times* said, "What I find in the feminist literature is a harangue about sexism, ageism, and greed on the part of doctors and pharmaceutical companies, which tells me little or nothing about the surgery I am about to undergo and leaves me feeling guilty for selling out the sisterhood by choosing to have it [hysterectomy]." One of the most important factors in helping you choose appropriate medical care is your comprehensive understanding of the reasons for treatment, the risks, and the potential benefits. This especially applies to hysterectomy.

Unfortunately, as physicians, we sometimes do not explain medical issues very well and often do not discuss the psychological or sexual aspects of hysterectomy at all. A patient education program about the risks and benefits of hysterectomy was introduced into a small town in Switzerland, and the hysterectomy rate was compared to a neighboring town that did not have this education program. At the end of a year, the rate of hysterectomies had decreased by 26 percent in the town with the educational program but had increased by 1 percent in the other town. If hysterectomy has been suggested to you as an option for your particular problem, you should carefully weigh the pros and cons, the alternative treatments, and the potential benefits and risks. We have tried to provide you with some of that information. Coupled with the personalized information you have gotten from your own doctor, we hope you will be able to make a comfortable and informed decision about whether hysterectomy is right for you.

The percentage of women who have had a hysterectomy has actually gone down slightly since 1975, when 725,000 women had a hysterectomy in the United States. However, despite efforts to educate both physicians and the public about the alternative treatments now available, hysterectomy rates have not changed at all in the last decade. Many gynecologists do not offer endometrial ablation to women who are bleeding, myomectomy or uterine fibroid embolization (UFE) to women with fibroids, or removal of an ovarian cyst rather than complete hysterectomy. As we discuss throughout this book, it is important for you to educate yourself about the alternatives available for any problem you might have and seek out doctors who are experienced with these alternatives.

The total number of women who will have a hysterectomy is expected to rise as the baby boom generation enters the ages when hysterectomy is most commonly performed. The number of women expected to have a hysterectomy in the year 2005 may approach 1,000,000. For individual women and our nation as a whole, hysterectomy is an enormous health issue.

What Is a Hysterectomy?

A hysterectomy is a surgical procedure that removes the uterus. The word is derived from *hyster*, the Greek word for uterus and the suffix for removal, *-ectomy*. It should be noted that the term *hysterectomy* denotes the removal of *only* the uterus.

Does Hysterectomy Include Removal of the Ovaries and Fallopian Tubes?

By definition, hysterectomy only refers to the removal of the uterus. The Latin word for removal of an ovary is *oophorectomy*. The word for removal of the fallopian tubes is *salpingectomy*. *Bilateral* means both sides. Therefore, the term *bilateral salpingo-oophorectomy* means the surgical removal of both fallopian tubes and ovaries (see fig. 12.1a). In the past, this procedure has been performed about 60 percent of the time when a hysterectomy was performed. However, for many women it does not need to be done, and the decision about removal of the ovaries should be separate and distinct from that of removal of the uterus (see page 340).

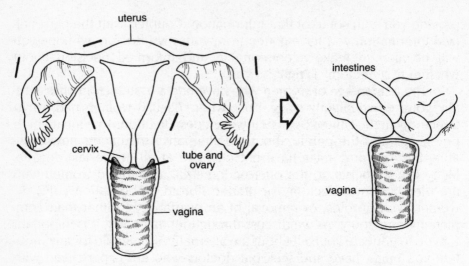

Fig. 12.1a.   Total hysterectomy and bilateral
salpingo-oophorectomy

What Are the Most Common Reasons Hysterectomy Is Performed?

The most common reason listed by American gynecologists for performing a hysterectomy is fibroids. This accounts for about 30 percent of all hysterectomies. The symptoms of fibroids that can lead to hysterectomy are pain or pressure, or abnormal bleeding (see chapter 4). Hysterectomies performed because of endometriosis have increased in the past thirty years and now account for about 19 percent of all hysterectomies. Prolapse, the falling of the pelvic organs into the vagina, is the reason for about 16 percent of all hysterectomies. Atypical endometrial hyperplasia, precancer of the uterine lining cells, accounts for about 6 percent of hysterectomies. Hysterectomies performed because of cancer of the cervix, uterus, fallopian tubes, or ovaries account for about 10 percent of all procedures.

In the past, sterilization was used as a reason for performing hysterectomy. However, female sterilization can be performed in a safer, quicker, and less expensive way by blocking the fallopian tubes with laparoscopic techniques. Therefore, hysterectomy is not recommended for sterilization. In addition, male sterilization (vasectomy) is even safer, faster, and less expensive than female laparoscopic sterilization.

Should Prevention of Cancer Be a Reason to Have a Hysterectomy?

Some women choose to have a hysterectomy, not because they have cancer but because they are afraid that they might get cancer and wish to prevent this from happening. Some doctors are aware of this fear and do recommend hysterectomy to prevent the formation of cancer. However, the risk of developing uterine cancer is extremely low; only 3 women out of 100 will ever develop this disease. Uterine cancer usually causes symptoms of abnormal bleeding in the early stages or even precancerous stages, when the disease is curable. Therefore, it does not make any sense to remove the uterus to prevent the unlikely future occurrence of uterine cancer.

Removal of the uterus also does not make sense if surgery is needed for the removal of an abnormal ovary. A recent study of women who had surgery for an abnormal ovary found that the risk of complications was much lower if just that ovary was removed than if both ovaries and uterus were also removed simply "because they were there." It also does not make any sense to remove the uterus and ovaries to prevent ovarian cancer. In the rare families (see page 282) where the risk of developing ovarian cancer is very high, removal of the ovaries by laparoscopy can be performed as an outpatient procedure; there's no need to perform a major operation to also remove the uterus.

It has been calculated that if every woman had her uterus removed at the age of thirty-five just to prevent the development of ovarian, cervical, and uterine cancer, the average increase in life expectancy would be only 2.4 months. And, as noted in chapters 10 and 11, both cervical and uterine cancer are easy to detect at a preinvasive or early stage, when they are easily treatable.

TYPES OF HYSTERECTOMY

Total hysterectomy, the operation that is most commonly performed, removes the entire uterus, including the cervix (see fig. 12.1b). *Subtotal or supracervical hysterectomy* removes only the upper body of the uterus, and the cervix is left in place, connected to the top of the vagina (see fig. 12.1c). If the hysterectomy is performed because of cervical cancer, then the cervix must be removed, and total hysterectomy is always performed. The same is true for uterine cancer, since the cancer can spread down the body of the uterus and involve the cervix.

However, if the hysterectomy is performed for uterine fibroids, abnormal bleeding, or pelvic pain, you have a choice as to whether the cervix should be removed. Some women feel that if the cervix is removed, they will have diminished sexual pleasure, while other women do not feel the cervix is part of their sexual enjoyment. Some doctors suggest that removing the cervix cuts some of the nerves going to

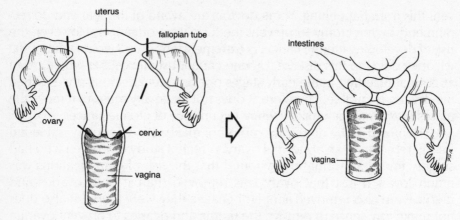

Fig. 12.1b.   Total hysterectomy

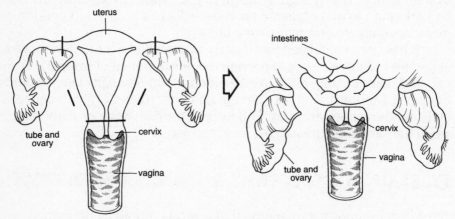

Fig. 12.1c.   Subtotal hysterectomy

the bladder and rectum and interferes with their function. This issue is discussed in detail on page 344.

If the cervix is not removed, you will need to have annual Pap smears to check for cervical dysplasia and cancer. Even if the cervix is removed, a Pap smear of the vagina should still be done to detect abnormal vaginal cells, but perhaps on a less frequent basis.

What Are the Different Ways to Perform a Hysterectomy?

There are presently three ways to perform a hysterectomy: abdominal hysterectomy, vaginal hysterectomy, and laparoscopic hysterectomy.

Radical hysterectomy, almost always performed through an abdominal incision, is necessary for some types of cervical or uterine cancer and includes the removal of lymph nodes from around the uterus and cervix in addition to the removal of the uterus. The different types of hysterectomy are discussed below.

What Is an Abdominal Hysterectomy?

Abdominal hysterectomy removes the uterus through an incision in the abdominal wall and is the type of hysterectomy performed in about 75 percent of women who have the operation in the United States. The abdominal incision may either be made from side to side ("bikini incision") (see fig. 12.2A) or up and down, from the pubic bone to just below the navel (see fig. 12.2B). After the incision is made in the skin, the abdominal muscles are stretched apart (not cut) so that the abdominal cavity can be seen. This stretching of the muscles causes some of the discomfort that follows abdominal surgery. The operation takes from one to three hours; the hospital stay is from three to five days; and the recovery until normal activity can be resumed is about six weeks.

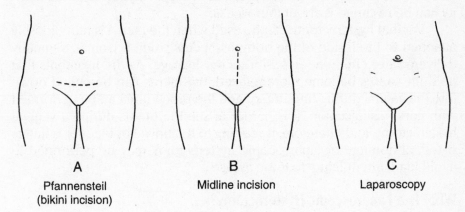

A
Pfannensteil
(bikini incision)

B
Midline incision

C
Laparoscopy

Fig. 12.2.   Surgical incisions

Abdominal hysterectomy may be utilized because it gives the doctor the ability to see and feel all of the pelvic organs during the operation. It is often used if the doctor expects the operation to be difficult because of scar tissue from previous surgery, previous infection, or endometriosis. It is usually the way a hysterectomy is done if cancer is present because it allows the doctor to remove all the cancer and inspect and feel inside the abdomen to make sure the cancer has not spread.

Laparoscopic hysterectomy techniques (see below) have been developed to deal with special situations such as scar tissue or fibroids and, in some cases, even cancer. However, because considerable laparoscopic training and skill are needed to do this safely and many gynecologists have not acquired these skills, it is likely that abdominal hysterectomy will have a continued role in the treatment of these problems.

What Is a Vaginal Hysterectomy?

The second most common type of hysterectomy is called vaginal hysterectomy because the surgery is performed through an incision made at the top of the vagina. The blood vessels and other connections of the uterus to the inside of the body are first cut and sutured through the vagina. Once detached, the uterus is removed through the vagina. Since the incision is made only in the vagina, there is no visible scar. The vaginal incision is small and heals quickly, and because the abdominal muscles are not stretched, less discomfort occurs than with abdominal hysterectomy. This procedure takes about one or two hours. The hospital stay lasts from one to three days, and the recovery until normal activity can be resumed is about four weeks.

Vaginal hysterectomy can be used when the uterus is more loosely attached to the inside of the body, as occurs when a woman vaginally delivered her children, and with increasing age. As the ligaments that hold the uterus become more relaxed, the uterus can be pulled down into the vagina during the surgery, and the procedure can be performed with good visualization. It is harder to see the uterus during a vaginal hysterectomy, and, therefore, if scarring to the bowel or bladder is anticipated, abdominal or laparoscopic hysterectomy may be performed to avoid inadvertent injury to these areas.

What Is a Laparoscopic Hysterectomy?

Laparoscopic hysterectomy is a relatively new surgical procedure, first performed in 1989, that allows the uterus to be detached from inside the body by laparoscopic instruments while the doctor is viewing the uterus, fallopian tubes, and ovaries through a camera attached to a telescope. After the uterus is detached, it is removed through a small incision at the top of the vagina. One advantage of laparoscopic hysterectomy is that the incisions are smaller (one-half inch) and much less uncomfortable than that of abdominal hysterectomy (see fig. 12.1C). Also, the hospital stay of one day and the ability to resume normal activity in about two weeks are substantially shorter than for abdominal hysterectomy and slightly shorter than for vaginal hysterectomy.

For patients who have known or suspected pelvic scar tissue or endometriosis, laparoscopic surgery allows the surgeon to remove the diseased tissue with the laparoscope before performing a vaginal hysterectomy, thereby reducing the risk that the intestines or bladder might be injured during surgery. For patients who have fibroids that are large and might otherwise be difficult to remove by vaginal hysterectomy, laparoscopic hysterectomy allows the surgeon to detach the blood vessels to the uterus while viewing them through the laparoscope. Then, the uterus can be removed through the vagina more easily and with less blood loss. For some women with large fibroids, new instruments permit laparoscopic subtotal hysterectomy to be performed more easily and safely than before.

However, it appears that vaginal hysterectomy is safer and less expensive than laparoscopic hysterectomy. It also has about the same hospital stay and recovery time. Therefore, a laparoscopic hysterectomy should not be performed if a vaginal hysterectomy is possible. However, if a vaginal hysterectomy might be difficult or an abdominal hysterectomy is needed for medical reasons, then laparoscopic hysterectomy may be considered as an alternative.

Laparoscopic hysterectomy is still being studied with regard to its overall risks and benefits. It does require considerable skill and experience on the part of the surgeon. You should ask your doctor what kind of training he or she has gone through and how many procedures he or she has performed with each technique. If your gynecologist is not comfortable or experienced with laparoscopic hysterectomy, then it may be best to have the surgery the way he or she feels is most appropriate, or you may ask for a referral to someone who is more comfortable performing laparoscopic hysterectomy.

Caroline Has a Laparoscopic Hysterectomy

Caroline, a thirty-four-year-old woman with two young children, had known she had uterine fibroids for one year. While fairly large when initially discovered, the fibroids had recently grown to the size of a large coconut. She had heavy bleeding with her periods, now requiring her to change menstrual pads every half hour for two full days. This heavy bleeding had made Caroline weak and irritable. When she had her period, her activity had to be severely limited. Both Caroline and her husband, Dan, were anxious and worried before the start of her period each month. Dan feared that she would begin to hemorrhage. He was insistent that she get immediate treatment.

Another gynecologist had recommended removal of the fibroids with both the resectoscope and laparoscope. Despite pressure from her husband and the strong recommendation of her gynecologist, Caroline could not commit to the surgery. She was uncertain about wanting more children and thus was ambivalent about a surgery that could compromise her fertility. She was desperate to have the bleeding end, yet wanted some other solution.

Based on my examination, I felt that removal of the fibroids as had been recommended would be extremely difficult, and that repair of the uterus through the laparoscope might not be safe for future childbearing. We discussed the probable need for myomectomy through an abdominal incision (see page 129). Because of the anemia, I recommended that she begin treatment with Lupron to shrink the fibroids (see page 122). In addition, this would stop her periods for the three months she was on the medication. Stopping the heavy bleeding would give her body time to make new blood and self-correct her anemia. In fact, this was just what happened, and she began to feel stronger and more energetic.

With a return to her usual strength and vitality, Caroline began to devote more time and emotions to her thoughts of having another child. Much to her surprise, she realized that she really did not want any more children after all. By the end of the three months, after careful consideration by herself and with Dan, she decided that she was sure she did not want any more children and requested a hysterectomy. We performed a laparoscopic hysterectomy, and Caroline had a one-day stay in the hospital and only two weeks to full recovery. She has done well since that time and is happy with the decision she made.

What Are the Types of Laparoscopic Hysterectomy?

Prior to 1989, a few skilled laparoscopic surgeons were performing *laparoscopic-assisted vaginal hysterectomies*. The laparoscope was used at the beginning of procedure to sever the upper part of the attachments of the uterus to the blood vessels and ligaments supporting it inside the pelvis. Following this, the remaining attachments of the uterus were severed through the vagina, and after removing the uterus, the vagina was sutured closed.

In 1989, the first hysterectomy was performed entirely using laparoscopic instruments and techniques. The uterus was pushed out of the pelvis through the vagina, and the top of the vagina was sutured closed with laparoscopic instruments. This operation is called *total laparoscopic hysterectomy*. Another variation of laparoscopic hysterectomy was difficult to perform until the recent development of special instruments called morcellators. *Laparoscopic subtotal hysterectomy* removes the body of the uterus, but leaves the cervix intact. A morcellator is placed inside the pelvis through the small laparoscopic incisions and cuts up the body of the uterus into small pieces. These pieces can then be removed through the small incisions. Because the cervix is left in place, no surgery is needed near the vagina, and no sutures are left near the vagina.

Are There Any Advantages to Subtotal Hysterectomy?

There has been a bit of controversy for the past few years over the advantages and disadvantages of subtotal hysterectomy. Subtotal hysterectomy was the most common type of hysterectomy performed before 1940. Leaving the cervix in place avoided some of the risk of injuring the nearby ureters, bladder, or intestines and also reduced blood loss. However, the remaining cervix was susceptible to developing cancer, a fairly common condition at that time. As surgical and anesthetic techniques became safer and antibiotics became available, doctors began performing more total hysterectomies to prevent the future development of cervical cancer. These changes all preceded the discovery of the Pap smear. Once the Pap smear became widely used as a means to find precancer, an easily curable condition, removing the cervix was no longer essential for all women.

Laparoscopic hysterectomy has been shown to be associated with a shorter hospital stay and recovery than abdominal hysterectomy. Women having laparoscopic subtotal hysterectomy may have an even faster recovery. The fact that no surgery is needed near the vagina and no sutures are left inside the vagina may be responsible for reducing discomfort during the recovery period. A few studies have shown just that, with return to work in one week, rather than the two weeks it may take after laparoscopic total hysterectomy. We have been performing laparoscopic subtotal hysterectomy, when indicated and requested by the patient, for the past few years and have seen the same excellent results—early recovery and return to normal activity—as reported in the medical journals.

Sandra's Subtotal Hysterectomy

Sandra is a forty-two-year-old chiropractor who came in for a second opinion regarding her fibroids. The fibroids had been diagnosed five years ago when they were quite small and not bothersome. However, over the past year they began pressing on her bladder. Most days she had to go to the bathroom every hour, and she had to get up about four times every night to urinate. In addition, the fibroids were causing discomfort in her lower abdomen. Her work was physically demanding, massaging and manipulating her patients, and she was finding work increasingly difficult and tiring. She was very active and ran about ten miles every other day but was also finding this uncomfortable. She wanted to get back to her work and exercise and activities. Her previous gynecologist had recommended abdominal hysterectomy because of the size of the fibroids. After looking into alternatives like UFE (see below) she decided that hysterectomy was right for her. However, she was unhappy about the long recovery. Sandra came in to see whether laparoscopic surgery was possible.

Her examination showed the fibroids to be about the size of a large cantaloupe. She had not had any children so the cervix was high up in the vagina, making a vaginal hysterectomy difficult. However, laparoscopic surgery certainly seemed possible. We discussed laparoscopic subtotal hysterectomy as a way to remove the uterus and have a short, two-week recovery. Sandra liked the idea of leaving the cervix, since she had never had any problems with her Pap smears. Since she was only in her early forties, leaving the ovaries also seemed like a good idea.

Surgery went extremely well, and she was ready to go home the next morning. She called a few days later because of gas pains, but she was thrilled with the surgery and already noted that her frequent urination and abdominal discomfort were gone.

At her two-week postoperative visit, I asked her how she was doing. With a sheepish grin she admitted to hiking two miles a few days after surgery and was now hiking seven miles a day to get back into shape. That was a bit more exercise than I had intended for her, but her exam was normal, and she felt fine. At the end of the visit, I gave her my okay to do what she was already doing and told her she could get back to work. Her parting words were, "I have a number of women patients with large fibroids who are afraid of surgery. I will be sending them all in to see you soon."

What Is a Radical Hysterectomy?

In addition to the removal of the uterus through an abdominal incision, a radical hysterectomy includes the surgical removal of the lymph nodes and other tissue surrounding the cervix and uterus. Radical hysterectomy is often recommended if a woman is found to have cervical cancer and may also be beneficial in some women with uterine cancer that has spread to the cervix. Lymph nodes are part of your immune system and cleanse the body of abnormal cells. They are linked together by a chain of lymph vessels that follow along the blood vessels in your body. By removing the lymph nodes and surrounding tissue, we remove any additional cancer cells. Moreover, the pathologist will be able to tell whether the cancer has already begun to spread, and this information will be helpful in planning further therapy.

After You Have a Hysterectomy, What Do You Look Like Inside?

The small intestines are about twenty feet long and normally curl up around the front and back of the uterus. When the uterus is removed, the intestines move into this spot, so that no "empty space" remains (see figs. 12.1a–c). If your uterus was a relatively normal size before surgery, you will probably not notice any difference in the way your abdomen feels. If you had an enlarged uterus from fibroids, you may feel less pressure in your abdomen, as the intestines can now move back to the area where they belong.

The top of the vagina normally attaches directly to the cervix, and both are covered with a continuous layer of skin. If a total hysterectomy is performed, the cervix is cut away from the vagina and the uterus removed. The remaining top portion of the vagina is closed together with dissolvable sutures. Very little of the vagina is removed, but the end result may be a slightly shorter vagina than before surgery. After total hysterectomy, when viewed through a speculum, the cervix is absent, and the top of the vagina appears as a continuous, closed layer of skin.

If a subtotal hysterectomy is performed, the attachments of the cervix to the vagina are not cut, and the length of the vagina is not altered. When viewed through a speculum, the cervix and vagina look the same as they did before the hysterectomy.

RISKS OF HYSTERECTOMY

Some books and magazine articles have quoted the risk of having a medical complication from a hysterectomy as being 50 percent. However, this is a distortion of the facts. The majority of these reported "complications" are mild fevers that result from easy-to-treat infections of the incision, the bladder, or, rarely, the lungs. Serious complications occur very rarely.

Bleeding that requires transfusion has been reported about 10 percent of the time. However, those statistics were collected before the awareness that HIV could be acquired from blood transfusions. Doctors are now much less likely to give a transfusion for just slight fatigue or mild anemia, as was often done in the past. Therefore, it is likely that the number of transfusions has already fallen, but the newer statistics have not yet been reported in the medical journals. In addition, blood transfusion is now safer than ever before. As a result of the careful screening of blood donors, the risk of HIV is 1 out of 1,900,000 units of blood, and the risk of hepatitis C is 1 out of 1,000,000 units of blood.

Other risks during hysterectomy include inadvertent injury to the organs near the uterus. The risk of injury to the bladder, ureters, or intestines is about 1 per 1,000 operations. The risk may be higher or lower depending on the reason for your surgery and the technical difficulty that your condition presents.

All operations have risks. But in general, the risk of a serious complication from a hysterectomy is very small. The risk to you will depend on the reason you need surgery, your medical condition, and your age, and the experience of your doctor and anesthesiologist. For women age thirty-five to forty-four, the risk of dying from this procedure is about 3 per 10,000 women. For women of all ages who are operated on for benign conditions, the risk of dying from a hysterectomy is 6 per 10,000 women. If a hysterectomy is performed because of cancer, it may be a more difficult operation, and sometimes the initial medical condition of the woman may be worse. For these reasons, the risk of dying from surgery when cancer is present is about 37 per 10,000 women. The Maine Women's Study, described in detail on page 348, recently reported that only 1 percent of women in their study who had a hysterectomy had a bleeding complication; 5 percent had a treatable wound or bladder infection; and the total complication rate was 7 percent. Of the 400 women in that study who had a hysterectomy, none had a serious complication, and none died.

Can Hysterectomy Affect Your Bladder Function?

A recent, well-conducted study compared bladder symptoms in two groups of women interviewed both before and after undergoing surgery. One group of women had a D&C performed, while the other group had a total hysterectomy performed. Both groups had an increase in reported frequency of urination, urgency to urinate, and incontinence. Still, there was no difference in symptoms between the two groups, except that the women who had a hysterectomy noted *less* incontinence. Another study precisely measured bladder function before and after hysterectomy and could not detect any adverse change in function after the surgery. Consequently, there is no evidence that hysterectomy leads to bladder problems.

For women who have fibroids pressing against their bladders, frequency of urination or even loss of urine during laughing, coughing, or sneezing can sometimes occur. For these women, hysterectomy may remove the pressure on the bladder and may actually improve bladder function.

Can Removal of the Uterus Increase the Risk of Heart Disease?

In the past, the uterus was not thought to produce any hormones or substances that were medically important. However, a few studies found that women who had only their uterus removed had a 4 percent increased risk of developing coronary artery disease, either in the form of chest pain or an actual heart attack.

Recently, it has been discovered that the uterus does produce a biochemical called prostacyclin that is able to dilate blood vessels and permit more blood, oxygen, and nutrition to reach the heart. Furthermore, prostacyclin prevents blood from clotting, thus discouraging the blockage of blood vessels to the heart that can result in a heart attack. While not yet proven, prostacyclin produced in the uterus may enhance blood flow to the heart and, thus, protect your heart. However, this effect on the risk of heart disease would be *very small* compared to the effect of exercise, diet, cholesterol level, and hereditary factors. Nevertheless, with the presumed increased incidence of heart disease so small, it would take a study of 10,000 women who had a hysterectomy (without removal of the ovaries) and 10,000 who did not, all of whom were followed until death, to prove if an increased incidence of heart disease had in fact occurred. Unfortunately, it is unlikely we will ever know the answer to this question.

Does Removal of the Ovaries Increase the Risk of Heart Disease?

The ovaries produce the main female hormone, estrogen, until the time of menopause. Estrogen has a beneficial effect on your heart and cardiovascular system, and we know that women who have their ovaries removed at an early age, or those who go into early menopause, have a higher risk of having a heart attack later in life.

The reasons for this protective effect of estrogen are not entirely clear. However, we do know that estrogen lowers the level of cholesterol in your blood, which reduces the risk of clogged arteries. Estrogen also acts directly on blood vessels to dilate them and allow more blood, oxygen, and nutrition to reach the heart muscle. Estrogen is an antioxidant and protects the vessel walls against damage. There are probably other effects of estrogen on the heart that are not yet known. Nevertheless, we do know that the ovaries play a role in the prevention of heart disease.

Therefore, the decision to remove your ovaries during a surgery intended to remove the uterus should be considered as a separate decision, as discussed in detail below. If you need to, or choose to, have your ovaries removed, you might consider taking estrogen replacement after surgery. Replacement estrogen, available in pills, skin patches, or creams, will then continue to provide the protective effect for your bones. To date, no independent beneficial effects of progesterone have been found other than the protection of the uterus from overgrowth or cancer of the uterine lining cells. Following hysterectomy, this protective effect is not needed and, therefore, progesterone does not need to be taken.

If You Need a Hysterectomy, Should You Also Have Your Ovaries Removed?

I have changed my view about this controversial subject since the first edition of this book was published. At that time, I suggested that women who were having a hysterectomy performed for appropriate reasons also consider having their ovaries removed after the age of about forty-five. My thinking at the time was that the ovaries would continue producing hormones for only a few years thereafter, and this advantage would be overshadowed by the benefit of removing the ovaries and eliminating the 1 percent chance of developing ovarian cancer in your lifetime. However, a number of issues have come to my attention since then, and I now believe that the ovaries should almost never be removed at the time of hysterectomy.

First, as noted on page 284, the risk of ovarian cancer goes down if the ovaries remain after hysterectomy. The reason for this is not clear, but it may be that the path for potential carcinogens from the vagina to the ovaries is interrupted when the uterus is removed. Thus, the risk of a woman developing ovarian cancer after hysterectomy is 1 in 300 rather than the 1 in 80 for women who have not had a hysterectomy. The benefit of removing ovaries for ovarian cancer prevention has been overstated in the medical literature and is, therefore, misunderstood by most physicians.

Significantly, the ovaries produce hormones long after menopause. Estrogen continues to be produced in small amounts, about 25 percent of normal premenopausal levels. Blood levels of estrogen in some post-menopausal women are equivalent to the levels attained by low-dose estrogen patches used for estrogen replacement in menopause. The circulating level of estrogen produced by the patch has been shown to be sufficient to prevent bone loss in clinical studies. Studies also show less bone loss in women who have ovaries than in women who have had their ovaries removed. Studies show that women who have had their ovaries removed (and have not taken replacement estrogen) have higher rates of heart disease than women the same age who still have their ovaries.

Testosterone is usually thought of as solely a male hormone. However, it and other androgen (male) hormones are produced by the ovaries from the time of the first menstrual period. These androgens continue to be produced by the ovaries after menopause. Testosterone has many direct and indirect benefits to your body. Some of the testosterone is converted into estrogen by your body, and it circulates in the bloodstream to all of your tissues where it has a direct effect on many organs. It helps to build bone and thus reduces osteoporosis. Its steroid features prevent muscle loss that often occurs with aging. Testosterone directly affects the brain and increases libido. Sexual feelings, desire, and arousal are all related to androgen levels. Testosterone also affects brain function and mood. Women with hormones from their own ovaries have a lower rate of depression than women who have had them removed, even if estrogen replacement therapy (ERT) is taken.

Some physicians have argued that women can replace estrogens and androgens with medications. However, less than 30 percent of women who have a hysterectomy and removal of their ovaries will actually take hormones. Therefore, 70 percent of women will not have the benefit of their own hormones. Some women do not take ERT because they feel fine and do not understand the benefits of taking estrogen for their bones. Some women are concerned about the still controversial issues surrounding estrogen and breast cancer, although it appears that the effect of estrogen on the risk of breast cancer may be very small. Some cannot afford the medication. For whatever reason, most women would be better off with their own supply of estrogen and testosterone from their ovaries.

Another problem with estrogen replacement therapy (ERT) is the dilemma that some doctors and women have as they try to find the right doses. Some women note that despite trying multiple regimens of ERT, they still do not feel right. Because hormone production and metabolism is a complex issue, it should not be a surprise that we are not able to mimic normal hormone levels in all women. For all the above reasons, I have recently started recommending that most women choose to keep their ovaries at the time of hysterectomy for uterine problems, regardless of their age.

However, there are a few situations where women may wish to have their ovaries removed at the time of hysterectomy. If the ovaries are affected by endometriosis or a woman has severe endometriosis and pelvic pain, studies show that removing the ovaries is associated with better long-term relief of pain than if the ovaries are not removed. Severe adhesions, or scar tissue, around the ovaries may also cause continued pelvic pain.

As noted in chapter 10, some women are at increased risk for developing ovarian cancer. If you feel your family history suggests an increased risk for ovarian cancer, you should see a genetic counselor to help evaluate your risk. The counselor may suggest you have BRCA (breast cancer) gene testing to determine if you have inherited the gene that increases your risk. If you have an increased risk, you should strongly consider having your ovaries removed. In this case, the benefits of removing your ovaries and preventing ovarian cancer should far outweigh the benefits of keeping your own ovarian hormones.

Some women are very uneasy about leaving their ovaries in because of the fear of ovarian cancer. They may have seen a friend or relative die of this terrible disease. As a result, some women may choose to have their ovaries removed at the time of hysterectomy. But for each woman, the risks should be weighed carefully against the benefits of having her own hormones from her own ovaries after menopause. Women tend to make very different decisions based on their particular circumstances, their feelings about estrogen replacement therapy, and their risk and fear of ovarian cancer. However, it is always best to make these decisions based on accurate and current medical information. This decision is yours to make and should be discussed in detail with your doctor. As always, if there are unanswered questions or concerns, get a second opinion.

What Happens to a Woman's Monthly Cycle After Hysterectomy?

After the uterus is removed, menstrual bleeding and cramping ceases. But if the ovaries are left in place, the hormones estrogen and progesterone continue to be produced in the normal cyclic fashion. As a result, any breast tenderness and bloating that you may have had prior to your period will likely continue. Some women find that headaches and PMS symptoms are lessened following hysterectomy, presumably because removal of the uterus eliminates prostaglandins and perhaps other substances that possibly cause these symptoms. However, in other women, PMS symptoms are unchanged. The ovaries continue to produce eggs as well. An egg is microscopic, and, after it is released during ovulation, it dissolves quickly within the body cavity.

If you have your ovaries removed at the time of a hysterectomy, your body will not have any natural source of estrogen or progesterone, and the monthly changes your body normally experiences will cease. For women who choose to take estrogen replacement therapy, the levels of estrogen are constant throughout the month, and these women will only rarely experience PMS or other cyclic changes.

Can Hysterectomy Lead to Psychological Problems?

Many women fear hysterectomy, and some will delay or avoid surgery even when it is medically necessary. Determining whether you should have a hysterectomy is a personal decision as well as a medical one. Some women have fears about the actual surgery, discomfort, and possible complications. Some women are concerned about the effect hysterectomy will have on their sexuality, on the way they will feel about their own identity, and the way others (especially their partner, if they have one) will view them. One study found that 16 percent of women had a negative psychological reaction to having had a hysterectomy. The women described feelings of sadness, grief, and lowered self-esteem. Some said that, even though they did not wish to have any more children, the finality of not being able to have more children was upsetting. Some women talk about an empty feeling following surgery. Some say they no longer feel like a woman or they feel like a different person. Some feel depressed or can't sleep. If a woman also has her ovaries removed, the resulting hormonal changes sometimes wreak havoc with her system. Some women note a lack of lubrication during intercourse, some a change in libido.

For other women, the relief from symptoms and worry may outweigh any depressing feelings they may experience. The attitudes and knowledge that a woman brings to surgery will often affect the way she feels after surgery. Therefore, it is important to give careful thought to whether a hysterectomy is the right thing for you. In addition to getting accurate and thorough medical information, it may be helpful to seek out an experienced therapist, preferably before surgery, to help provide some clarity with these important emotional issues.

Can Having a Hysterectomy Lead to Psychological Problems for Your Partner?

Some women may find that their partners have a hard time after a hysterectomy. Partners may also experience a sense of loss or sadness that having biological children is no longer possible, and perhaps that middle age has arrived. They may worry about your lack of strength and your need to recover. They may also be afraid of hurting you during sex or be uncertain about how you feel about sex after the operation. These feelings can be found in both heterosexual and lesbian relationships. Anticipating these feelings for both of you and talking about them before, or at least after, surgery, will probably go a long way toward resolving these issues. Talking to a therapist oftentimes helps if either of you has a difficult emotional time.

Can Having a Hysterectomy Affect Your Sexuality?

There is much that is not known about sexuality after hysterectomy. Most of the research available is poorly done. Some current research is directed at finding out more about women's sexuality in general, and other researchers are trying to understand what happens specifically after gynecologic procedures such as hysterectomy, myomectomy, and uterine fibroid embolization. Ultimately, hysterectomy should be a well-considered choice after looking at all of your alternatives.

In the medical community itself, a number of factors cloud the issue of sexuality and hysterectomy. First, most doctors do not ask about sexuality before or after hysterectomy (or any treatment, for that matter) and therefore do not really know what happens to their patients. Women who try to discuss sexuality with their doctors often get dismissed because the doctors (even women doctors) do not know much about women's sexuality in the first place and do not know what to say.

Other women do not feel free to bring up sexuality issues with their doctor, even with women doctors, so physicians are often not made aware of problems that do exist. A recent online survey found that 25 percent of women having UFE declined to answer questions about sexuality even though the survey was entirely anonymous. It may be that one of the reasons doctors think sexuality is better after surgery or UFE is that these are the women most likely to tell us, and these are the women we are most likely to listen to.

Some women are not attuned to their own sexuality and may not notice a difference. Orgasm is experienced differently by different women. Many women reach orgasm by stimulation of the clitoris, other women by vaginal stimulation, and still others by a combination of the two. Some women have cervical or uterine contractions with orgasm, while other women do not and will not miss these contractions if the cervix or uterus is absent. Some women also feel that pressure against the cervix during intercourse is pleasurable and is important to their sexual experience. Removal of the cervix may change this sensation and decrease the sense of pleasure. In some women, hysterectomy can result in the formation of scar tissue where the sutures are placed at the top of the vagina. The scar tissue may be less elastic than normal tissue and may lead to discomfort during intercourse. For some women, laparoscopic subtotal hysterectomy might be considered in an attempt to avoid these problems.

Other women have so much discomfort from their fibroids, endometriosis, or adhesions that removal of the uterus actually can make intercourse pleasurable again. One study of women with gynecologic problems found that following removal of the uterus, 75 percent of the women noted that sex was better, and only 10 percent of the women felt that it was worse than before surgery. Another study found that the best predictors of sexuality after hysterectomy were the frequency of desire, intercourse, and orgasm prior to the surgery, as well as the woman's feelings about her partner. And, lastly, some women report that hysterectomy actually increases their enjoyment of sex by eliminating the fear of pregnancy.

Debbie's Problem After Hysterectomy

Debbie is a forty-nine-year-old woman who was seen at a well-known medical clinic for a complete physical. She felt fine and was surprised when the gynecologist at the clinic found uterine fibroids on her pelvic examination. Despite the fact that Debbie lived in another town about two hours away, the doctor recommended that she have surgery immediately. Even though she is a high-level executive used to making quick and weighty decisions,

Debbie felt flustered, indecisive, and afraid. Feeling she was already in the best of hands, she chose not to seek a second opinion and had a hysterectomy performed that week. The surgery went well, and she left the hospital five days later feeling relieved that it was over and that she could return to her normal life.

I first saw Debbie a year later. Following the surgery, she had found that intercourse was very uncomfortable. This was very upsetting to her since she and her husband, who had met in high school and been married for thirty years, had an active and wonderful sex life. The discomfort she felt made intercourse difficult and had strained their relationship. Debbie returned to see the gynecologist who had performed the surgery, but the doctor dismissed the problem as psychological and had not been of much help to Debbie.

When I examined Debbie, as the speculum was inserted toward the top of her vagina, she moved away in pain. I was able to see an area of scar tissue where the sutures had been placed during the surgery. The area seemed thicker than expected for a year after surgery. On the manual part of the examination, this area was extremely tender to the touch. I reinserted the speculum to get a better look at the tender area and was surprised to find an area of raw and unhealed skin at the point of tenderness. This delayed healing is not uncommon and is called granulation tissue, or "proud flesh." It is formed when new blood vessels begin to grow in a wound, but are not covered up by skin when the tissue heals. Sometimes the granulation tissue is discovered because it starts to bleed and sometimes, as in Debbie's case, because it is tender.

I felt happy that the problem appeared to be such a simple one, which could be treated by placing a chemical on the affected area to encourage proper healing. This treatment was mildly uncomfortable but took less than a minute. When I saw Debbie three weeks later to check the area, it appeared to have healed well, but it was still uncomfortable. We decided to allow a couple more months for the healing to be complete.

Two months later, when I examined the area, it appeared healed but was slightly thickened from scar tissue, and it was still tender. Debbie was upset, and I was disappointed because what I thought was an easy problem to treat had not gotten better. I felt the next step was an attempt to cut away the scar tissue and repair the vagina in the hospital under anesthesia. I hoped this would allow new tissue to start the healing process over again, this time with more success. Debbie was anxious to try anything and agreed. The surgery was not difficult; the scar tissue was cut away, and the healthy tissue sutured back together. I saw Debbie every few weeks following surgery, and the tissue appeared to be healing fine. About six weeks after surgery, Debbie and her husband had intercourse for the first time in many months. While still mildly uncomfortable, Debbie felt much better than she had since before her hysterectomy had been performed. By the time of her next visit, six months later, Debbie reported no discomfort during intercourse and was back to full enjoyment of sex.

There are a number of lessons to be learned from Debbie's story. First, if you are not sure about what has been recommended to you, there is always time to get a second opinion. Do not rush. Second, if you are having problems after surgery, be evaluated to see whether there is a medical, and correctable, reason for how you feel. And, lastly, even if problems do occur after surgery, many of them can be corrected.

Can Removal of Your Ovaries Affect Your Sexuality?

Some of the other inferred effects of "hysterectomy" on sexuality are actually related to the removal of the ovaries and subsequent hormonal deficiency, rather than the removal of the uterus. If the ovaries are removed and no hormonal replacement is started, then sexual enjoyment may be altered. Without estrogen to maintain the health of the vaginal tissue, the vagina may become thinner, drier, and inelastic, often leading to pain with intercourse. Also, estrogen and testosterone, both produced by the ovaries, are needed to maintain libido and normal sexual feelings.

Testosterone, the main hormone produced by men, is manufactured in small amounts by your ovaries, and it increases libido, or sexual desire. Some women will note a decrease in libido after removal of the ovaries, even if they take estrogen replacement. If this happens, you might consider taking testosterone in pill form. In large doses, testosterone can cause side effects such as weight gain, change in the texture or amount of body hair, acne, oily skin, or, very rarely, deepening of the voice. These side effects can be avoided by taking very small doses. One study found that women with their ovaries and uterus removed noted a decrease in the frequency of intercourse and orgasm if no hormone replacement were given. But women who subsequently took estrogen had a twofold increase in the frequency of intercourse and orgasm, and women who took both estrogen and testosterone had a sixfold increase. Testosterone may also improve mood, and some women who take testosterone feel better in general, in addition to having a return to normal libido.

What Can Be Done If Hysterectomy Has Caused Sexual Problems?

One thing to do is understand that you are not alone and help is available. First, you should be evaluated physically to make sure your hormone levels are normal or scar tissue hasn't formed to cause you pain. If you feel that your emotions are part of the dilemma, and if you would like to improve your sex life, help is also available. Probably the best place to start is by explaining to your partner how you feel about the change in your sexuality. Hopefully, your partner will be understanding, and the two of you can explore different ways of having sexual pleasure. This may be an opportunity to experiment. The goal is for sex to be pleasurable, even if it may feel different.

Psychological counseling, especially sexuality counseling, may also be very helpful. Most doctors are not skilled in dealing with issues of sexuality, but your doctor may be able to direct you to the appropriate therapist.

ARE THERE ANY BENEFITS TO HYSTERECTOMY?

It seems clear that too many hysterectomies are performed in this country every year and that some women could have avoided surgery had they been aware of other alternatives and treatments. However, it is also clear that some women benefit from having a hysterectomy. Not many would argue with the usefulness of removing the uterus for cervical, uterine, or ovarian cancer, where hysterectomy can be lifesaving. But many other women have symptoms that, while not life threatening, do affect their general physical and emotional health and their ability to perform normal activities. Is there any evidence that a hysterectomy can be of any benefit to these women?

An important study was published in 1994, the Maine Women's Health Study, that examined how women felt both physically and emotionally before and after hysterectomy. This is the largest study of its kind concerning hysterectomy. More than 400 women were interviewed before they had a hysterectomy and then followed for a year after their surgery. The study included half of the women who had a hysterectomy in the state of Maine during that time. Likewise, a separate group of 380 women who had similar gynecologic problems, but chose not to have a hysterectomy, were interviewed. Even though the group of women who chose to have a hysterectomy had somewhat worse symptoms than the women who chose nonsurgical treatment, the large number of women interviewed makes the results interesting.

What is especially noteworthy is that the study found that after hysterectomy a substantial number of women had a marked improvement in their symptoms, which included pelvic pain, urinary problems, bleeding, fatigue, and psychological and sexual problems. They also reported a significant improvement in mental health and general health at the end of one year. Many of the women reported a marked improvement in the quality of their lives. Therefore, for some women, especially those who had significant symptoms as a result of gynecologic problems, hysterectomy may be beneficial. The details of the study are outlined below.

Can Hysterectomy Help Relieve Gynecological Symptoms?

In the Maine study, 93 percent of the women reported "some" or "a lot" of discomfort or limitation of their activity before surgery. The reasons for hysterectomy included fibroids, endometriosis, heavy bleeding, prolapse of the uterus, and chronic pelvic pain. The women studied noted significant symptoms that had a substantial negative effect on the quality of their lives. After hysterectomy, the vast majority of these women noted an improvement in their symptoms. For example, of the 85 percent of women who had pelvic pain "frequently" before surgery, only 13 percent complained of this problem after surgery. While 70 percent of the women had pain with intercourse before surgery, only 30 percent had this problem after hysterectomy. And, while 60 percent of the women had diminished enjoyment of sex before surgery, only 15 percent complained of this after surgery. Therefore, the Maine study showed that for women who are significantly affected by gynecologic symptoms, hysterectomy might be helpful.

Can Hysterectomy Improve the Way You Feel?

In the Maine study, 72 percent of the women felt "much better" and another 16 percent felt a "little better" after they had a hysterectomy performed. Only 3 percent of the women interviewed felt worse than they did before surgery. Remember that most of these women had a significant degree of symptoms before surgery, and therefore would be expected to benefit more from surgery than someone with only mild symptoms. Also, despite some other accounts to the contrary, only 3 percent had a negative feeling about themselves as women as a result of having their uterus removed.

Can Hysterectomy Improve Quality of Life?

Women entering the Maine study had lower scores in tests of their quality of life than the general population but had improved scores equal to the general population after their hysterectomies. This improved quality of life was expressed as less pelvic and back pain, less pain with intercourse, less abdominal swelling, and less fatigue. Significant improvement in activity, general health, and mental health was also seen in women who had a hysterectomy. The Maine study found that the women who had a hysterectomy were much more able to go where they wanted, do things for fun and recreation, and work after surgery than they had been able to do before surgery.

While improvement in quality of life can be expected once recovery from surgery is complete, one study found that in the short term, at least for the first few months following hysterectomy, women suffer from fatigue that interferes with daily activity. However, fatigue is not unique to hysterectomy and has been reported after all types of surgery and uterine fibroid embolization.

Jane's Hysterectomy

Jane is a forty-four-year-old woman who had known that she had uterine fibroids for about three years. They never caused her any problems until recently, when she felt fairly constant abdominal pressure and discomfort during intercourse. When she was examined, I noted the fibroids to be larger than they had been before. Since the symptoms were not severe, Jane decided to be reexamined in three months to see if the fibroids continued to grow.

At the follow-up visit, the fibroids were the same size, but Jane felt more disturbed by the symptoms they were causing. She no longer wanted to have intercourse and found herself in pain and irritable most every day. She asked about the possible treatments. We discussed the possibility of no treatment until menopause, when the fibroids would most certainly shrink. But Jane felt that this was too far off. The second option was to perform a myomectomy, which involves removing the fibroids but leaving the uterus. Since the fibroids were very large, the myomectomy would need to be performed through an abdominal incision. The last option was hysterectomy, which would also require an abdominal incision. Jane felt that if she was going to go through an abdominal incision and the needed recovery, she probably ought to have her uterus removed so that she would not have to deal with fibroids in the future. But Jane was concerned about hysterectomy because she had heard that the surgery might affect her sexuality. After a long discussion about the risks and benefits of each option, Jane decided to think about it and wait a little longer.

Three months later, Jane was ready to do something about her fibroids. The constant pressure was interfering with her job and daily activities, and intercourse was totally unenjoyable. We went over the options again, and Jane was fairly certain that she wanted a hysterectomy but was still worried about the effect it might have on her sexuality. We discussed the possibility of performing a subtotal hysterectomy and leaving the cervix in place, but after much thought, she decided to have a total hysterectomy without the removal of her fallopian tubes or ovaries.

The surgery went well, as did her recovery. At her appointment six months after her hysterectomy, I asked Jane how she was doing. She said she no longer had discomfort during the day, and the pain with intercourse had disappeared. Intercourse was now totally enjoyable. She was surprised at how much discomfort she had learned to live with and was relieved that it was over. She felt certain that the hysterectomy had been the right thing for her to do.

Can Medication Relieve Pelvic Pain or Bleeding?

The second part of the Maine Women's Study was an evaluation of the symptoms of women who chose to be treated with medication for their problems. These women were then compared to women who chose to have a hysterectomy for similar problems. For many of the women, medication was effective and allowed them to avoid surgery. The two groups of women were not entirely similar because the women who chose surgery had worse symptoms than those who chose medication. But the authors of the study felt the results were valuable because there were significant similarities between the two large groups of women.

The study reported that, of the 85 percent of women who complained of significant pelvic pain before treatment with medication, 50 percent still had this problem after treatment. For women who had a hysterectomy, 95 percent complained of pain before surgery, but only 3 percent had pain after the hysterectomy. For women who had pain from fibroids, 50 percent were better following medication, while 85 percent reported feeling better after hysterectomy. For women who had abnormal bleeding, 60 percent were better following medication while, as would be expected, 100 percent of women had no problems with bleeding following their hysterectomy.

The study found that more women in the hysterectomy group were satisfied with the relief of symptoms they achieved and were ten times more likely to have a positive feeling about how they felt following hysterectomy than those who chose medication.

Although the results of this study should be interpreted with care, it does appear that hysterectomy may provide relief for women who have a *significant* degree of symptoms, especially if other treatment has failed. As new developments come along, the need for hysterectomy should decrease. However, hysterectomy does appear to have a place in the appropriate treatment of some medical problems.

Will Hysterectomy Become a Less Common Operation?

New treatments for fibroids and abnormal bleeding, two of the most common reasons for hysterectomy, should decrease the need for hysterectomy. Recent studies of women with fibroids have shown that the medical risks of no treatment, even with large fibroids, have been overstated in the past. Therefore, for many of these women, no treatment may be needed. If treatment is necessary, myomectomy by hysteroscopy, or laparoscopy, or abdominal surgery can often be used to remove fibroids and alleviate symptoms without removing the uterus (see page 129). Myolysis, a new procedure described on page 137, uses a laparoscopic technique to destroy fibroids without removing them at all. To date, the results have been promising. Uterine fibroid embolization (UFE), as described on page 140, has been a very successful nonsurgical treatment for some women with fibroids. With continued experience in the performance of the procedure, better understanding of the women for whom the procedure is likely to be successful, and more cooperation between gynecologists and interventional radiologists, the procedure will become available to more women. Medications used to shrink fibroids have been developed but are only effective in the short term because of their solely temporary benefit, their side effects, and their expense. Newer medications are in the experimental phase and may, hopefully, provide long-term relief for women with fibroids and allow them to avoid surgical or embolization procedures altogether.

Abnormal bleeding may now be treated by endometrial ablation and/or resectoscope myomectomy with 90 percent of women reporting excellent results, allowing them to avoid hysterectomy (see pages 89 and 138). Endometriosis, the third most common reason for hysterectomy, may be treated by medical therapy, although the side effects and expense of the medications limit its use at the present time. Laparoscopic techniques that remove scarred or diseased tissue short of hysterectomy may also be used to alleviate pelvic pain associated with endometriosis (see page 223). Hysterectomy, for most of these conditions, should be a last resort, not the first one.

Despite the development of many such alternatives to hysterectomy, a disappointing tally of hysterectomy rates in 2002 showed no change in the number of hysterectomies performed per capita in the United States in the last ten years. To find what is available and best, you will need to educate yourself. You may also need to see more than one doctor and get a second or even third opinion to find alternative treatment options for your problem, in addition to hysterectomy.

Mary's Fibroids

Mary is a forty-seven-year-old woman who knew that she had fibroids for about five years. At first, the fibroids had been small, and she was not bothered by them at all. After a few years, they began to grow little by little, until they were the size of a four-month pregnancy. She had been told by a number of doctors over the past few years that surgery would be necessary. However, Mary was afraid of surgery, afraid of being in a hospital, and afraid of any of the possible risks to her health. She had wanted to avoid surgery if at all possible. She had been very active, playing tennis and exercising regularly, and while the fibroids had slowed her down a bit, she was still able to do these things.

I was the fourth doctor to see Mary for her fibroids. By this time, she had started to have heavy and irregular bleeding, but otherwise she felt fairly well. Her examination showed that the fibroids had not grown any further. To make sure that there was no reason for the abnormal bleeding other than the fibroids, I recommended that she have a D&C and hysteroscopy (see page 86) in the office. Mary was relieved that she did not have to go to the hospital and agreed. The procedure went well, and no abnormal cells were found, suggesting that the bleeding was from the fibroids. In addition, based on a blood test (hematocrit) done prior to the D&C, Mary was not at all anemic. Therefore, the amount of blood she was losing did not seem to be harming her.

In the weeks following the procedure, Mary and I had two long discussions about her options. These included follow-up with pelvic examinations to monitor any further growth of the fibroids, myomectomy to remove the fibroids, myolysis to shrink the fibroids, or hysterectomy. Mary once again chose the option of careful follow-up with pelvic examinations every three months. I felt totally comfortable with her decision. There was nothing wrong with her medically, and she was able to live with the fibroids comfortably enough to do the things she wanted to do.

Now, two years later, Mary continues to do well and has avoided surgery. We are both aiming toward her menopause, when the fibroids will be expected to shrink down to about half their present size (even if she chooses to start HRT). Mary is totally comfortable with her decision, and, for her, it is clearly the right one.

QUESTIONS TO ASK YOUR DOCTOR ▨

It is important for you to understand the reasons that your doctor has suggested a hysterectomy as treatment for your gynecologic problem. The best way to help you make a decision as to whether the procedure is right for you is to ask your doctor the right questions.

The most common reasons for surgery are pain, bleeding, or symptoms from fibroids. You know the reason you went to see the doctor in the first place. The first question that you should ask is, "What exactly is causing my pain?" Sometimes the reason will not be entirely clear to the doctor. In particular, the cause of pelvic pain may originate in the intestines or the bladder and not from the uterus. You should ask if there are other tests that can be done to make the diagnosis more apparent. The decision whether to have these tests should be yours and should be balanced with their side effects and cost. For example, laparoscopy can help to make a diagnosis of the cause of pelvic pain, but you may or may not wish to go through an operation to have an exact diagnosis made.

Once a diagnosis, or probable diagnosis, has been established, you should also ask what the consequences to your health will be if you do not have surgery, either at all, or at this time. For non–life-threatening problems, one option is always to do nothing. However, doing nothing often means more frequent visits to your doctor to monitor your problem.

The next question to ask the doctor is, "What are the nonsurgical alternative therapies available to treat my condition?" For every condition, there are usually alternatives of varying degrees of effectiveness. As described throughout this book, medications, pain management, even homeopathics or other alternative therapies may sometimes be tried to alleviate symptoms. But again, I would advise you to continue to see your doctor regularly to detect any changes in your condition.

You should also ask about your doctor's experience doing the operation that has been proposed. You should feel comfortable with the number of procedures he or she has performed for problems *like yours*. If the doctor's experience is limited, you may ask who the assistant is going to be and how much experience the assistant has had. Additional training and experience must be acquired before some of the newer procedures, such as endometrial ablation, laparoscopic surgery, or laparoscopic hysterectomy, can be safely performed. The same questions should be asked of an interventional radiologist regarding uterine fibroid embolization. Some hospitals have strict requirements for training before a doctor is allowed to perform these operations or procedures, while other hospitals have no such requirements. Therefore, it is important for you to ask about surgical training and experience.

Should You Get a Second Opinion?

You should also ask your doctor whether obtaining a second opinion would be a good idea. Most doctors will welcome the idea of a second opinion. If they have done a complete job on the diagnosis and on the explanation of the problem to you, then they should feel confident about the range of options they have suggested to you. In addition, no doctor knows everything, and your doctor may welcome any other new ideas about your problem. This is your body and your life, and you deserve to know everything you can about all the options available. Other thoughts on second opinions are discussed on page 360.

What Is Right for You?

The decision to have a hysterectomy should not be taken lightly. There are medical conditions that require treatment—cancer, prolonged heavy bleeding to the point of severe anemia, or incapacitating pain. However, as outlined throughout this book, all medical conditions have more than one option for treatment. Medicine is an evolving art as well as a science. Recently, with more open attitudes toward women's opinions and feelings, and with the advent of new technology, doctors have been looking for new medical treatments for gynecologic symptoms in order to avoid hysterectomy. As discussed above, there are possible side effects of hysterectomy, none of which is entirely predictable for each individual. But for some women, hysterectomy will be the right treatment.

As with most decisions, you should carefully consider the pros and cons of hysterectomy as they relate to *your particular* medical situation and emotional well-being. On one hand, you should weigh the degree of discomfort that your gynecologic problem presents to you, the ways in which it interferes with your health, both emotionally and physically. On the other hand, weigh the potential risks of the operation, including the possible physical and emotional side effects of having a hysterectomy. There are women who happily choose to live with fibroids the size of a five-month pregnancy despite the fact that they have some daily discomfort and look pregnant. Other women choose surgery for small fibroids because they are distressed by symptoms or by worry and don't wish to live with the problems any longer.

The universal indications for hysterectomy have not been defined. Ultimately, each woman needs to make the final decision about the appropriateness of hysterectomy for herself. That is what this book is about.

REFERENCES

Avis, N., D. Brambilla, S. McKinlay, and K. Vass. 1994. A longitudinal analysis of the association between menopause and depression: Results from the Massachusetts Women's Health Study. *Annals of Epidemiology* 4: 214–20.

Bachman, G. 1990. Hysterectomy: A critical review. *Journal of Reproductive Medicine* 35:839–62.

Broder, M., D. Kanouse, B. Mittman, and S. Bernstein. 2000. The appropriateness of recommendations for hysterectomy. *Obstetrics and Gynecology* 95:199–205.

Burger, H., E. Dudley, J. Hopper, J. Shelley, A. Green, A. Smith, L. Dennerstein, and C. Morse. 1995. The endocrinology of the menopausal transition: A cross-sectional study of a population-based sample. *Journal of Clinical Endocrinology and Metabolism* 80:3535–37.

Carlson, K., B. Miller, and F. Fowler. 1994. The Maine Women's Health Study: I. Outcomes of hysterectomy. *Obstetrics and Gynecology* 83:556–65.

Carlson, K., B. Miller, and F. Fowler. 1994. The Maine Women's Health Study: II. Outcomes of nonsurgical management of leiomyomas, abnormal bleeding, and chronic pelvic pain. *Obstetrics and Gynecology* 83:566–72.

Centerwall, B. Premenopausal hysterectomy and cardiovascular disease. 1981. *American Journal of Obstetrics and Gynecology* 139:58–61.

Coulter, A., K. McPherson, and M. Vessey. 1988. Do British women undergo too many or too few hysterectomies? *Social Science and Medicine* 27:987–94.

DeCherney, A., G. Bachman, K. Isaacson, and S. Gall. 2002. Postoperative fatigue negatively impacts the daily lives of patients recovering from hysterectomy. *Obstetrics and Gynecology* 99:51–57.

Dionne, C. 2001. Sex, Lies and the Truth About Uterine Fibroids. New York: Avery.

Dranov, P. 1990. An unkind cut. *American Health* 9:36.

Farquhar, C., and C. Steiner. 2002. Hysterectomy rates in the United States 1990–1997. *Obstetrics and Gynecology* 99:229–34.

Gambone, J., R. Reiter, and J. Lench. 1992. Short-term outcome of incidental hysterectomy at the time of adnexectomy for benign disease. *Journal of Women's Health* 1:197–200.

Griffith-Jones, M., G. Jarvis, and H. McNamara. 1991. Adverse urinary symptoms after total abdominal hysterectomy: Fact or fiction? *British Journal of Urology* 67:295–97.

LaLonde, C., and J. Daniell. 1996. Early outcomes of laparoscopic-assisted vaginal hysterectomy versus laparoscopic supracervical hysterectomy. *Journal of the American Association of Gynecologic Laparoscopists* 3:251–56.

Langer, R., M. Neuman, R. Ron-el, A. Golan, I. Bukovsky, and E. Caspi. 1989. The effect of total abdominal hysterectomy on bladder function in asymptomatic women. *Obstetrics and Gynecology* 74:205–7.

Munro, M. 1997. Supracervical hysterectomy: A time for reappraisal. *Obstetrics and Gynecology* 89:133–39.

Parker, W. 2000. Laparoscopic hysterectomy. *Obstetrics and Gynecology Clinics* 27:431–40.

Raisz, L., B. Witta, A. Arthis, et al. 1996. Comparison of the effects of estrogen alone plus estrogen and androgen on biochemical markers of bone formation and resorption in postmenopausal women. *Journal of Clinical Endocrinology and Metabolism* 81:37–43.

Ryan, M., L. Dennerstein, and R. Pepperell. 1989. Psychological aspects of hysterectomy: A prospective study. *British Journal of Psychology* 154:516–22.

13

IF YOU ARE FACING SURGERY

In some situations, your physician may recommend surgery. Although many people around the world walk into hospitals each day to face an operation, very few of us can do it without some fear. It is always a step that requires a great deal of thought and consideration since it involves some discomfort, some risk, and some disruption of one's life.

I strongly feel that the decision to have surgery is always up to the patient. It is your body and your life, not your doctor's. Do everything you can to understand your condition and the surgical and medical options available to treat that condition. Take charge of your medical care by educating yourself. Knowledge is often a good antidote to anxiety. Any medical problem, particularly one that seems to be pointing toward surgery, is anxiety producing. You will begin your own healing and recovery by taking charge of the decisions that need to be made.

What Should Happen During the Doctor's Consultation?

When one of my patients needs surgery, I like to set up a consultation visit to discuss all the available options; even the ones I may not feel are entirely appropriate for that particular woman. The role of a physician at this point is to provide information so that you can make the decisions you need to get well. Diagrams or photographs of anatomy and surgical procedures are always a part of my consultation visit. Understandably, most of us are not familiar enough with anatomy or medical terminology to get a genuine understanding of a problem or the surgical options from just a verbal explanation. Being able to visualize the problem through diagrams or photos helps to make all the options and procedures clear. During this long talk together, we discuss the risks and benefits of each possible solution to the problem.

We also talk about the recovery period after surgery and predict, as best we can, how long it will take to get back to work and normal activities. People seem most comfortable with decisions made when all information available is understood and carefully considered. If you know and understand the whole story, your head and your heart will lead you to the best decision. The notion of physician as educator and the patient as an active participant in the decision process is one that is very important to me. When this relationship works well, I feel comfortable that the patient will make a decision that is right for her. My patients tell me that these appointments are worth their weight in gold when choices need to be made.

Should You Bring Someone to the Doctor's Office?

If I needed surgery, I would not want to be alone at the time decisions were being discussed or made. I have found it very helpful for the woman facing surgery to have a family member or friend accompany her to the consultation visit. You will often feel calmer with a loved one near, and you will be better able to take in the information discussed. Sometimes your companion is able to listen when you are too anxious to do so or will simply pick up something you missed. Often your companion is able to hear the optimism and reassurance in the words spoken when you may only be able to hear your own fear. Having another person hear the information at least ensures that there will be someone knowledgeable for you to talk to after the appointment is over. Having a loving, trusted, and informed companion on the ride home may be the nicest gift you could give yourself.

After all the options, both surgical and nonsurgical, are presented and understood, I will then make some recommendations based on my best medical judgment. Often women will ask, "What would you do if you were me?" I always find this a difficult question to answer because so many nonmedical factors need to be considered. Ask yourself: How much discomfort am I in because of this condition? Can I or should I tolerate that discomfort? Can I afford, both emotionally and physically, not to have surgery? Can I afford the time off work to recuperate if I do have surgery? What are my emotions about my condition? How do I feel about having surgery? How will my choice affect my family? These are questions only you can answer. If medically appropriate, I always like to offer at least two possible treatment options. This helps to ensure the possibility that each woman will have a comfortable choice.

When Should You Make a Decision About Surgery?

I don't think any decision should be made about surgery at the initial consultation visit. You should think about the information and options for a while in a relaxed environment. Be sure to call the doctor back with any questions that you may not have thought of before, or for questions that were not completely answered during the visit. Almost all women call me back within a few days with a few more questions. This is your body; do not be afraid to ask questions.

Should You Get a Second Opinion?

If surgery has been recommended to you, I think a second opinion is an excellent idea. Very few things in medicine are black or white, and there is a lot of room for differences of opinion. A number of possibilities exist after a second opinion. First, the physician you see for the second opinion may give you the exact same options as your original gynecologist. This may put your mind at ease in that you will feel sure that nothing has been overlooked. Second, the new physician may bring up other options that are available to you or give you more information to think about. Or, the physician giving the second opinion may disagree with what you have been told or even disagree with the diagnosis. For my patients who seek a second opinion, I always ask them to call and talk to me about the results of that consultation. This allows me to answer any new questions and respond to any suggestions the other physician has offered. I never feel offended if a patient wants a second opinion.

When a new patient comes to see me for a second opinion, our office asks them to bring all the physician's notes from previous medical appointments and any test results that are relevant to the problem. If an ultrasound or MRI has already been performed, I like to look at the films myself so that I can come to my own conclusions about the diagnosis. While we both sit comfortably in my office, I ask the patient to tell me what her concerns are. Whether the concerns are medical or emotional or of some other nature, they should be an important part of the discussion. I ask questions to clarify my impression of the problem. Then the woman proceeds to an exam room, where I perform a complete examination. If a family member or friend is present, they are welcome into the exam room if the patient wishes.

Once the exam is completed, the patient gets dressed, and we meet back in my office. I will show her what I have seen on the ultrasound or MRI and review the findings of the examination. I often use illustrations to demonstrate what those findings are. At this point, I make a list of one or more possible diagnoses and outline the treatments available for each problem. To be complete with this list, I usually include even those treatments I would advise against or those the patient has eliminated. Together we then go through the list and come up with a short number of options that are both medically sound and personally acceptable to the patient. I encourage her not to decide on any specific course at this time. I think these decisions are usually best made in the comfort of home, when there is time to think. I tell them to call me with questions in the next few days.

One of the issues that sometimes comes up during a second (or third) opinion visit is the question of which doctor will care for the patient. This is a difficult issue for both patient and doctor because patients sometimes worry about hurting a doctor's feelings. I think it is best to deal with this dilemma in a straightforward manner. At the beginning of the consultation, I ask the patient in what capacity she would like me to serve. Is she seeking only a second opinion, or is she looking to change doctors? Some women are clear that they are happy with their own doctor and want to see if I agree with what has been recommended. Some women are clear that they are unhappy with their doctor and are definitely seeking a new doctor. Most women are happy enough with their doctor but feel they have not been given all the options available. They are seeking more information first and may wish to switch doctors if they find a more reasonable option or are more comfortable with the new doctor. If an explanation of the goals of this consultation is clear at the beginning of the appointment, the course of the discussion is easier, and each woman will get what she is seeking.

Many of my colleagues and I encourage seeking second opinions, particularly when the patient is unsure of what is best for her. This is your body and your health. Do not be afraid to get another opinion.

Who Should You Go to for a Second Opinion?

It is probably *not* a good idea to ask your gynecologist which doctor you should see for a second opinion. Despite a high degree of honesty in the profession, your doctor may refer you to someone he or she knows well, who may be less likely to disagree with the diagnosis or proposed treatment. There are a number of good sources available to you to suggest the name of a doctor for your second opinion. Your family doctor or internist will know other gynecologists in the community who are knowledgeable, honest, and provide good care. Another possibility is to call the gynecology floor of your local hospital. The head nurse may be able to suggest doctors for you who have experience with your particular problem. Nurses have a unique vantage point since they see physicians interact with and care for patients and also know how each doctor's patients do following surgery. Nurses are a good source for a physician referral. You may also consider calling a teaching hospital near you and asking for a faculty member with expertise in your area of concern.

I do think, however, that you should tell your gynecologist that you are going to get a second opinion. This will maintain the trust and honesty in your relationship. You should also consider telling him or her who the doctor will be. There may be doctors in the community who are well known but who may not have knowledge about the specific procedure or problem you are faced with. This will give your gynecologist an opportunity to voice any concerns about the doctor you have chosen. This need not dissuade you from using that doctor for a second opinion, but you will at least be prepared for any differences of opinion.

What If You Decide Surgery Is Right for You?

If you decide that surgery is right for your situation, you will need to choose the doctor to perform your surgery. There are a number of factors that should influence your decision. The first is to choose a doctor who will perform a procedure that fits your particular situation and problem. In most cases, you should have more than one option from which to choose.

The next concern is the skill of the surgeon. How many procedures does the doctor perform a month? How many procedures like the one you are requesting? How many of these procedures has the surgeon performed in women with problems like yours? How many complications has the doctor had and what kind of complications were they? Studies show that experience makes a surgeon better. Surgeons who perform procedures frequently have lower rates of complications. But surveys show that many gynecologists perform less than one major operation a month. Choose your surgeon carefully.

It is also important to feel comfortable with your doctor. Do you get an opportunity to ask questions and are they answered? Is the doctor available?

If you decide to have surgery, another visit should be set up with the doctor you have chosen, to go over the specific details of the procedure you are to have performed. Again, it is nice to have someone accompany you. Once a decision has been made, we go over a paper called the Informed Consent. Filling out this form, if properly done, encourages a frank discussion of what you should expect from surgery. It allows the doctor and patient to go over the details of the operation to be performed, the specific risks of the procedure, the alternatives to the surgery, and the possible consequences if the surgery is not performed. Basically, this is the time when you will hear all the risks and possible complications during and after your surgery. This is difficult and may feel as if it's the last thing you want to hear, but ultimately it is quite helpful to you. I see this form as part of my job as an educator. I choose to fill out the form by hand in the patient's presence and make it specific for each woman's situation. I am available to answer any questions related to the risks of the procedure. Doctors are certainly not trying to erode your confidence at this point, but we are legally and morally bound to tell you about all the things that could happen. Most people's emotional reaction to this form is fear, which is understandable. Just remember to be sure to hear the optimism in your doctor's message. This is another opportunity for you to inform and educate yourself. Learning as much as you can will help, not hurt, you.

How Do You Schedule Surgery?

The next step is to schedule the surgery based on the urgency of the problem, your schedule, the availability of your family or friends who may be helping you out after surgery, your doctor's schedule, and the availability of the hospital operating room. In our office, we have a person who sits down with the patient and helps them through this process. Scheduling the date of surgery, blood donation appointments (see below), laboratory test appointments, and appointments with a primary care doctor can all be arranged at this time. We like to write all this information down so that you can refer to it later. Again, planning can go a long way toward reducing anxiety. We also tell our patients to stop taking any products containing aspirin for the two weeks before surgery, since they can lead to more bleeding during the operation. You will also be instructed to not eat or drink anything for at least eight hours prior to your surgery. Anything in your stomach at the time of the operation could cause vomiting and aspiration of food into your lungs—a serious problem. And last, but certainly not least, if you smoke, you should stop at least a few weeks before surgery to allow your lungs to clear and reduce your risk of breathing problems after surgery.

Should You Donate Your Own Blood Before Surgery?

While the risk of needing a blood transfusion because of an operation is usually small, give some thought to this issue while you are planning your surgery. Consider these three options: You may accept blood from the blood bank if necessary; you may donate your own blood prior to surgery; or you may refuse to accept blood under any, including life-threatening, circumstances. You need to know that screening of blood donors has become very strict and includes detailed personal questions regarding risk factors for infectious diseases. If the answers suggest that the potential donor is low risk, a sample of blood is drawn and tested for HIV, hepatitis B and C, HTLV (a rare form of viral infection), and syphilis. At some hospitals the donor is given a form and an addressed envelope to take home. If there were something the donor should have told the blood bank—possible risk factors or exposure, but were reluctant to mention because he or she was in the presence of friends or relatives, the donor has a second opportunity to respond.

Due to this careful screening, the risk of acquiring HIV from a blood transfusion is now 1 out of 1,900,000 pints of blood. The risk of hepatitis C is 1 out of 1,000,000 and hepatitis B is 1 out of 135,000. Blood transfusion is safer now than ever before.

The second option is to donate your own blood before surgery. Autologous transfusion, as this process is called, is not entirely without risk. Very rarely, the blood bank gives blood intended for one patient to another patient, and a reaction to the blood can occur. A variation of self-transfusion is called directed donor transfusion. A directed donor is someone, usually a friend or a relative, who has volunteered to give blood specifically for you. However, it turns out that the risk of infection is just as great in these donors due to unsuspected infections with HIV or hepatitis.

If you choose to donate your own blood, the process of giving blood is very much like having a blood test taken. A needle is inserted into a vein in your arm and attached to a plastic bag. You may be asked to open and close your fist to help pump the blood out of the vein. The entire procedure takes about forty-five minutes, and there is no discomfort other than the initial stick of the needle. Before you leave the blood donation center, you need to drink some juice and have a snack—all provided for you by the blood bank.

If you are going to donate your own blood, you will be advised to take iron pills to build up your blood prior to donating the first pint of blood. Sometimes iron pills can cause stomach upset, but taking them with food often prevents this from happening. The iron should be continued until after you have surgery. First, one pint of blood is taken, and then another pint is taken a week later. After another week to allow you to rebuild your blood, surgery can be performed.

We used to encourage women to give their own blood before surgery. However, now that blood from the blood bank is so safe, the need for other sources of blood has become less important. Discuss these issues with your doctor before making a decision.

Some women, usually for religious reasons, will not accept blood even if their lives are in danger. It is extremely important that you discuss this issue with your doctor well before surgery is planned. Some physicians are not comfortable with this situation and may chose to refer you to another doctor for surgery. Other doctors may be comfortable with the situation but will want to know about this choice before a problem develops. Again, the more you discuss with your doctor, the better.

What Other Tests May Be Needed Before Surgery?

A few days prior to your surgery, blood tests will be performed to check your blood count. Depending on your age and medical history, other tests—an EKG to check your heart, a chest X-ray to check your lungs, other blood tests to check the kidneys or liver, or a blood sugar test to check for diabetes—may be needed to be sure that all bodily functions are strong. Your surgeon and anesthesiologist review these test results prior to your surgery.

If you have had problems with your heart or lungs before, your doctor may want you to set up an appointment with an anesthesiologist before your surgery so that these problems may be discussed and any further tests or preparations ordered ahead of time.

What Should You Do to Prepare for Surgery?

You may find that this time prior to surgery can be useful to get ready in other ways. If you can, take care of any business that may cause you anxiety. Make arrangements for child care, pay your bills, and get someone to water plants and take care of your pets. Also, it's a good idea to inquire about disability benefits at work so that you know in advance how much time off you will be allowed and how much money you will receive. Try to tie up loose ends at home and at work. Taking care of details will give you peace of mind during your hospital stay and recovery period.

If you have the luxury of free time before your scheduled surgery, use it to be nice to yourself and to stay in a positive frame of mind—visit friends and family, write letters, listen to music, see a movie. Concentrate on building up your confidence and optimism. Picture yourself getting well and getting strong. Try to keep your attitude about your surgery and your health positive and healing. Know that there are good times and good health in front of you. Enter the hospital as confidently and as peacefully as you can. A positive outlook can aid in your recovery.

AT THE HOSPITAL

What Happens When You Get to the Hospital?

Hospitals are generally large places with lots of rules and red tape. I hope that a friendly and helpful hospital staff member will greet you when you arrive for admission. A smile from a staff member can go a long way toward making you feel welcome and safe. That smile and courteous help in filling out forms cannot, of course, be guaranteed. Here is another instance where taking a trusted companion with you can help ensure your comfort. They can do any running around that needs to be done, can help listen to instructions, and can give you the much needed smile that a harried clerk may not manage.

You are usually asked to go to the hospital two to three hours before surgery. Generally, you go to the admitting office where admission and insurance forms will need to be filled out. You should remember to pack your insurance information the night before so that it will be readily available. You should also be sure to leave all your valuables at home. Hospitals usually have a place to store valuables, but it is better not to have to worry about them. Once the paperwork is complete, you will then be escorted to your room in the preoperative area that is usually right near the operating room.

If you didn't believe you were going to have an operation before, the reality begins to hit about now. You change into a hospital gown. Many people begin to feel as if they are sick the moment they don this particularly unattractive piece of clothing. Contrary to popular belief, the gown was not designed to humiliate you and keep you uncomfortable. It is completely functional for surgery in that it is easy to put on and take off and gives the doctors and nurses quick access to you. But since the back of the garment usually leaves parts of your body exposed, it is not especially pleasant for you to wear.

The nurses will ask you about the reason you are in the hospital, your allergies to any medications, and any other medical problems you may have. You may be asked some of these questions repeatedly by a number of nurses or doctors during the time prior to your surgery. You will also need to sign another surgical consent form for the hospital, much like the one you signed in the doctor's office. Be reassured this is all for your safety to eliminate any confusion or mistakes. Because of these safety systems, I have never seen a case of mistaken identity occur.

Do You Need an IV?

Prior to surgery, a small needle is inserted into one of the veins of your arm, and a plastic tube is attached to the needle. A bag of fluid is attached to this tube and run into your vein. This IV, which means intravenous, provides you with the necessary water, salt, and sugar during the operation. It also provides access to your bloodstream for your anesthesia and any other medications you might need. While having an IV started is not fun, there is only minimal discomfort associated with inserting the needle and no discomfort thereafter.

Will You Need an Enema?

Before some types of surgeries, an enema is given to clean out your intestines. This empties the lower intestine and keeps it away from the uterus, fallopian tubes, and ovaries so that the surgeon can see the pelvic area more clearly. Discuss the need for an enema with your doctor. If it is necessary, some women prefer to give themselves one in the privacy of their own home before going to the hospital.

When Do You See the Anesthesiologist?

On the day of surgery, your anesthesiologist will visit you to review your medical history and your allergies to any medications and will discuss your options for anesthesia. The type of anesthesia used will depend on the type of surgery, the expected length of the surgery, your medical condition, your preference, and the comfort and experience of the anesthesiologist with different techniques. This is the time to ask any questions and express any preferences regarding anesthesia that you may have.

By this time, you are usually ready to have the surgery over. The anesthesiologist will generally have some kind and comforting words for you and often will also give you some medications to help you relax before taking you into the operating room.

Is It Normal to Be Nervous About Anesthesia?

Over the years, as I have listened to people's concerns regarding surgery, it seems to me that one of the issues that causes a great deal of anxiety is the idea of general anesthesia, or being "put to sleep." The loss of control inherent in being put to sleep is a very powerful notion. We all try to retain as much control as we can over our own lives. Once again, education and a positive attitude can help to allay your fears and give you more of a sense of control. Anesthesia, like most fields in modern medicine, has made great strides in providing safe and effective care. Your anesthesiologist is a highly trained specialist, skilled in providing a safe and painless experience. Complications are extremely rare. In some cases, there will be anesthesia options available to you. Following is a brief overview of what we can do to ensure that your surgery is safe and pain free.

What Is General Anesthesia?

General anesthesia is actually a combination of liquid medication injected into your IV to induce sleep, plus the administration of a medication that you breathe to keep you asleep. Initially, a clear plastic mask will be placed over your face to give you oxygen. This may feel a little confining, and the rubber may smell funny, but it is not at all uncomfortable. At this point, a medication is given in the IV that will put you to sleep. It takes less than a minute, and most patients do not find this unpleasant. I usually stay with my patients as soon as they are brought into the operating room. You will probably not know anyone else in the room, and I think the presence of your surgeon is comforting. I like to talk to my patients to help them relax. While they are falling asleep, I will tell them to think about something pleasant, such as a trip to Hawaii or the Caribbean. As they drift off to sleep, I tell them, "Everything will be fine—we'll take good care of you." Besides making the experience more pleasant, there is even some evidence that this encouragement will actually help you recover faster.

After you are asleep, the anesthesia gas will be passed through either a mask over your mouth and nose or a tube placed through your mouth into your windpipe. The gas then seeps through your lungs and dissolves into the bloodstream. This dissolved gas reaches your brain, and in ways that are not totally understood, keeps you comfortably asleep for the duration of the operation. You will not feel any of the surgery.

What Is Epidural Anesthesia?

We experience physical pain because our nerves transmit this sensation from the site of the pain up to our brains. Nerves communicate with each other by sending chemical signals to the next nerve along the line. The brain soon gets the message, and we know that we're hurting. Local anesthetic, like the type your dentist uses, works by preventing the release of these chemical signals. When this happens, the nerves can't relay the message up to the brain to tell it that you hurt, and so you do not feel the pain.

Epidural anesthesia uses the same principle. After local anesthesia is placed in the skin, a small needle is guided into your back. A small plastic tube is placed through this needle into a space right outside your spinal cord. The needle is removed, but the plastic tube is left in place outside the spinal cord. Liquid local anesthetic is then dripped through the tube, which numbs the pain-sensing nerves and the motor (movement) nerves of your spinal cord. The anesthetic prevents these nerves from sending the brain any pain signals. At the same time, the anesthetic prevents the nerves from making your muscles move. As the anesthetic begins to work, you may feel warmth and tingling in your legs and feet and then, within about fifteen minutes, you will be unable to feel or move anything from your abdomen to your toes. Because the numbing medication is confined to a localized area, your brain remains awake and alert, and you are able to breathe on your own. You are also able to speak, hear, and answer questions. In addition to the epidural anesthesia, some patients choose to have Valium or another type of sedative given through the IV to help them relax during the surgery.

For abdominal surgery, some women prefer epidural anesthesia because they are concerned about the sense of losing control during general anesthesia. Others may prefer general anesthesia, since they may not want to "be awake" during the operation.

Are There Advantages to Epidural Anesthesia?

An advantage of epidural anesthesia is that it blocks the brain's perception of the initial pain signals from surgery. Even though you are asleep during general anesthesia, the nerves in your skin and body are able to send signals to your brain, which are perceived subconsciously. It appears that these signals program the brain to be more sensitive to pain and, after you wake up, you may feel more postoperative pain. If these initial signals are blocked before you are operated on, which epidural anesthesia does, postoperative pain seems to be diminished. Some studies have shown that patients who have epidural anesthesia have less pain following surgery than those given general anesthesia.

Why Must General Anesthesia Be Used for Laparoscopic Surgery?

If your operation is being performed with the laparoscope, general anesthesia is almost always used. During laparoscopy, carbon dioxide gas is put into your abdomen to form a bubble. This bubble pushes the intestines away from the uterus, fallopian tubes, and ovaries so that the pelvic area can be seen, and the surgery can be performed. But the bubble of gas also pushes the intestines into the upper abdomen and against the diaphragm, the muscles that push and pull on your lungs allowing you to breathe. Let's say you wanted to remain conscious during laparoscopic surgery and requested an epidural or spinal anesthesia. As the gas was pumped into your abdomen to enable us to do the surgery, you would begin to feel the pressure on your diaphragm. You would soon feel as if you were unable to breathe. Needless to say, this would be terrifying. Also, you might inadvertently move around in an attempt to breathe more deeply, and this could be dangerous in the middle of your surgery. For this reason, when you have laparoscopic surgery, general anesthesia is more pleasant and safer.

What Type of Anesthesia Can Be Used for Abdominal Surgery?

Most abdominal surgery, other than laparoscopy, can be performed with either general or epidural anesthesia. You should discuss the options with your surgeon prior to the day of surgery. On the day of surgery, and while you are still alert, your anesthesiologist will also discuss the appropriate choice of anesthesia with you based on your medical situation and your own preferences.

When Do You Go to the Operating Room?

About fifteen minutes before surgery, you will be wheeled on a gurney (a bed on wheels) to the operating suite. Some hospitals kindly allow your family to accompany you to the door of your operating room. You will then be wheeled to the hallway outside the operating room. For some people, this causes some anxiety because strangers (surgeons, orderlies, and nurses) may be walking by as they go about their business. Hopefully, the relaxing medications you have been given should be working pretty well by now. Besides making you relaxed, you may also feel a little light-headed and have a dry mouth. These are normal side effects of the medication and are nothing to worry about.

Before being taken into the operating room you will be checked in by the nurse. They will ask you some seemingly ridiculous questions such as your name, what is wrong with you, what operation is to be performed on what part of your body. These questions avoid the wrong patient ending up in the wrong operating room or with the wrong operation. Again, in my eighteen years of practice, I have never seen an error made.

What Happens in the Operating Room?

Next you will be wheeled into the operating room. An operating room looks like it does in the movies, but it is always a little intimidating when it's real and you are the patient. Large lights are on the ceiling, and the room looks sterile and impersonal. It usually feels cool because the rooms are kept at around 65°F. During surgery you will be covered with sterile sheets; the surgeons will be wearing sterile gowns, and everyone will be under hot lights. If the room is kept warm, the surgeons tend to sweat and fatigue easily, so the room is kept cool.

You will be helped onto the operating table, and a few small stick-on pads and wires will be put on your chest to monitor your heartbeat. More relaxing medication is given in the IV, which usually feels very pleasant and reduces much of the anxiety you may be feeling. Again, you may feel a little light-headed, but it's not bothersome. Some patients anticipate feeling uncomfortable and have a fear of losing control in the operating room. I find that quiet conversation with my patient goes a long way to avoid this fear. At this point, the anesthesia is given as described above.

Are There Better Ways of Starting Anesthesia?

The hospitals in England have a better way of starting general anesthesia. Patients are admitted to a small room next to the operating room, where they are prepared for surgery, and the medications are given. The family can be present until just before surgery. After the family leaves, the patient is given anesthesia in this comfortable and now familiar room and then wheeled, while asleep, into the operating room. The patient never sees the starkness of the operating room. This certainly seems a more humane way to take care of someone facing an operation.

Why Is a Bladder Catheter Used?

After you are anesthetized, a small rubber tube called a catheter is often placed in your bladder to allow urine to drain during surgery. This keeps the bladder from pushing on the uterus, fallopian tubes, and ovaries during surgery and also prevents the bladder from overstretching with urine during surgery. If you are leaving the hospital the same day, the catheter is usually removed before you wake up. If you are staying in the hospital, it is usually left in overnight so that you don't have to get out of bed to urinate during the night. The catheter may cause a sensation of pressure, but it is not painful. If you feel alert and well enough to get out of bed and go to the bathroom by yourself, you may ask to have the catheter removed right away. But most patients would rather not have to get up at night and choose to leave the catheter in until the morning. After the catheter is removed, you may notice some mild discomfort when you urinate. This sensation results from stretching and irritation of the urethra (the tube through which the urine leaves the bladder) by the catheter. This irritation is not worrisome, and the feeling will go away in a day or two. If the irritation gets worse rather than better, let your doctor know so that your urine can be tested to check for a bladder infection. If so, the infection can be easily treated with antibiotics.

What Other Preparations Are Made in the Operating Room?

After you are asleep or sedated, your abdomen and vagina are washed with iodine to remove bacteria from the operative area. If you are allergic to iodine, let the nurses know, and they will use a different solution. Before the surgery actually begins, sterile paper sheets are placed over your body to keep bacteria away from the surgical area and reduce the risk of infection. Now the operation can begin.

What Is Everyone Doing During Surgery?

During the operation, the doctors and nurses often talk to one another to ask for instruments or to describe what is happening. Many anesthesiologists will play music during surgery. I find the music relaxing and am always glad when an anesthesiologist plays a tape or CD. There is evidence that the patient actually "hears" the music and that this is soothing and helps the recovery process.

In the movies, you probably have seen doctors and nurses talking casually about sports or the weather during surgery. This does happen, but generally only during the more routine, easy parts of the surgery. When the operation gets to a more difficult part where concentration and complete attention is necessary, most surgeons and operating room staff get very quiet. They know they have an enormously serious job to do, and everyone concentrates on their area of responsibility. Once the difficult portion of the surgery is finished and we know that the patient is doing well, the mood in the room relaxes again.

During the entire surgery, the anesthesiologist will monitor your heartbeat, your breathing, and the amount of blood lost and will advise the surgeon if anything appears abnormal. The different types of surgery and techniques are described in the other chapters of this book.

What Happens Immediately After Surgery?

If you have had general anesthesia, the anesthesiologist will begin to decrease the amount of anesthesia just before the end of the operation so that you will start to wake up just after the surgery is over. You will be fairly groggy and won't remember much of what happens at this point. If you have had an epidural anesthetic, you will be fairly awake and alert but will be unable to move your legs. Next, you will be taken to a recovery room nearby, and the nurses will take your blood pressure, pulse, and temperature (with a sensor placed on your skin). The anesthesiologist will tell the nurses the type of operation you have had, any problems that may have occurred during surgery, any medical problems you may also have, and any problems they should look for. The nurses then take over your care and will call your doctor or anesthesiologist for any problems or questions.

How Will You Feel Immediately After Surgery?

When you are in the recovery room, you will slowly start to awaken and be able to talk to the nurses taking care of you. It will probably be an hour before you feel fairly alert and able to stay awake without dozing off. Depending on the extent of surgery, you may begin to feel some soreness or pain at this point, and pain medication will be given to you if you need it. General anesthesia can make you queasy, and if you have any nausea or vomiting, medication can be given to relieve the feeling. You may also feel cold or get the chills, and the nurses will bring you some warm blankets. This part of the recovery is not pleasant because you feel somewhat disoriented, possibly nauseous, possibly in pain. The recovery room nurses will be helpful and reassuring during this time.

When you are awake, alert, and your heart and breathing are stable, you will be wheeled in your bed to your room. The nurse on your floor will get a status report on your surgery and condition. You will have your blood pressure, pulse, and temperature taken on a regular basis, and you will be given medication for pain and nausea as needed. At this point, you will probably be annoyed from having been poked and prodded when you don't feel well. Please understand, though, that your condition right after surgery is very important and needs to be watched closely, at least hourly, for the first few hours. If you need something, ring the bell that is provided at the side of your bed to call for a nurse.

How Soon Can You See Your Family and Friends?

Your family will be asked to wait in the surgery waiting room or hospital lobby during your surgery. After you have been transferred to the recovery room and all the nurses' orders have been written, I usually go out to talk to family and friends to tell them how you are doing. It is a good idea to tell your doctor ahead of time what, if any, information should be told to whom. Certain information may be appropriate for some of the people close to you but not for all. It is also helpful for your doctor to have one main person to communicate with, who then can pass the information on to others.

Following most procedures, you will stay in the recovery room for about two hours and then be moved to a hospital room. At this point, your family and friends are welcome to be with you. They should be prepared for you to look a little pale, and you may be too groggy to talk much, but at least you may be heartened by being together. In some situations, the nurses or doctors may ask your visitors to leave the room for a while so that they may care for you. Certain hospitals may also have visiting hours or limit the number of visitors that may be in your room at one time. These rules are good to know before your surgery so that everyone can plan accordingly. It is probably a good idea to limit your visitors early on because you will find even short visits to be quite tiring.

Is There Anything New for Postoperative Pain Relief?

The first few days after surgery are the hardest, and research is always being done in an effort to ease postoperative pain and soreness. The standard method of giving pain medication is by injection. This is done when you request something to reduce the pain. With injections given this way, the amount of pain reliever in your system is very high initially and then wears off to almost nothing. The high initial dose of injected medication is often sedating and makes a person groggy. Many of us won't like this feeling and will put off the next dose of medication until we are in pain just to avoid feeling useless and groggy.

However, if you wait too long and develop severe pain, your brain becomes sensitized to the pain, and it will take more medication to stop it. Also, after the first time or two of feeling pain, you may begin to antici-pate its return with each passing hour. Many people find themselves anxiously awaiting their next shot. This anxiety and tension actually in-creases the pain, and higher doses are needed for pain control. Thus, the whole process becomes ineffective.

A recent and quite effective innovation is called patient-controlled analgesia (PCA). With this method, a small pump is attached to the IV you already have. The pump contains pain medication that is allowed to go into your system at a very controlled, slow, and steady rate. With a constant *low* level of medication continuously bathing the area of your brain that perceives pain, you do not develop significant pain. Because the doses are so small, the total amount of medication necessary per day is much smaller than with shots. You will not feel as groggy, and the pain relief is much better.

Since we each feel pain as individually as we feel pleasure, you may need to adjust your medication dose at times. There will be a small button located at your bedside that can be pushed to give you a little ex-tra dose of medication if needed. To make sure that no one uses the extra doses so much that they endanger themselves, the entire pump is under the watchful eye of a computer programmed per your doctor's in-structions. The computer only allows a predetermined small dose of medication to be given during a predetermined time interval. Extra push-ing of the button does nothing. If you feel you need more medication, tell your doctor, and the pump can be reprogrammed.

Some women have been concerned that the pump might malfunc-tion and cause a large dose of medicine to be given by mistake. In mil-lions of uses of this pump, that has been reported to happen only once. That is not a statistic worth worrying about. If your hospital offers PCA, discuss this form of pain relief with your doctor.

What Is Epidural Morphine?

If you have had epidural anesthesia, you may have the option, following the completion of surgery, of having a small dose of morphine injected through the plastic tube that was placed in your back. Although the exact mechanism of its action is unknown, this small dose of morphine can often provide excellent pain relief for the next twenty-four hours without any need for additional medication. Some patients, however, experience bothersome nausea or itching as side effects of the epidural morphine. If so, other medication can be given to relieve these symptoms. If you are going to have an epidural anesthetic, you can discuss this type of postoperative pain relief with your anesthesiologist before your surgery.

When Will You Use Oral Pain Medication?

If you have had PCA, you will be switched to pain medication in pill form after you feel better, which is generally in about two days. If you have had epidural morphine, the pain relief lasts for about twenty-four hours, and pain pills can be started at that time. These pills should be taken regularly every few hours while you are awake to prevent the pain from becoming bothersome. Don't wait until the pain is severe before taking the medication because you will then require higher doses, and the pills will not work as well. Studies have shown that patients who wait too long to take pain medication, because they want to avoid taking too much, end up taking a greater amount of medication to relieve the stronger pain.

Generally, people find that by the time they go home, pain medication is only needed rarely. I usually send people home with a mild medication that can be taken for soreness or discomfort. It is a great feeling to know that you are feeling better and stronger each day, as the pain medication becomes a thing of the past.

RECOVERY

How Soon Can You Eat After Abdominal Surgery?

If you have had major surgery, you usually will not be allowed to eat until the next morning. Most of my patients have not cared about this, since the surgery and anesthesia may cause nausea. In addition, most women need a great deal of sleep right after surgery and are not usually very hungry. Every morning after surgery, your doctor will listen to your abdomen with a stethoscope. If your doctor hears gurgling, this signifies the intestines have recovered from surgery, and you will be able to start drinking liquids. Usually, this happens the first morning after surgery. If your intestines sound quiet, you are not yet ready to digest food. And if you eat too soon, nausea and vomiting may result. At this point, you have had enough discomfort and aggravation, and the last thing you'd want is to feel nausea or to start to vomit. You will feel stronger as the days pass. Once your intestines recover, they will begin to push gas through the rectum. By then you will be able to eat and digest regular food.

What Activities Will You Be Able to Do in the Hospital After Abdominal Surgery?

The morning after major abdominal surgery, you will be able to get up out of bed and sit in a chair next to the bed. You should also be able to walk, with some assistance, to the bathroom. You may be sore, and the incision may be uncomfortable, so you should start out slowly until your body tells you how much you can do. By the second day, most women are up and around for short walks down the hall. You will probably find this tiring, but it is important to walk and keep your circulation going. By the third day, most women are able to get up periodically, walk for about fifteen minutes at a time, and take a shower.

What Activities Will You Be Able to Do at Home After Abdominal Surgery?

If needed, you will be given pain medication to take at home. For the first week or so, physical activity should be limited to walking to meals, to the bathroom, and short walks (fifteen minutes) inside or outside. Because an abdominal incision needs six weeks to heal fully, you should not lift, exercise, have intercourse, or do anything that puts stress on your incision for that time. Walking is fine, and stairs are okay but should be taken slowly. As you feel stronger, you can increase your walking. When you feel up to it, probably after a few weeks, you can go outside to visit friends, eat, shop, or see a movie.

You will feel exhausted after surgery, and too much activity will actually make you feel sore. Most women need to sleep a good part of each day, and the simplest activity will leave you winded. The fatigue is not harmful, so do not let it worry you. Your body has undergone an enormous stress and needs time to recuperate. You will return to a good energy level in about six weeks. Some women need more time, others less. Just give yourself adequate time and care.

Will You Feel Fatigued After Surgery?

Fatigue is a very common consequence of surgery. In general, the amount and duration of fatigue will be related to the extent of surgery, the length of time you spend under anesthesia, the amount of pain you experience during recovery, and your general health and well-being. The amount of blood you lost during surgery and your blood count at the time of discharge from the hospital will also influence the way you feel. Oral iron tablets can help raise your blood count more quickly and help alleviate fatigue. A recent study found that 75 percent of women who had either a myomectomy or a hysterectomy (with an abdominal incision) had significant fatigue lasting up to a few months after surgery. Sixty percent of women noted fatigue for six months. Based on studies that show a faster return to normal activity after laparoscopic surgery, it appears that fatigue may be less persistent after laparoscopic surgery. However, a study comparing abdominal surgery to laparoscopic surgery has not been done.

In general, doctors do not ask patients about the amount of fatigue they experience after surgery. If you are bothered by significant or prolonged fatigue, let your doctor know.

How Is Recovery Different If You Have Laparoscopic or Other Outpatient Surgery?

Outpatient surgical procedures require a shorter hospital stay and less recovery time. Often if a catheter was placed in your bladder during surgery, it will be removed before you wake up. Pain medications may be given through your IV at first but can be given by mouth once you are able to drink water. Once you are alert, and your heartbeat and breathing are fine, you will be helped out of bed and asked to go to the bathroom. The nurses will want to see that you can walk and will want to know that you can urinate by yourself before they let you go home. If you can't urinate because of the anesthesia or irritation from the catheter, they may want you to stay longer. You will be allowed to drink water when you feel ready and will be allowed to eat as soon as you are able. Once you are stable, totally alert, and able to urinate, you will be allowed to go home. However, you may not drive at this time, so plan on getting a ride home. If you plan to or need to stay overnight, you will be moved to a regular room in the hospital.

When Can You Return to Normal Activity After Laparoscopic Surgery?

Most patients recover quickly following laparoscopic surgery because the incisions are small and cause little discomfort. There also tends to be less irritation to the inside of your abdominal cavity than with major abdominal incisions, so you will be able to eat a few hours after surgery. You should be able to be up and around by the morning after surgery. Discomfort is usually minimal, and oral pain medication should be adequate for relief. Depending on the type of surgery performed, you may be able to return to work, exercise, and activity within a week or two. We recommend increasing your activity slowly over the first few days. While the incisions from laparoscopic surgery are small, it is important to remember that surgery, possibly major surgery, was performed through those small incisions. It is best if you allow your body to recover gradually.

What Should You Watch Out for at Home?

After surgery, you can expect some discomfort, some occasional light-headedness, some vaginal spotting or light bleeding, and some occasional queasiness. Most doctors will instruct you to call them if you notice an increase in pain, any vomiting or persistent nausea, any temperature over 100.4°F, heavy vaginal bleeding, or a feeling of faintness that persists for more than a few minutes. Redness or drainage from the incision should also be reported to your doctor.

When Will You See Your Doctor After You Go Home?

Most physicians will want to see you back in the office at two weeks and at four or six weeks after your surgery. At your two-week office visit, your incision will be checked, and you may have a pelvic exam to make sure that there is no infection and that healing is proceeding normally. This visit also gives you an opportunity to ask your doctor any questions that have come up about your activity, stamina, emotional well-being, or return to work. Usually after this visit, you can slowly increase your activity. If all is well after abdominal surgery, I usually will let women drive a car following the two-week visit. Prior to this, you may become weak or light-headed while driving, and that might be dangerous. After laparoscopic surgery, many women will be well enough to drive after one week.

At your six-week postoperative visit following abdominal surgery, a full pelvic examination is performed to see if your healing is complete. None of this should be uncomfortable. If all is back to normal, you should be able to resume full activity at this point, including a return to work. Following laparoscopic surgery, most women will be able to return to full activity after about two weeks. Of course, every patient and situation is different, and all the above should be discussed with your doctor.

HOW YOU CAN BE SURE TO GET GOOD CARE

We have tried to provide you with descriptive and intelligent coverage of gynecologic problems and state-of-the-art information regarding a range of solutions. We have focused on the common gynecologic problems that are sometimes difficult to understand and often not adequately covered during doctor's visits or in magazines. We want to foster an empowering, compassionate view of the doctor-patient partnership, something we believe is vital to good care. It is in your best interest to be educated about the health-care decisions you make. If you need more information, seek it out. Read more; get a second or third opinion. Ask all the questions you need to, until you feel comfortable with the answers. Seek out information about possible alternatives. When it comes time to make any decisions, you will then have the peace of mind that you have done your homework and are making the right choice for you.

REFERENCES

DeCherney, A., G. Bachman, K. Isaacson, and S. Gall. 2002. Postoperative fatigue negatively impacts the daily lives of patients recovering from hysterectomy. *Obstetrics and Gynecology* 99:51–57.

Flood, A., W. Scott, and W. Ewy. 1984. Does practice make perfect?: The relationship between hospital volume and outcomes for selected diagnostic categories. *Medical Care* 22:98–114.

Mais, V., S. Ajossa, S. Guerriero, M. Mascia, E. Solla, and G. Melis. 1996. Laparoscopic versus abdominal myomectomy: A prospective, randomized trial to evaluate benefits in early outcome. *American Journal of Obstetrics and Gynecology* 174:654–58.

INDEX